'When we meet a fact which contradicts a prevailing theory, we must accept the fact and abandon the theory, even when the theory is supported by great names and generally accepted'

'What makes a scientist important is how well he or she has penetrated into the unknown. In areas of science where the facts are known to everyone, all scientists are more or less equal—we cannot know who is great. But in the area of science that is still obscure and unknown the great are recognized: they are marked by ideas which light up phenomena hitherto obscure and carry science forward'

Claude Bernard

## About the Authors

**Elena Ewing (Dr)**

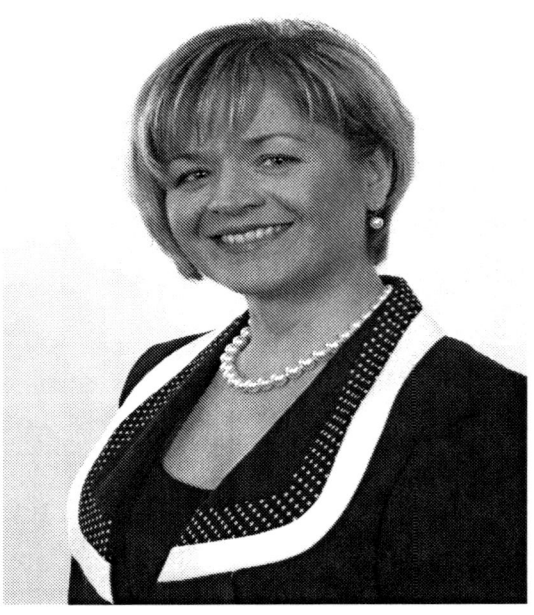

Elena Ewing (Dr) is 40 years of age and is a qualified doctor.

During her career in Russia she practiced for 10 years as an ophthalmic surgeon and also spent several years practicing as a dermatologist, venereologist and as an environmental hygienist.

For several years she appeared regularly on Ural TV and radio as a medical consultant.

Elena is a trained Virtual Scanning practitioner and is the only person, located in the EU, who is qualified to train Virtual Scanning practitioners.

**Graham Ewing B.Sc.**

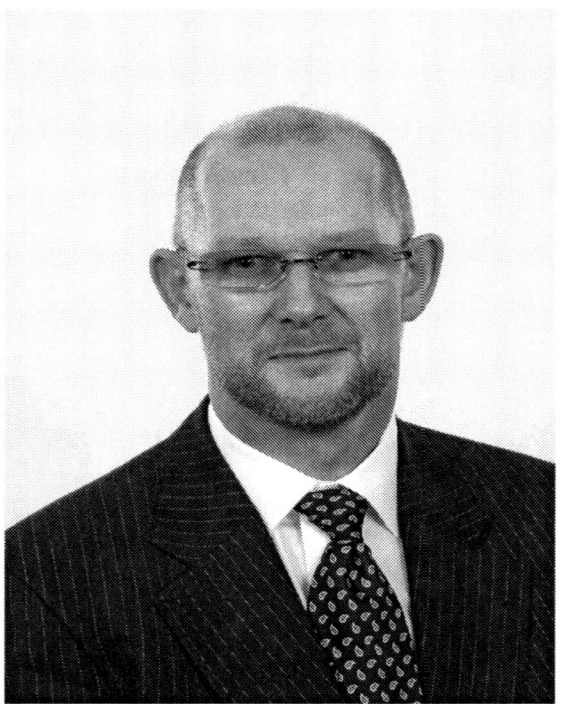

Graham Ewing is 55 years of age, a qualified industrial chemist and has a 23 year history in international sales and marketing.

Graham is the founder and Chief Executive of Montague Healthcare, a UK-based business, which provides technical and medical expertise in the use of Virtual Scanning technology.

This book is the product of over 4 years research into the origins, theoretical concepts and market potential for Virtual Scanning technology.

**Publisher**

Montague Healthcare books, Mulberry House, 6 Vine Farm Close, Cotgrave, Nottinghamshire NG12 3TU, England

Tel: 0115-9890304/9899618/Fax: 0115-9899826

Orders: enquiries@montague-diagnostics.co.uk

Email: graham.ewing@montague-diagnostics.co.uk

elena.ewing@montague-diagnostics.co.uk

ISBN: 978-0-9556213-0-7

# Contents

iv

## Clinical Trial Status

Virtual Scanning is an approved technology in Russia where it is approved by the Russian Health Authorities. It is also approved for use in Ukraine and other of the former Soviet republics. Montague Healthcare is the only company in the EU which is authorised under the Medical Devices Directive to supply CE-marked Virtual Scanning software.

Whilst it is intended to commission the first clinical trials of Virtual Scanning during the period 2007-8 it is necessary to specify that, at the time of printing the first version of this book that no clinical trials have been conducted which comply with western requirements i.e. of double-blind clinical trials.

All claims which are provided in this text are based upon studies from credible Russian medical doctors, articles from credible medical researchers, of articles provided by Dr I.G.Grakov, and of case studies from its use in Russia or the UK.

## Non-disclosure of Intellectual Property

The unique mathematics of the programme which is used in the software is the property of Dr I.G.Grakov of the company MIMEX.

In order to protect his intellectual property Dr Grakov has designed the technology in a manner which prevents access to the intellectual property i.e. key mathematics and algorithms, by separating the test programme from the server unit which processes the data.

## Illustrations

Illustrations are the work of Keith Bullock.

## Acknowledgements

My thanks to the many researchers who have, through their work, contributed to this book and to Dr I.G.Grakov of MIMEX, developer of Virtual Scanning and his colleagues Julia Borovleva (Dr) and Yuri Spassky (Dr).

My thanks also to the many people who have contributed to the text including Alex Hankey (Dr), Elena Nikolayevna Ewing (Dr), Vysochin.Y (Dr), Fiona Simpson.

Thanks to all those who have in their own ways contributed to our lives and hence have made this book possible including Norman and Lillian Forster, Sam and Olive Ewing, Professor J.Hankinson, and to those patients who have authorised the use of their results in texts and articles.

# Preface

This book is the first comprehensive guide to Virtual Scanning, the first of a new generation of medical technologies, which links our psychology to our physiology using concepts involving cognition and mathematical modelling. These are typical of approaches used in psychology, neuroscience, and computational neuroscience.

**Everything that we think, how we perceive our world, everything that we do, and the precise ways that act, are the product of our unique biochemistry.**

The result is a technology, seemingly unprecedented in modern medicine, which is precisely able to relate the function of our mind to our body and hence is able to provide the first broad-spectrum diagnosis of a person's mental and physical health AND forms the basis of a highly effective light therapy.

Russian researchers have demonstrated that Virtual Scanning is more accurate than most diagnostic technologies thereby indicating its value as a broad-spectrum medical screening technology. As a therapy it has been shown to be very effective when treating illness, often better than drugs. The existence of this technology enables us to make world-leading conclusions which sweep away the sceptical criticisms of many about the dubious nature of complementary therapies.

Virtual Scanning casts light upon principles, long considered to be the domain of psychology or complementary health, which highlights the limitations of the biomedical approach. It presents concepts which extend our understanding of how the body functions. It shows how complementary health principles form the basis of possibly the most progressive medical technology since the isolation of penicillin in the 1930's heralded the advent of the biochemical era in medicine. It illustrates that sensory stimulus and the sensory therapies use mechanisms which regulate our health and wellbeing.

This book provides an introduction and guide to Virtual Scanning technology. It discusses the origins of the technology, how the technology has been developed since its first introduction to the market in 1998, how results are reported and their significance, the medical precedents for a technology of this nature, the diagnostic & therapeutic scope of the technology, a summary of available data, the limitations of current medical technologies, the scope for a technology of this nature. Finally, we summarise why Virtual Scanning technology is truly a world-leading technology with the potential to revolutionise the future provision of healthcare.

This book will be of interest to the general public and patients; complementary health practitioners, nurses, and therapists; medical researchers, doctors, consultants and psychologists; members of government throughout the world; and international health organisations.

"It is arrogant of us, as scientists, to claim that because we cannot precisely define a problem it doesn't exist."

Dr. Daniel J. Clauw

# Summary of Contents

**Chapter 1:**

**Introduction to the Concepts and Precedents involved in Virtual Scanning.**

- How We React With Our Environment
- Our Brainwave Frequencies
- What is the Significance of Sleep?
- The Effects of Drugs on the Brainwaves
- How we receive Sensory Data
- The Influence of Age upon our Physiological Function
- The Difference between Men and Women
- The Influence of Stress upon our Physiology
- Stress Affects the Brain
- Stress Affects the Body
- Stress Influences our Sleeping Patterns and Weight
- It is a Fact that our Health is Inversely Proportional to our Weight.
- What is the Evidence for the Body's Physiological Systems?
- The Influence of the Body's Physiological Systems on our Health
- The Biological Limits of our Health and Behaviour
- How these Regulatory Mechanisms Function?
- Are the Systems which Regulate our Physiology responsible for Brain function?
- The Brain Expands Through Use.
- The Senses, Complementary Health and the Body's Processes of Compensation.
- The Negative Effects of Electromagnetic Radiation
- Could a Person's Personality Change as a Result of an Organ Transplant?
- How we Absorb Data in the Form of Colour.
- The Mind-Body Connection

**Chapter 2:**

**What is Virtual Scanning?**

- The Test Procedure and Report

- Virtual Scanning version 4 (1998-2002)

- Virtual Scanning version 7 (2002-    )

- Virtual Scanning version  4 psychological profile

**Chapter 3:**

**How Virtual Scanning Works**

- Why do we get ill?
- What evidence is there to relate our cognition to our psychology?
- Grakov's Work
- Extracts of Articles by Russian Medical Researchers
- Homeostatic and Behavioural Limits Change with Age
- The Justification for Physiological Systems
- The Holistic Nature of the Human Physiology
- How Stress Affects our Health.
- How Nutritional Deficits can Cause or are Related to Behavioural Problems
- Why did the symptom occur?
- How does our Behavioural Disposition Change as we Grow Older?
- Is it Right to Trust Purely Biomedical Conclusions?
- A Summary of Current Research
- Virtual Scanning
- The need to understand the implications of change in our Society
- The Limitations of Biomedicine
- Complementary Health
- How can we Explain the Relationship between Cognition and Health?
- If Physiological Systems Exist What Do They Control?
- What Is the Structure of Each of the Physiological Systems?
- Does This Explain the Function of Other Complementary Health Therapies?
- Placebo effect & Positive thinking
- What Proof Can be Offered for the Fundamental Concepts Outlined?
- The Influence of Light and Colour upon our Health

**Chapter 4:**

**The Available Evidence**

- Government Approvals & Certifications

- Performance of Virtual Scanning

- Assessment and Treatment of Migraine

- Assessment and Treatment of Dyslexia

- Assessment and Treatment of Chronic Fatigue Syndrome

- Assessment and Treatment of IBS

- Assessment and Treatment of Stroke

- Assessment of Ulcerative Disease

- Assessment of Diabetes

- Assessment of Breathing Dysfunction

- Health assessment of a Professional footballer

- Assessment of Depression

- Assessment of Heart Problems

- Assessment of Psoriasis

- The Effects of Virtual Scanning Therapy

- Further Case Studies:

- Typical Comparative Analyses before and after Treatment

- Use of Virtual Scanning to monitor various influences on a person's physical and psychological health

- Weight Loss

- Discussion

- Accreditations

**Chapter 5:**

**The Value of Virtual Scanning to the Medical Profession**

### Defining the Need for improved Medical Technologies

- What do you want to achieve when you visit your doctor?

- What Does the Government Expect from the Medical Professions?

- Medical Diagnosis is Fraught with Errors.

- How Can a GP Improve the Services Which They Offer?

- The Evidence-based Requirement

- How Likely is a doctor to Make a Mistake?

- Do Biomedical Researchers Understand the Influence of Age upon the Effectiveness of a Drug?

- Are Drugs Able to Treat the Medical Condition?

- Does the Medical Condition Need to be Treated by a Drug-based Intervention?

- How safe is the Medical Technology/Therapy?

- How necessary is the Surgery?

### Virtual Scanning - Fullfilling the Need

- What Value does Virtual Scanning Have to the Medical Profession and the General Medical Practitioner (GP)?

- Where does Virtual Scanning fit into the Medical Spectrum?

- The Scope of the Technology

- The Placebo Effect

**Chapter 6:**

**The Implications of this New Generation of Medical Technologies**

- Biomedicine

- Vaccines

- The Future Provision of Healthcare

- Could Diabetes and Obesity be due to the Destabilization of the Body's Physiological Systems?

- Medical Insurance

- Education

- Delinquency & Criminality

- Sporting Achievement

- Military & Performance-related Professions

- Recruitment

- Detection and Treatment of Mental Health Issues

- Industry

- Beauty and Wellbeing

- How can we use this information to improve the quality and quantity of our lives?

# Chapter 1

# Introduction

Introduction to the concept, biomedical precedents, which are involved in Virtual Scanning technology

by

Graham Ewing

# How We React With Our Environment

*Everything that we see, hear, smell, taste, touch or 'sense' in our lives is the result of input of data from our external environments.*

It is a fundamental human trait that sight is our dominant sense. This includes our perception of colour [1], light intensity, the shape of items [2,121] and rate at which we process data. Light is estimated to comprise c85-90% of sensory input and is therefore the most important sense which we use to interact with our external environment. Without vision we become significantly less effective.

To illustrate the importance of vision - our eyes and brain require 25% of our nutritional intake yet represent only 2% of our total body weight. The eyes use more oxygen than the heart [1, 120].

## Figure 1

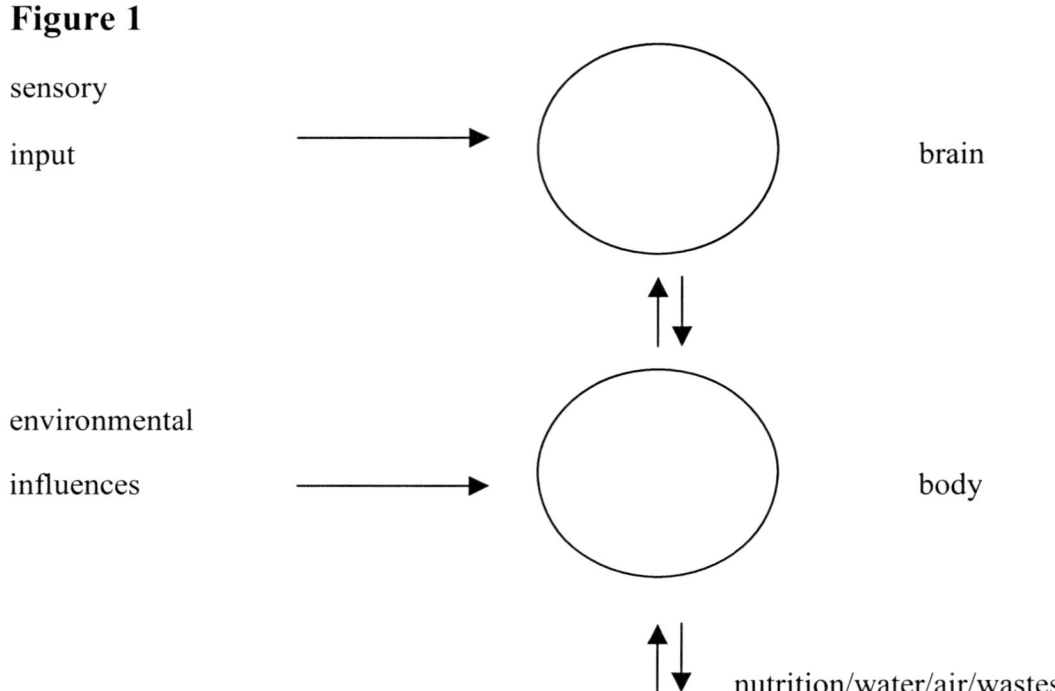

sensory

input    →    ○    brain

environmental

influences    →    ○    body

nutrition/water/air/wastes

From the sensory point of view, our body's functioning state is defined by the accumulation of our sensory input comprising light, sound, touch, smell and taste, each defining aspects of how we perceive ourselves.

Everything that we do is influenced by our sensory input; by air, water and by food; and also by less obvious sensory influences such as electromagnetic radiation, microwave radiation, etc; thereby illustrating that we react to our environment in a multiplicity of ways as a complex organism.

OTT [3] illustrated how the quality of light affects the growth of the living organism. He exposed plants to blue and red filtered light and recorded how these plants grew in a deformed manner and/or died. The same is true of the human being where, through the seasonal exposure to summer or winter light, our health and behaviour is affected. Recent studies have shown light therapy to be more effective than Prozac [4]. More than 100 medical conditions are known to respond positively to the therapeutic use of light [5-38], (table 1).

**Table 1:**     The Therapeutic Benefit of Light

Condition:                              Arthritis
                                        Cancer
                                        Depression
                                        Diabetes
                                        Eczema
                                        Hyperbilirubinemia
                                        Jaundice
                                        Migraine
                                        Psoriasis
                                        Seasonal Affective Disorder (SAD)

Documented effects upon:                Blood Pressure
                                        Breathing rate
                                        Growth
                                        Immune System
                                        Longevity
                                        Mood
                                        Motor Activity
                                        Pulse rate
                                        Reproductive function
                                        Sleep
                                        Tumour Growth

The effect of light and of colour upon our physiology was studied by Berezin and Martinek [39] who identified that the function and activity of proteins and enzymes can be variously affected by the influence of light of different colours.

Most drugs are accompanied by changes to sensory perception and aspects of our behaviour usually noted as side-effects. Viagra which affects sensory perception to such an extent that those taking the drug see the world as if through a blue-green filter. This is due to the effect of Viagra upon the enzyme PDE VI [40] which is involved in the process of transduction (signal processing) in the retina. This illustrates how changes to our physiology affect our sensory perception. In fact over 60% of drugs are known to influence our visual perception.

Accordingly, changes to our sensory perception and in particular to our visual perception relate (directly or indirectly) to biochemical changes which are linked to the various processes of transduction in the retina. Absorption and transmission of light/colour changes in a manner depending on the nature of drug-substrate reactions in blood - not dissimilar to the technique of 'immunofluorescence' - which uses fluorescent substrates to identify the presence of antibodies or proteins.

Changes in blood flow, blood volume, blood pressure, blood cell content, etc; influence our sensory organs and affect their function. Such changes can be produced by health changes such as are experienced in illness or by drugs for which they are noted as side-effects.

Another possible mechanism involves GPCRs (G-protein coupled receptors) which are an important class of cellular receptors. Over 50% of drugs function by interacting with them. These influence our sensory perception and act upon the regulation of our visual processing, odour/smell processing, behaviour and mood, inflammatory mechanisms, immune system, and the autonomic nervous system which is responsible for control of many automatic functions of the body such as blood pressure, heart rate and digestive processes. This establishes the relationship between sensory perception and our biochemistry from a deeper perspective.

The body's workings can be monitored and/or described in many ways:

1.  anatomically – through the ever greater level of sophistication of techniques which are able to study our function at the physical level i.e. of organs and physiological systems.

2.  biochemically – through the ever greater level of sophistication of techniques which are able to study our function at the molecular and cellular level.

3.  electrochemically – through the passage of electrical responses which, directly and/or indirectly, are involved in the processing of data which flows between the brain and organs

4.  physically – through the approach of structural mechanics and fluid mechanics which describes our function in terms of our skeletal structure and of the flow of bodily fluids

5.  psychologically - through sensory input at the conscious and subconscious level

6.  magnetically – using the body's response to magnetic influences

7.  electromagnetically – using the body's response to the wide range of radiation such as x-rays, microwave radiation, ultrasound, etc

Though this explains our body's function(s) and describes our structure, and how we react to the various types of stimuli, this approach is comparable with how we could

4

investigate the structure of a computer and of the flow of electrical impulses, but tells us little about what how we actually work i.e. our 'software'.

This can only be explained by noting how we react to receipt of sensory stimulus i.e. of data; which affects our function at the level of the systems, organs or cells of the body.

Each year many of us recognise the positive therapeutic benefit, of relaxation and enjoyment; and getting away from the stresses which affect each of us in our daily lives; which we get from a summer holiday in the sun. Light and colour gives a significant and positive therapeutic benefit.

As living organisms we are dependent upon sensory stimulus mainly in the form of light, sound, and touch for the quality (and perhaps also for the quantity) of our future lives. The study of the neurological development of orphans under the Ceaucescu regime in Romania [41] illustrates how insufficient sensory stimulus affects our physiological development i.e. we shrivel up, are inadequately developed, and may die.

Sensory stimulus is therefore necessary for our physiological and mental development. Continuous exposure to positive sensory influences enhances our health whilst exposure to negative sensory influences weakens our health and wellbeing.

# Our Brainwave Frequencies

*The brain is an electrochemical organ which functions in characteristic ways. Electrical activity emanating from the brain is displayed in the form of brainwaves but what is their function?*

Our brain waves, which are measured by ElectroEncephaloGraph (EEG), decline with age until our deductive capabilities decline [42]. As beta and alpha frequencies are largely dormant during the night, and as delta and theta frequencies function throughout the 24 hour cycle, we conclude that the beta and alpha frequencies are related solely to daytime activities i.e. our active behavioural function; and that the delta and theta frequencies are related to the regulation of our health and behaviour during the complete day/night cycle.

The delta waves [43] are associated with periods of deep sleep, except in conditions such as coma, epilepsy, encephalitis, narcolepsy and brain tumours; and hence are associated with the natural processes of diagnosis and repair. They are also seen in the infant and in most individuals throughout the day; begin to increase about noon in normal men and women between 19-39 years; and attain a peak around 4:00 pm. This increase is not considered to be related to sleep and is also considered to be independent of alertness. In addition delta wave intensity [44] is known to decline with age – e.g. by up to 50% between ages 10 years and 20 years, and by up to 25% between ages 11 years and 14 years – apparently representing changes associated with physiological development and the ageing process.

The human brain scans and receives data, in at least four frequency ranges - beta, alpha, theta and delta - which function between frequencies of 0.2 and typically 40 hz (figure 2. This appears to be the neural equivalent of having four interlinked data-processing programmes – perhaps similar to that of a computer programme comprising for example 'access' and 'excel' – each handling different functions.

It is having to cope with the influence of modern electronic devices which deliver data at frequencies of 25 hz and upwards. This influences the function of the brain and the biochemical processes controlled by the brain.

An illustration of how this affects our sensory input and neural processing is by considering how subliminal messages [126] can be delivered in a film or how hypnotic effects, or of migraine and/or epileptic occurrences can be induced by exposure to specific frequencies of flashing lights. Subliminal messages are designed to pass below normal limits of perception and consciousness but to be perceived by the subconscious mind and hence influence our emotions, opinions, purchasing patterns, etc. They have been used in advertising of soft drinks and, allegedly, in the delivery of political propaganda.

In the 20th and 21st centuries we are being forced, as a result of new technologies, to adapt to a huge range of external influences yet our body is only able to adapt at a relatively slow rate. Our bodies interact with our environment as a result of inherited traits and of our experiences and learning processes but, in general, we are unable to identify the effects of new technologies upon our bodies except through monitoring the illnesses which develop.

**Figure 2**

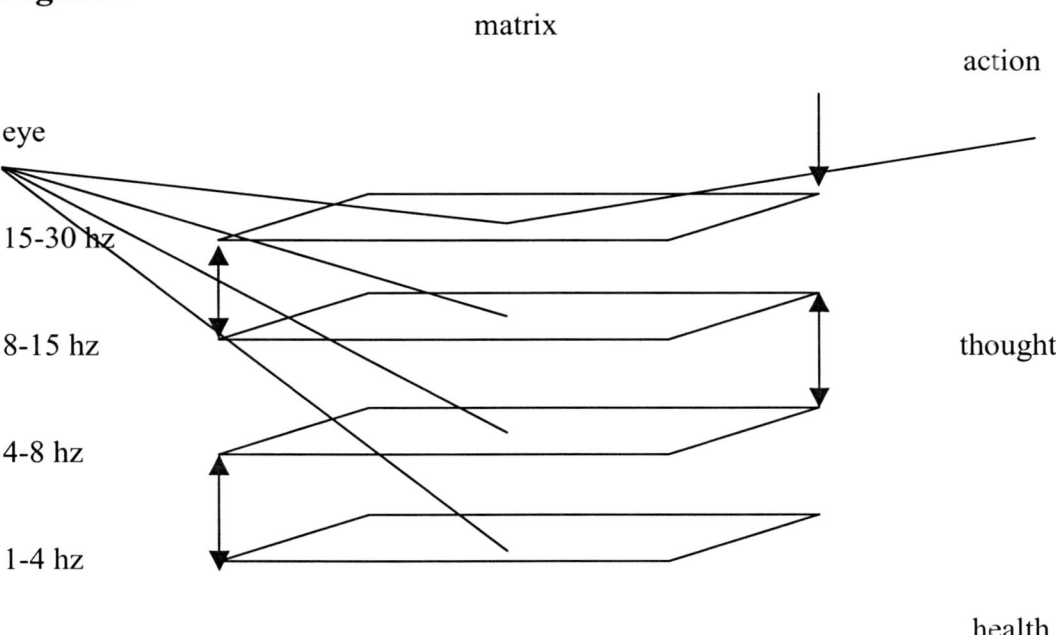

The developer of Virtual Scanning, Dr I.G.Grakov, identified that medical conditions arising from alterations to the neural programmes which affect the body's stability. This results in changes to bio-chemical processes inducing the release of stress-chemicals and subsequently by their manifestation as pathological processes. This is not an entirely new concept. All physicians will accept that illnesses are made worse by stress - a line of logic which Grakov has merely extrapolated.

Most stress is experienced visually. Visual data is processed by the beta wave and hence by the associated data processing matrix (figure 2). Depending upon the precise nature, magnitude or longevity of the stress event the data is fed through the alpha frequency, theta and delta frequency; thereby affecting our thought processes and finally the stability of the physiological systems which regulate organ and cell function.

The release of stress-chemicals can be initiated by a wide range of environmental factors including excess exposure to Televisions (60-80 hz), Cinema (24-48 hz), Computers (60-90hz), Fluorescent lights (125-150 hz), Microwaves and Mobile phones; Air, Rail and Car travel; Music, Sound and Vibration; X-rays in medical applications; intra-family and inter-family social unrest and violence (in the social and work environment); etc. Our bodies are not designed for this exposure.

The diagnostic technology to prove their damaging effects is limited and insufficient results have been published. We can only speculate upon the damage or changes being caused to our brains and bodies by these new technologies. Indeed could society, as we know it, exist without these technologies?

Rather than a Luddite approach intended to reverse technological progress it seems more logical to develop a strategy which would limit the alleged damage caused by these technologies, establish means to quantify risk and limits of exposure, and improve the technologies in order to reduce the risk. Finally, we can treat people who are suffering from the adverse effects due to overexposure.

Sensory input influences our health. Modern technological devices and associated influences cause stress reactions which provoke pathology. We need an approach to health maintenance which reverses the damage they cause.

# What is the Significance of Sleep?

*The vast majority of us sleep at night and hopefully awake refreshed. We appreciate the value of sleep but not even sleep researchers know how sleep benefits us.*

The most plausible explanation for sleep 45 is that during waking hours when the brain is active the brain cell metabolism produces chemical by-products which need to be excreted otherwise they accumulate and get in the way of normal neurotransmitter activity. This may be what causes the sensation of tiredness. Without sleep, the brain has difficulty functioning and our function is affected. Interestingly, the brain can become larger with use – like a muscle. The body requires rest in order to regenerate.

The autonomic nervous system, comprising the sympathetic and parasympathetic, is associated with our processing of red and blue light signals 128. It is considered that both cannot be active at the same time i.e. when one predominates, the other is switched off. When we're active and coping with challenges and stressful situations, we're using our sympathetic nervous system and hence the human organism uses energy. When we're calm and passive, the parasympathetic nervous system becomes active and the body repairs and restores itself. Without rest, the immune system is lowered, we heal more slowly and become more vulnerable to disease. When we are ill we take to our beds and sleep. Sleep is important because it reduces our physical and mental activity for a significant period.

As beta waves are related to our active behavioural state lowered frequency brain waves e.g. in the alpha frequency range, are associated with deductive processes and learning, and are essential for good mental function.

Memory formation involves a process called long-term potentiation (LTP) involving electrical and chemical changes in the neurons associated with memory. Without LTP, incoming information is not stored and is forgotten. At the University of California 46 neurophysiologists have discovered that the key to LTP is the theta brain wave pattern which is considered to be the natural rhythm of the hippocampus which is essential for the formation and storage of new memories and the recall of old memories.

Without good physiological function new memories and the recall of old memories becomes inhibited and progressively more difficult.

Caffeine (which raises the brain frequencies) is recognised to have a negative effect upon concentration and illnesses such as schizophrenia are associated with significantly raised brain wave activity in the gamma brain wave frequency range which exists at typically 30-100 hz. By contrast alcohol lowers our brain wave frequencies and puts us to sleep but not necessarily at a frequency appropriate for our reparative and restorative functions. Moreover small doses of alcohol may have a stimulating effect.

The importance of delta sleep is that it involves various reparative and growth processes including the release of growth hormone by the pituitary gland and hence that repair functions, including those associated with the immune system, become more active [47].

As we age our physiological functions of repair and regeneration decline; the regulation of the physiological systems and hence of organ and cell function declines; the production of growth hormone declines and hence the creation of new memories and the recall of old memories becomes progressively more difficult.

Accordingly good physiological function appears to be essential for the creation of new memories and for the recall of old memories.

Memories are not just limited to that of behaviour and experiences of our external environment but also of our internal environment.

# The Effects of Drugs on the Brainwaves

*Few researchers understand the significance of the brain waves and the relationship between the brain waves and our biochemistry.*

Most drugs that affect the central nervous system, particularly those designed for neurological or psychiatric conditions, have an effect on brainwave activity. In many cases the effect is dependent upon the concentration of the drug and low concentrations of a drug may exert the opposite effect on brainwave activity compared to a higher dose.

Differences may be caused by other factors e.g. age, nutrition, drug/drug interactions, and/ the presence of brain injury.

- Hypnotics, antidepressants and sedatives increase the delta and theta wave activity in the brain and also cause an increase in beta wave activity and a decrease in alpha wave activity.

- Anxiolytics increase beta wave activity and decrease alpha wave activity

- Stimulants such as caffeine and cocaine increase beta wave activity

- Marijuana, linked with incidences of euphoria after smoking, is associated with an increase in alpha wave activity

- Barbiturates increase alpha, beta and delta wave activity

- Benzodiazepines increase the beta waves and decrease delta activity

- Prednisone, a steroid, increases theta wave activity and may cause deterioration in cognition as well as mild behavioral side effects.

- Morphine and the opiates slows alpha wave activity

- Corticosteroids are known to produce euphoria and other behavioral abnormalities, including psychoses.

Mori [48] studied the impact of video games on children's brains, noting a lack of beta wave activity in frequent players which is considered to be indicative that the gamers were hardly using the frontal regions of their brains, which are considered important for emotional processing, planning and self-control. "If levels of beta waves are very low, people get angry easily and have difficulty in concentrating," he commented. His conclusions were based upon the analysis of EEG traces of 240 people, of typically 6-29 years of age, and compared the amount of alpha and beta wave activity of people who rarely played video games, those playing for 1-3 hours per day for 3-4 days per week, and those who played for up to 7 hours per day.

The existence of the alpha waves is generally considered to be indicative of a relaxed thoughtful state and beta waves are thought to represent active neural and physical activity. Mori noted that the beta waves were almost absent even when the regular gamers were not playing games.

Drugs affect your brainwaves which in turn govern how we function. A drug will alter our behavioural potential, disposition and performance which is not surprising when considering that this is the function of your body's natural drug substances i.e. proteins, hormones, endocannabinoids, endorphins, etc. The same is true of stress chemicals in the blood stream which influence brain wave levels and also the levels of the various immunochemicals. The result is that feedback loops between brain waves and biochemistry can give rise to stable pathological states.

**Whereas conventional thinking is based around the concept that the brain waves are the product of our collective biochemistry the complementary or unconventional approach appears to be the reverse i.e. that the brain waves regulate our physiology.**

Let us explore these issues further.

If the body's processes of diagnosis, reparation and preparation take place mainly during the periods of sleep then the delta frequency range is associated with the maintenance of health. This is confirmed when we note the faster rate of healing and recovery from illness which occur during sleep. The theta frequency range may have a similar function, in relation to the delta frequency (health/systems), as the alpha frequency range has to the beta frequency (behavioural). This is consistent with the phenomena of CAP (cyclic alternating pattern) and how adverse changes to CAP influences quality of sleep. Greater CAP instability 127 would be reasonably expected to affect the function of the body's physiological systems, the quantity of delta sleep and hence the body's regeneration.

There may be simplistic links between the alpha and theta frequency ranges which might explain how a person can remain aware of their environment when in the deepest stages of sleep. This would link the various stages of neural function from the delta range – to the theta range – to the alpha range – and to the beta range. A good example is of a mother who can be aware of her baby's breathing at all times despite being in the deepest sleep or a father who wakes due to some perceived threat e.g. of someone or something unexpectedly walking around in or near the home during the night. It is difficult to conclude anything other than that the brain waves are functionally inter-connected e.g. figure 3.

**Figure 3**

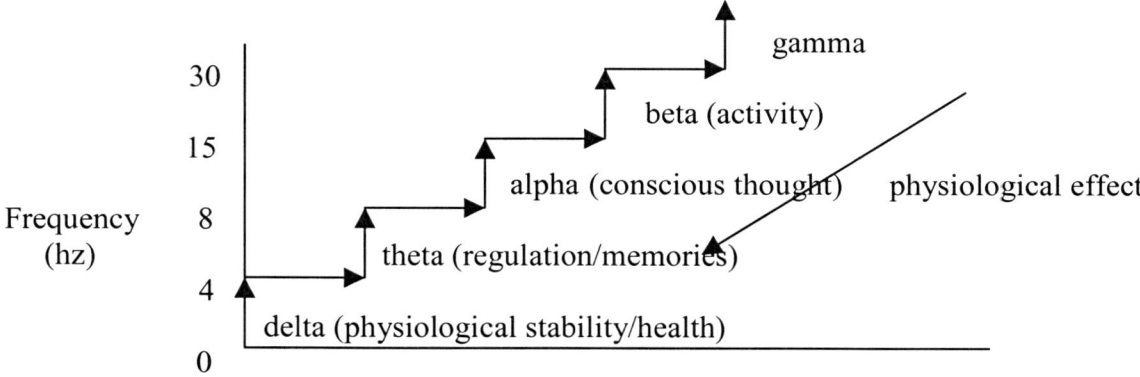

Every visual experience in our lives (estimated to be typically 20-30 times per second) is the accumulation of life experience data upon which we base our daily decisions. This coincides with the beta wave (EEG) frequency which functions at typically 15-30 hz. Accordingly consider the possibility that the various brain wave frequencies constitute the brain's main data processing programme(s), which function simultaneously, and that they regulate differing aspects of our physiology and health.

As we age the speed of our processing abilities declines and the related content of the lower brain waves i.e. of the alpha frequency range, increases and the beta wave content decreases.

To illustrate how flashing light frequency i.e. exposure to flicker or flashing rates, affects our health we can note at least two examples from our modern lives e.g. (1) in Japan a television programme which featured rapid flashing images at typically 6-8 television frames per second induced a mass occurrence of epilepsy and migraine in the children who were watching the programme – hundreds of children were affected - and (2), in France, people driving through the long tree-lined vistas were found to be at greater risk of crashing because of the combined and potentially hypnotic effect of speed and distance (100-140 kph) between the trees which, depending upon the distance between trees, is typically 4-8 trees per second.

Further clues as to the functional role of the brain waves comes from comparative studies of the brain waves in the animal kingdom. Bullock 49 noted that the brain waves of species higher on the evolutionary ladder have a higher frequency whereas mammalian brain waves are at the lower frequencies. It seems reasonable to conclude that lower frequency brain waves are in fact related to a more complex and sophisticated neural function i.e. of the ability to process more information and to relate it to memories, rather than just reacting to a external stimulus.

# How we receive Sensory Data

*Consider how we experience sensory input and how this affects our cognition.*

Although we measure our experiences mainly through vision, assessing the visual changes in our environment, each visual experience is accompanied by input from the other senses i.e. of sound, smell, taste, touch and sensory input. Our sensory perception is therefore the result of a multidimensional sensory neural network of data processing (see fig 4).

## Figure 4

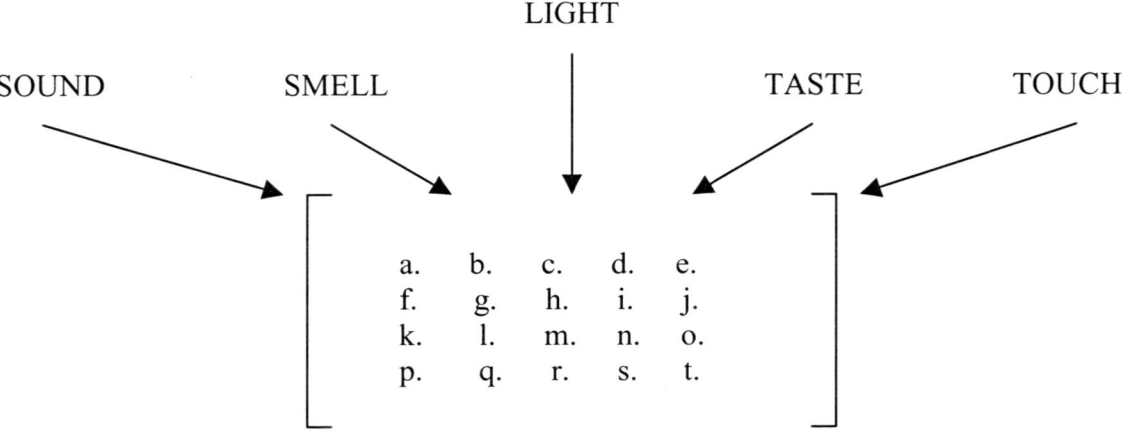

The implication is therefore that this could trigger memories by the association of sensory data or combination of sensory data with a past event.

We function as a complex data processing entity. Our ability to survive is based upon our abilities to grow; provide warmth, remain dry and protected from the elements; procure food; breed and raise our progeny. All of which is based upon our ability to understand and manipulate our environments. Our lives therefore comprise elements of learning, memory, adaptation, deduction, associative thinking, co-operation, and decision-making.

Generally, in childhood greater sensory stimulus (i.e. of a varied life) stimulates a positive outlook including reward, compliance, orderliness, happiness, good memory and attention, success, etc; whereas lack of sensory stimulus is associated with a negative outlook including e.g. disobedience, mischief, lack of attentiveness, poor memory, disorderliness, rejection, etc. These elements are largely related to our physiological development and age.

The brain doesn't work in a reductionist manner with isolated functions working separately. It functions as a coordinated whole and requires wholistic stimulation to function effectively.

# The Influence of Age upon our Physiological Function

*Consider how our age affects our physiology, our behaviour, our ability to do things, and ultimately our health and wellbeing*

The relationship between mind and body embodies all of the mental and physical changes which we experience during our lives. From birth, if not before, we undertake a short period in which as a child we seek first of all to survive i.e. the period of neurogenesis, whilst in the care of our mother and in preparation for the first significant period in our lives of childhood in which **'perception'** is our dominant neural function.

Copying is completely natural. This process of copying or learning is the most fundamental function for the human child without with we are unable to survive. **REPETITION, REPETITION, REPETITION.**

Nobel Laureate Susumu Tonegawa [50] states: 'Although baby animals are born with a handful of neurons tuned to respond to edges of light at specific orientations, the ability to detect these orientations improves with experience. The more the animal is exposed to shapes, objects and light, the better it can perceive them'.

The discovery by researchers of 'mirror neurons' [51,52] gives us insight into how the brain is able to reflect or copy acts and store memories. It forms the basis of our learning activity. This discovery enables us to understand how the body works at the sensory level and how we are able to memorise sensory stimuli. It also enables us to comprehend how 'the jig-saw like function of our brain' affects how we empathise and relate to our own experiences. In addition it conceivably affects our perceived emotions, and (immediate or otherwise) anticipation of events.

Researchers in the UK [53] have identified pathways connecting certain brain regions which continue adding layers of a fatty layer known as the myelin sheath onto neurones well into the adolescent period of development. As the myelin sheath speeds up the passage of nerve impulses to and from the brain, this shows that adolescents continue building their processing capacity as they move into adulthood.

REPETITION or TRAINING is the single most important factor in our lives and affects ever facet of our lives – from birth until our ultimate demise. Learning processes do not just affect our behaviour but also affect subtle aspects of our health and hence our ability to learn. Our health also learns to **adapt** to new circumstances through processes which maintain our stability or enable us to adapt to new circumstances.

Conversely, exposure to stress of sufficient magnitude or time, to which we cannot adapt, impairs mental and physiological development, learning abilities, immune system function, coordination and health.

The rate of physiological development varies from child to child. For some their immune system develops at a slower rate, or they may grow more slowly than average. Factors may include stress in their environment (variable temperature, a stressed mother (and of 'stressed' mother's milk) and dietary factors. This is not unusual. Some children are late developers whilst others have earlier or later experiences of development.

From childhood we steadily build muscle which enabling us to wriggle our arms and legs then, by a process of experimentation and of ' trial and error', learn to use our arms and legs, roll over onto our stomach, crawl, grasp and hold onto things, stand, walk, run, etc. This is the logical, cumulative process of learning which is consciously and subconsciously used throughout our adult life. We learn the basic routines necessary to control our function and then ever increasing sub-routines, and sub-sub-routines, as our lives become ever more complex in family, social, educational and work environments.

Everything which we do in our lives is based upon such processes of learning; of experimentation; of learning from experiences, of positive activities we enjoy and from which we derive benefit; and those negative activities which we do not enjoy and from which we derive no benefit or may even be punished. Such activities have a positive or negative effect and hence on our psychological and psycho-emotional profile, upon our biological function, our health, and our behavioural disposition.

If as a child we are suitably stimulated **this period of 'perception' which lasts until circa 15 years** is our dominant neural function and forms the period in our lives of most rapid learning i.e. the period of the greatest absorption of data and the period in which for example the most intricate issues related to balance and coordination can be most easily mastered.

We are born with a virtually empty brain (effectively devoid of memories from our short lives outside of the womb and of a limited number of memories and associations from our short time within the womb) and an **'operating program'**. During the first 15 years in our lives we steadily accumulate data which forms the basis for our lives. Our experiences from the very earliest days create the cumulative database upon which all other life experiences are compared. Traumas experienced in early life can therefore have a very much greater significance.

Each and every experience is compared with a previous experience(s) which explains the lingering memory of your first love, your reaction to your upbringing, your education, etc.

If we are lovingly nurtured we have a greater sensory receptiveness whilst if we are born into a turbulent or stressed environment we are subjected to the many stress effects influencing our mental and physiological development.

Accordingly the first memories of our lives become the dominant memories to which all our subsequent experiences and memories are compared and judged. Moreover our inherited genetic profile determines our key behavioural characteristics (including personality, attitude, etc) AND our predisposition to future health issues/ailments.

**The second period in our lives is at the point where our physiology changes from that of childhood into adulthood and lasts from c15 years until c30 years.** In this period in our lives our sensory perception is complemented by that of **'imagination'**, which becomes our dominating neural function, in which we relate our life experiences to our physical capabilities. We imagine how our lives should be, based upon our family model and the experiences of our lives gained to date, and we seek to implement this new model.

Consider this as the equivalent of moving from the simplistic model to one of the first grade of complexity e.g. from windows 95 to windows 98.

We move from the stage of learning and rehearsal i.e. of pre-puberty and adolescence; to the next stage of life in which we exercise the increasing physical capabilities of maturity and post-puberty; adapt to the greater social order of the adult work environment; create our lives in the manner which we have learned, or rejected, through our formative years; etc.

**By the end of this period we are nearing the end of our period of 'physical peak' and reach the third stage of our physiological development**, that of physical maturity, which lasts from the age 30 years until age 50 years in which **'memory and associative thinking'** becomes the dominant neural function.

For many this is the most productive period of our lives. We have energy and the product or memory of the issues which we have learned over the past 30-50 years which enable us to be accomplished in the more strategic and organisational aspects of our lives [54].

Continuing with the software analogy, it is the point where windows 98 gives way to windows millennium.

**And finally we reach the fourth and final stage in our lives in which at c50 years** we are in physical decline and we base our neural functions upon **'decision-making'**. The cynics would refer to this as 'been there, seen it, done it, got the t-shirt'. This explains the inflexibility or scepticism of the older generation when their production of neurons is no longer sufficient to expand their neural capabilities, to compensate for the loss of neurons, and the ageing brain goes into decline. We become steadily less energetic, less perceptive, less imaginative, and less able to associate facts. Our decision-making becomes based primarily upon our life's experiences and involves less integration of new facts/data. Associated with the menopause which affects both the male and female, this is the equivalent of where the brain's software programme becomes increasingly obsolete. These changes are supported by research conducted at Harvard Medical School [55], which has identified that a protein *PirB* that stops new neural connections forming in adult brains explaining why our brains become less flexible later in our lives.

The relationship of REPETITION with associative thinking lead to habits which become increasingly prevalent with age. It is the logical result of the accumulation of data, and associative thinking. We do things habitually because we have learned, rightly or wrongly, that this way is the least problematic and least stressful way.

The more that we see something, the more we expect to see that something, the more we consider it to be normal, the more that we consider it to be a true reflection of reality.

For example think about how a child raised in a difficult environment can become used to violence and consider it as normal in their world. Consider how someone raised in a violent environment gets used to handling knives and guns. Similarly consider how attitudes can be manipulated by continual exposure to programmes of advertising or brain washing. We are more susceptible to such influences in our youth, before we have had sufficient life experiences which enable us to formulate a balanced viewpoint.

We recognise how we go about our lives and do things out of habit. We use the same ways to travel to work; select our favourite foods, have the same breakfast. Each week our shopping bears an uncanny resemblance to that of the previous week's; we watch the same sports, the same television programmes, and have the same interests; we are drawn to films with our favourite actors, and to the same types of films or theatre presentations; we prefer the same types of car; etc. As we age it is surprising how predictable our lives become. We become creatures of habit.

As a young child we sought to conform yet as teenagers we actively sought and embraced change and looked for new experiences and new thrills. By contrast, with advancing years we avoid change because it represents the 'unknown'. The need to make decisions on these 'unknown' matters is increasingly stressful because our neural physiology finds it increasingly difficult to adapt.

Various psychologists have addressed the relationship between psychology and age. Grakov [56] has related our psychology to specific physiological changes in our lives, consistent with the mind-body philosophy, and appears to have based his work upon the findings of Carl Gustav Jung [57]. Other development psychologists have developed their own unique and often similar explanations of how behaviour changes with age [58].

While biochemists refer to the biological 'wet ware', computational neuroscientists increasing refer to the need to establish the right 'software' as the basis for the regulation and control of our physiology [64-67].

The phenomenon of age-related cognitive decline is generally accepted but there are studies suggesting that its onset is not solely related to age and that other factors can be used to slow its progress [62, 63].

# The Difference between Men and Women

*Many books have been written about the difference between Men and Women. Can these be explained by our differing biochemistry?*

Whereas a man's biochemistry remains relatively stable throughout each month a woman's changes throughout the menstrual cycle. A man's behaviour, attitude and mental outlook remains relatively stable whereas by contrast a woman's attitude, emotional profile, behavioural predisposition and health, varies throughout their monthly cycle - a product of their biochemistry – until in later years they encounter the menopause.

Women have greater sensory perception and sensory awareness whereas, by contrast, men are more functional and have less sensory awareness and sensory 'skills'. An estimated 10% of women are tetrachromic [59] whereas most men and the balance of women are trichromic.

[72, 73] One MRI study of males showed dominant activity in the left hemisphere of the brain. The MRIs of the female participants had heightened activity on both sides of the brain! It was evident that while men focused on processing the content they heard in a logical, linear way, the women were also using non-language based processing that included sensory perception, emotion, imagination, and experience.

Women - have 400% more connections between the left and right brains. They find it much easier to transfer data from one side of their brain to the other - as well as to absorb and process a wider range of information. Women have a "naturally ambidextrous brain," capable of enhanced perceptual speed, fine motor skills, and a higher degree of verbal fluency accounting for their ability to multi-task at an extremely high level.

Men are adept at concentrating, analysing, and working in a linear fashion which involves one mode at a time i.e. 'single-tasking'. This is most appropriate for tasks requiring speed of thought, action, and strength. They are good at transferring information from one region of the brain to another as they analyse something explaining how a man is generally more proficient at driving a car, reading a map, building a house, or logical processes of deduction.

Women are more efficient at processing information in general and are incredibly flexible and able to adjust to change. This appears to a man to be excessively complicating a simple process but explains why a woman appears to be less decisive, may be less proficient at driving a car, and would for example drive a car more carefully - than a man.

A man will spend time deliberating over a decision, reviewing the facts and evidence, whereas women will often make decisions based upon their interpretation, of what they perceive to be the issues based upon their complex biological function.

Women recover from strokes more quickly than men, with less damage to their ability to speak. It is conceivable that this ability is enhanced by the level of interconnection between right and left hemispheres of the brain.

Whereas a man's brain will function at the same rate as a woman's brain, the woman's brain will make decisions more slowly than a man because of its more complex decision-making process.

In September 2006 a leading academic [60,61] concluded from a study of the IQ of several thousand participants that men were more intelligent than women. Of course the IQ test was designed to assess linear thinking meaning that the study is biased towards men. This is in disagreement with the physical findings outlined above.

How would men would cope if the test was designed to assess their ability to deal with a women-oriented IQ test?

## The Influence of Stress upon our Physiology

*Everyone recognises the effect of stress upon our lives. To what extent does stress affect our emotional stability, behaviour, health and wellbeing?*

Whereas western researchers consider that stress merely exascerbates an established illness, Russian researchers have established since the 1970/80's that stress is actually the fundamental cause of illness 56.

### Figure 5

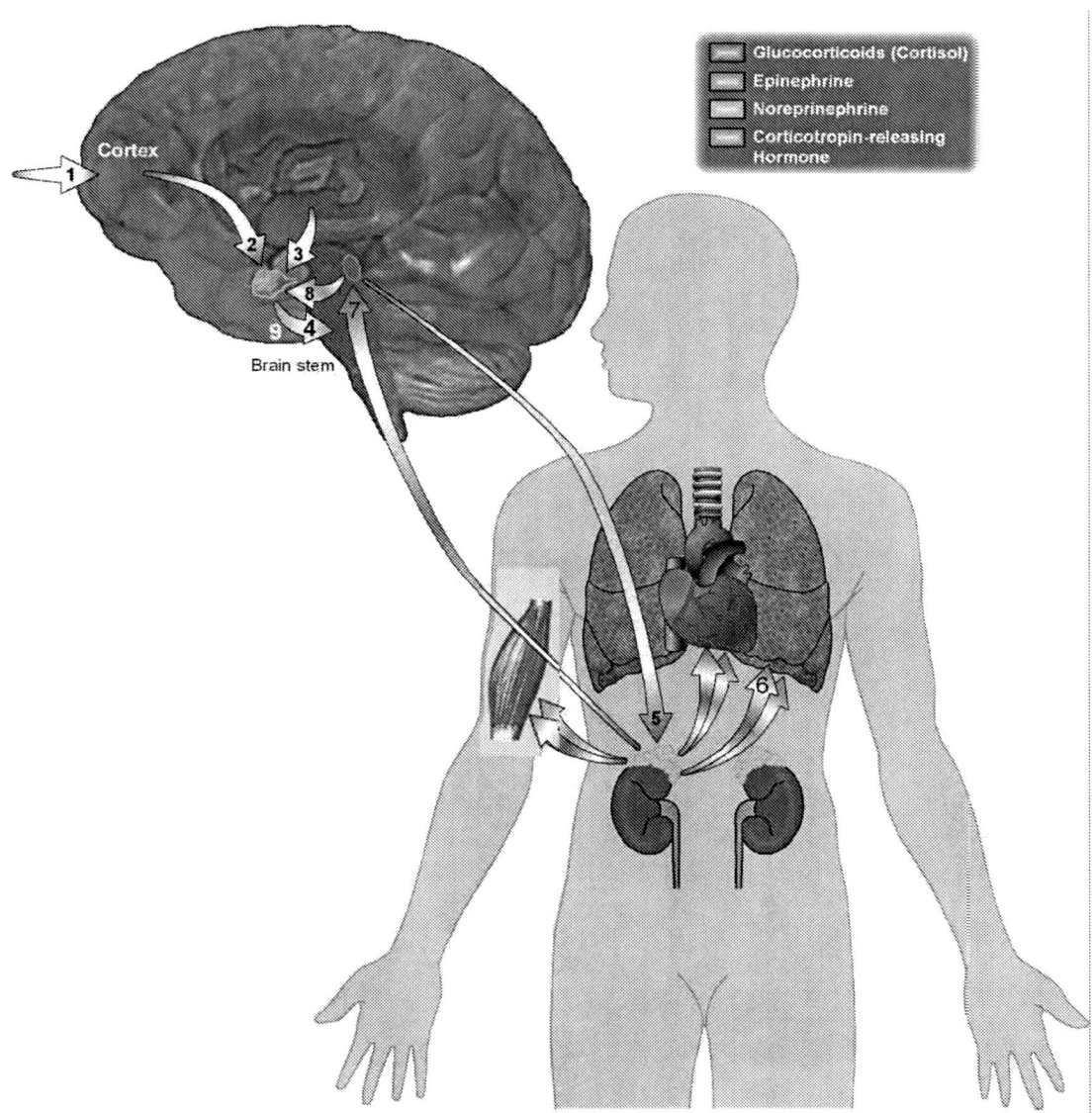

As illustrated in figure 5 stress depresses our immune system and destabilises all aspects of our physiology. In the most severe cases becoming manifest as chronic illness. If the exposure to the stress effect continues long-term or to extreme levels the body's natural mechanism for controlling stability (long-term memory and homeostasis) is overridden and a pathological functional system becomes established. Chronic illness manifests as pain and/or inflammation (thereby exascerbating the situation), as further stress factors, and hence create the conditions for a 'stable' pathological functional system.

Stress is accompanied by the production of adrenocorticosteroids by the adrenal glands which depress our immune system, thereby affecting our colour perception, our biochemical profile, and hence affects the coherence of the brain waves which regulate our physiological systems. As it depresses the immune system it also affects the production of Human Growth Factor and other related biochemicals which stimulate growth and cell reproduction thereby explaining how long-term exposure to stress can inhibit a child's mental and physical growth.

**Figure 6**

## The Effects of Depression

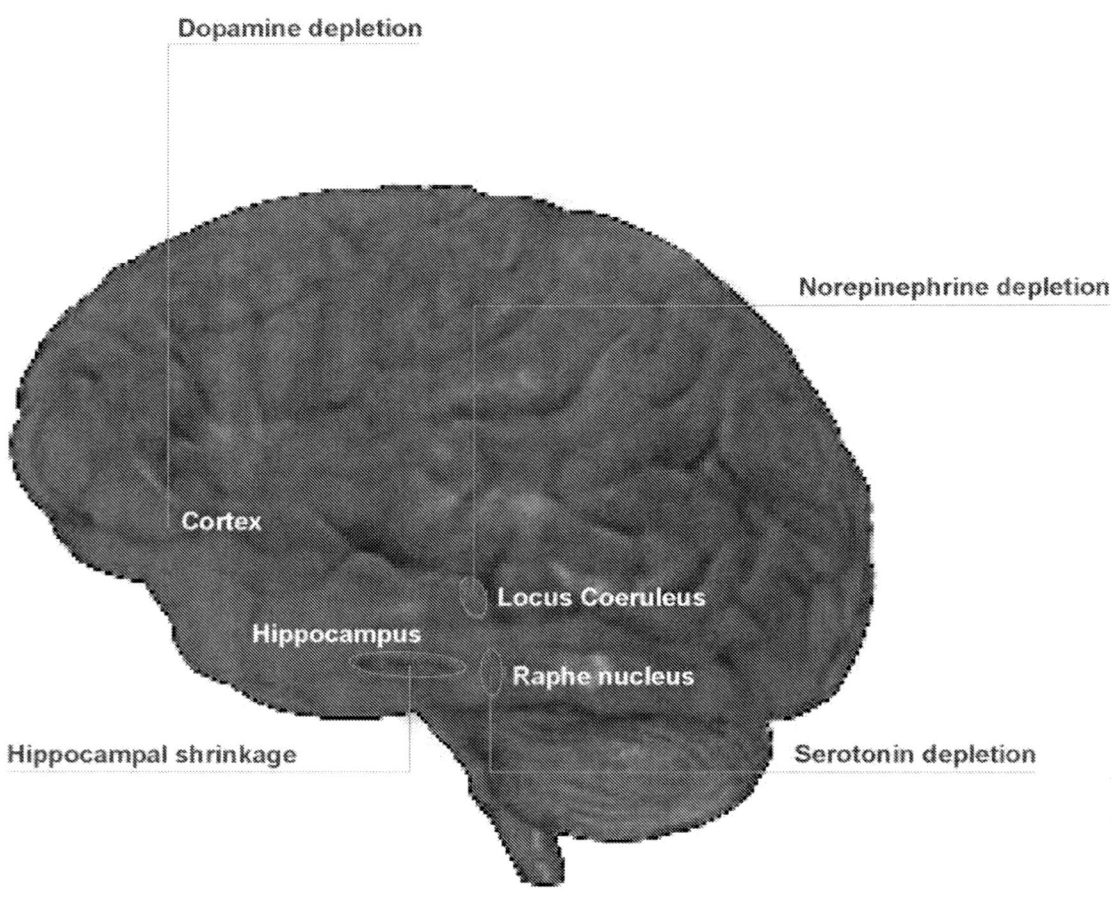

Stress factors include any influence demanding a physiological response beyond (either above or below) the body's normal physiological limits of operation, threatening the basic physiological requirements for warmth, food, drink, air, happiness, prosperity, mating, breeding, etc. Stress may arise for many reasons e.g. pollution; anxiety, violence or the perceived threat of violence; loud noise or excessive quietness, vibration; changed diet; rapid speed (car), jetlag, changing airpressure; heat or cold; imprisonment; drugs, vaccines, poison; tiredness and exhaustion; electromagnetic radiation; underachievement in education, sport or work, etc. Stress affects our pleasure response, attentiveness, memory, sleep, etc (see figure 6). Anything which changes our body's biochemistry is a stressor.

# Stress Affects the Brain

*Consider how stress affects the brain and how this results affects our physiological stability, mental health and wellbeing.*

Upon receipt of data the brain cortex sends signals to the amygdala, the organ of the brain considered to be the principal mediator to stress (figure 5). If the signals are of sufficient magnitude and significance, a stress response manifests releasing Corticotropin-releasing hormone (CTH) which, in turn, stimulates the brain stem and activates the sympathetic nervous system in the spinal chord.

The adrenal glands produce epinephrine and cortisol to produce the short-term stress response which stimulates the heart, lungs, etc.

**If the stress becomes a long-term issue the adrenal glands stimulate the locus coeruleus to produce norepinephrine which induces acceleration or long-term stability of the stress pathways.**

Long-term exposure to stress (figure 6) leads to effects which depress the levels of neurotransmitters such as dopamine. As dopamine is an integral component of the pleasure reflex the loss of dopamine can lead to lesser levels of pleasure and hence to depression.

Stress reduces the production of serotonin by the raphe nucleus and hence interferes with the communication between the locus coeruleus and the cortex. The locus coeruleus produces less norepinephrine and hence levels of concentration are reduced.

Stress interferes with the function of the raphe nucleus thereby creating depression and reducing happiness.

Stress inhibits the function of the hippocampus which is manifest finally by the loss of hippocampal cells and tissues which are essential for memory formation.

# Stress Affects the Body

*Consider how long-term exposure to stress affects our health.*

- When a person is stressed their blood pressure increases, the heart pumps faster, adrenal glands secrete adrenaline and cortisol. Too much stress leads to endocrine system disorders, excessive cortisol levels and a suppressed immune system.

- Excessive production of cortisol suppresses the immune system causing a drop in levels of dehydroepiandrosterone (DHEA) which is considered to be the body's anti-aging and immune-enhancing hormone.

- Stress is considered to increase the body's acidity (see chapter 3) and consequently leaves the body more prone to infections.

- Continued stress keeps the body remains in a constant state of alarm.

- Stress interrupts sleep and inhibits the regeneration of the body.

- By disturbing the quality and quantity of sleep, stress disturbs the levels of the proteins ghrelin and leptin involved in the regulation of appetite and satedness.

- Stress inhibits production of serotonin and is associated with onset of depression.

- Stress has been linked to most conditions with a psychosomatic basis including heart disease, cancer, gum disease; autoimmune diseases such as lupus, MS, rheumatoid arthritis; chronic fatigue syndrome and fibromyalgia, irritable bowel syndrome, skin inflammations (psoriasis, hives, eczema, herpes outbreaks), etc.

- Stress accelerates the brain's aging processes and affects learning and memory.

- Cortisol reduces production of NK cells - which kill cancer cells - therefore too much cortisol in the body increases the risk of getting cancer.

- Stress suppresses Natural Killer (NK) cell function and other aspects of immune function. The body compensates by increasing production of antibodies and specific hormones, which helps for short periods. When stress is severe or of long duration, inflammatory cytokines suppress NK cell function and the condition becomes self-perpetuating. This happens when several stresses occur simultaneously or coincide with NK cell suppression that naturally occurs at the time of ovulation in women.

The link between stress and ill-health appears indisputable.

# Stress Influences our Sleeping Patterns and Weight

*Consider how stress influences the quality and quantity of our sleep and how this subsequently affects our ability to regulate our weight.*

Stress manifests itself in ways which affect our function. It affects our sleeping patterns and hence affect the levels of proteins regulating appetite and feelings of satedness [71], which subsequently manifest through excess weight and in some cases the reverse i.e. too little weight. Inadequate duration, quality of sleep or disturbed sleeping patterns have a significant effect upon our ability to regulate our weight.

Excess weight affects our ability to control our body temperature, blood glucose, blood pressure, blood cell content, blood volume, and hence affects our processes of pH, digestion, excretion, sleep, etc. It even affects posture and places severe pressure upon our joints and our ability to pump blood to our extremities. Excess weight also affects our ability to regulate the levels of oxygen in our blood, and hence affects the function of all systems in the body including our ability (this applies equally to male and female) to have children.

Excess weight affects our cognitive function [68] with subsequent effects including mood swings, temper and aggression, lack of energy, poor memory and inadequate levels of concentration, depression, speed of response, etc.

Our ability to cope with stress declines with age. It is associated with lesser levels of health and wellbeing and at the end of our working life is associated with the quality and quantity of life expectations in retirement i.e. for males retiring at the age of 60 years there is a life expectancy of a further 20 years however for males retiring at age 65 years there is a life expectancy of less than 5 years.

# It is a Fact that our Health is Inversely Proportional to our Weight.

*Our quality of life is affected by our weight. Here we discuss how it affects our health, wellbeing, attitudes and ultimately our longevity.*

An international team of scientists [69] found that losing at least 5 kgs between 18 and 30 reduced the risk of cancer by up to 65%. They also showed gaining 5 kgs increased women's risk of developing cancer before the age of 40.

Simple logic makes us realize that excess weight limits our ability to exercise which subsequently affects a sequence of body functions including our muscle tone, our ability to breath/the function of our lungs, the quality of our blood, blood pressure, our ability to regulate our body temperature, our ability to fight illness, the level and function of our immune system, etc, etc.

Excess weight affects all aspects of life. Our vitality and quality of life are related to our physical capabilities which in turn are related to our weight and age. As our weight increases fat affects the function of every cell in the body. Our blood cholesterol levels are likely to increase, which make it more difficult to pump blood around our systems which in turn affect our blood pressure, and other aspects of our function including sleeping patterns, fertility, sexuality, appearance, posture, mental function, and wellbeing.

As we age our energy requirements decline; we need less food to fuel our lives; and our ability to burn off excess weight declines.

We look at a shapely, and fit, man or woman and consider their apparent health, beauty and vitality. It is not a coincidence that the fashion industry uses shapely fashion models to display the latest clothes. In general, we associate fitness and shapeliness and vitality with fertility and the ability to procreate a fit and healthy family.

Every kg of excess weight on the body places a disproportionately greater loading on the skeletal structure. In the most extreme cases this can result in curvature of the spine e.g. in a woman with heavy breasts; aches and pains throughout the skeletal structure; deprivation of blood supply to the joints resulting in arthritis-type symptoms; increased cholesterol and related components in the blood which affects the ability of the heart to pump blood thereby resulting in cold hands and feet and inadequate blood supply to the brain; difficulty raising the chest cavity to enable the lungs to inflate; inhibition of the processes of digestion and excretion; lack of energy; loss of participation in social events, reduced enjoyment and reduced quality of life; increased levels of anger, frustration; etc.

All these affect cognitive processing which shows that weight is a fundamental factor to be taken into account in any cognitive test [70].

# What is the Evidence for the Body's Physiological Systems?

*A physiological system is an inter-related set of organs that regulate a particular aspect of physiological function. If a system exists it will be identifiable and will have a dynamic range which has higher and lower levels of function.*

Examples of the more obvious of these functions, including useful supportive references extracted and edited from medical reference texts which refer to the existence of the body's physiological systems, are as follows:

**Blood pressure:**     which can be too high or too low

Blood pressure is regulated throughout the day and night by the autonomic nervous system which uses a network of receptors, nerves and hormones to regulate our blood pressure within accepted limits which, for most, is typically 135/90mm Hg.

Biomedicine appears not to understand why the body is driven to maintain high or low blood pressure Moreover, whereas in the UK high blood pressure is considered to be a significant problem and low blood pressure is largely ignored, in Germany low blood pressure is associated with impaired blood flow to the brain. Medications which thin the blood and stimulate blood flow (incl aspirin, ginkgo biloba and caffeine) are amongst the best selling products on the German pharmaceutical market.

**Body Temperature:**  which can be too high or too low

If the body is unable to remain at a normal temperature and it increases above normal (37C), this is hyperthermia; whereas when body temperature falls below normal levels, this is hypothermia.

**Sleeping pattern:**     sleep too little or too long

In general people sleep for around 8 hours per day. It is considered normal for those recovering from illness to sleep longer in the processes of recuperation from illness however there are recognised medical conditions insomnia and narcolepsy which are indicative of the high and low levels of the sleep system.

**Breathing:**          hyperventilation or dyspnea

Hyperventilation or tachypnea, illustrates the hyper function of our breathing system and is often associated with stress whereas dyspnea, or bradypnea, is indicative of the underperforming breathing system. If not regulated they would result in impaired absorption of oxygen and emission of carbon dioxide, reducing the CO2 concentration in blood below normal or increasing the concentration of oxygen above normal.

**Blood Glucose:**     too high or too low

Blood sugar concentration, or serum glucose level, is tightly regulated in the human body and stays within narrow limits throughout the day: 4 to 8 mmol/l. Medical conditions such as diabetes and excessive alcoholic consumption can affect the levels (referred to as hypoglycaemia or hyperglycaemia).

**Digestion:**

Digestion is separated into the processes: Ingestion and mastication, digestion, absorption and excretion. It involves the precise synchronisation and smooth operation of components in the digestive system.

**Excretion:**                 too high or too low/diarrhea or constipation

Ranging from constipation to incontinence

## pH:

It is considered that no matter what you eat, the food in your stomach is acidic and the food in your intestines is alkaline. You cannot change the acidity of any part of your body except your urine. Your bloodstream and organs control acidity in a very narrow range and anything that changed acidity in your body would make you very sick and could even kill you – by contrast, a child's pH is considered to be slightly more alkaline than an adult's!

All chemical reactions in your body are catalysed by enzymes which function in a very narrow range of acidity therefore if blood pH is changed for any reason, it is quickly regulated to the normal level or enzymes would not function and necessary chemical reactions would not proceed in your body e.g. when you hold your breath, $CO_2$ accumulates in your blood which turns acidic which may make you lose consciousness. If you do not rapidly recover this can result in damage to your kidneys which inhibits regulation of the blood pH with the consequences that chemical reactions in the body slow or stop, poisons accumulate in your system, and you may die.

Whilst the body's pH is homeostatically controlled to remain within strict limits there can be localised changes of pH associated with cancers, infections, our breathing system and hence of changes to the levels of oxygen and $CO_2$ in our blood, blood flow to the digestive system, and various medical conditions such as diabetes. It appears reasonable to consider that the body's pH system has subtle limits of operation.

## Blood Cell Content: too low or too high

anaemia or polycythemia are characteristic of illnesses caused by any deficit or excess of iron in the blood.

## Blood Volume: too little or too much

**Reduced blood volume**, called hypovolemia, is the most common mechanism producing hypotension. It can result from blood loss; insufficient fluid intake (starvation); or fluid losses from diarrhea or vomiting.

## Sexual Function: too high or too low

ranging from hypoactive sexual disorder to hypersexuality

## Skeletal Structure & Locomotion:

in which a person's locomotion or communication can be impaired or over stimulated (hyperactivity disorder)

## Osmotic Pressure

Osmosis regulates fluid retention and provides the primary means for the transport of water into and out of cells. It is essential for the flow of nutrients and minerals to the cell, the levels of minerals (incl sodium) in the cell and the removal of waste products.

# The Influence of the Body's Physiological Systems on our Health

*The body's physiological systems regulate all aspects of our health and function. Note how our exposure to environmental factors and influences subsequently affects the way which we do things, our energy levels, sensory perception, behaviour and ultimately our physiological stability.*

If the pH of our blood is destabilised, perhaps as a consequence of stress, this affects the pH in our digestive tract and hence the absorption of minerals, vitamins, etc. **If unduly acid this is manifest as indigestion and may be treated by antacids.** Unstable gastric acidity facilitates the growth of gut organisms which, although normally present in most people in small amounts, when the digestive acidity changes due to the onset of stress effects can result in significant growth of the organism e.g. helicobacter pylori, which is recognised to be responsible for processes of ulceration in the duodenum.

The level or ratio of mineral absorption may be affected; for example magnesium may be absorbed in preference to calcium, or potassium to sodium. This may affect the strength of the bones leading in the most severe cases to breakages or it may reduce the amount of haemoglobin in our blood affecting the efficiency of all physiological processes **involving the quality (cell content et al), quantity and pressure of our blood** i.e affecting all aspects of our physiology and mental function.

If we have too little blood volume, or our blood pressure is too low, or our **blood cell content** is deficient (and our immune system is compromised), or our **peripheral blood vessels** are in poor condition, this will affect our ability to regulate our **body temperature thereby** creating the conditions for the development of skin ailments such as eczema, psoriasis, etc. This may also leave us vulnerable to bacterial or viral infections.

Destabilisation of our **digestive system** may result in food arriving in the duodenum before the introduction of bile acids or after the introduction of bile acids. Either way this can result in the passage of undigested food, irritation of intestinal mucosa, build-up of digestive gases thereby leading to flatulence, diarrhea, or constipation. If constipation arises this will lead to the accumulation of toxins which should have been removed by the natural passage of the waste. If diarrhea arises this could lead to the lack of absorption of minerals and other nutrients.

If our **excretory system** is destabilised, involving the function of our digestive system, lymph nodes, kidneys, spleen, urinary tract, etc; this can lead to a build-up of toxins and to the establishment of pathological processes affecting our excretory function e.g. urinary tract infections, gastritis, colitis, irritable bowel syndrome, etc.

For this reason **nutritional supplementation** has only limited success. Similar to the adage 'you can take a horse to water but you cannot make it drink', you can give the body nutritional supplements but if it is not predisposed to absorb the nutritional supplement; perhaps due to adverse pH, insufficient blood supply, low blood pressure, poor blood cell content, etc; then they will not have the desired effect.

Nevertheless in the event that the body's systems have become destabilised it is important to consider a programme of mineral, vitamin or nutritional supplementation in the event that this condition has existed for a long period.

Nutritional supplements are not just limited to minerals or vitamins. Many significant medical conditions such as diabetes, pancreatic insufficiency, hypothyroidism, Cushing's syndrome (underfunction of the adrenal gland), are due the body's inability to produce (or to use) the required natural substances which are required for normal function. Accordingly the ability to restabilise the body's natural function and functional systems can support the various programmes which involve nutritional/drug supplementation e.g. of insulin, thyroxine, etc.

If we do not get sufficient **oxygen to our brain**, which is the most important organ (or collection of organs) in our body, our mental function will be impaired. Memory, concentration, and coordination are affected. Lack of oxygen can lead to migraine, epilepsy, stroke, hearing loss, alzheimers disease, parkinsonism, etc.

If we do not get sufficient flow of good quality blood to our sensory organs this will affect our ability to deal with inflammatory reactions and will affect our cognitive process including our sensory functions of hearing, smell, taste, vocal abilities, visual perception, and skin/touch.

If we do not get sufficient **sleep** the body's natural regulatory processes will be affected and the natural and normal level of proteins involved in daily function will be inadequate to regulate our function 71. As a result we will lack energy, be lethargic, mental processing will be dulled, appetite will be dysfunctional, feelings of satedness will be affected to the extent that we will eat too much (or, in the case of anorexia , too little).

Watching television too late; drinking too much beer, too often; all affect the quality and quantity of our sleep and hence can have a negative effect upon our learning abilities (memory, concentration, hearing, coordination, etc); upon our **sexual function**; upon our diet and hence upon our weight; upon our work; our health and safety in the work environment; upon the quality of our work and hence upon our promotional prospects, etc.

We should not ignore the effect of our **diet** upon our function although this has less to do with the functional systems. Any diet must comprise a balance of carbohydrates, protein and catalysts in the form of minerals and vitamins. Carbohydrates are essential for energy, proteins for the regulatory function, and minerals and vitamins as essential catalysts for our function but this excludes the reaction conditions (functional systems) of temperature, pressure, volume and pH. Stress, which can influence body temperature, blood pressure, the quality and quantity of the blood and body/digestive pH; can have an adverse affect upon the value of diet.

Nevertheless diet is known to affect our behaviour. Research [74] has established that DHA is structural to the brain and foresaw that deficiencies would lead to a surge in mental health and behavioural problems. Various studies have shown that adverse behaviour can be moderated by diet [73] although it appears certain that diet alone is unable to resolve the behavioural anomalies.

The ability to regulate our diet can also affect our digestion. If we eat carbohydrates the body releases the appropriate digestive enzymes for this task, and if we eat protein the body releases the appropriate digestive enzymes for this task however if we mix wildly differing diet comprising slow release foods and fast release foods it is clear that the digestive tract may not, especially in the older person, be sufficiently flexible and hence the accumulation of gaseous by-products could result in stomach aches and pains, diarrhoea, constipation, and other issues which we experience as part of the 'western diet'. Various dietary approaches consider the need to select the order in which we eat our food and, of course, the need to reduce carbohydrates in our diet as we become older – because we need brain food and not energy-creating foods.

In youth we require our mothers milk which provides valuable components for growth. Thereafter we require a balance of components which are appropriate to the stage of our lives. In general, up to 30 years of age we require fuel from carbohydrates and protein which is provided in and by nuts, pulses, meat and fish. Beyond 30 years of age we require less carbohydrates and greater levels of protein. As our age increases, our need for carbohydrates and fats declines significantly. Those who do not recognise this basic requirement suffer from increased weight, and place themselves at risk of declining health, poor mental health, decreased quality of life, decreased longevity, etc.

Our body's **skeletal structure** is an often undervalued component of our physiology. If the flow of blood to the spine (through low blood pressure, low blood volume, low blood cell content, etc) is affected this will have an effect upon our physical structure and of the function of the spinal region resulting in spondylosis (curvature of the spine), impaired flow/circulation of spinal fluid, impaired flow of blood to the brain, impaired cerebral circulation, inadequate flow of oxygen to the brain, etc. Further symptoms arising from spinal problems include myelitis, osteochondrosis, radiculitis, disc problems, headaches, migraine, stroke, etc.

If we are in good health our **sexual function** is good. We are more aroused and inclined to partake in the sexual act, our sexual organs have better blood flow, improved blood pressure, and hence are more sensitive. By contrast if we are in poor health we are less inclined to sex, our function is less satisfying, our fertility and productivity is poor, and the intensity of our love-making can be reduced.

**Osmotic pressure** is essential for the intracellular processes in our cells and blood. This affects the levels of white and red blood cells, function of the immune system, water retention of the cells, level of minerals in the cells, flow of signals to and from the cells, etc. These important factors affect our health, behaviour, speed of response, etc.

# The Biological Limits of our Health and Behaviour

*What is the implications of having biological limits?*

We must surely have limits of biological function which regulate the function of our physiological systems and which at the extreme will result in stress(es) which are subsequently manifest as medical conditions. Ultimately this may even threaten our existence. Such limits must be regulated by a mechanism which monitors and processes all physiological data. The medical profession refers to the function of these regulatory systems and associated limits as homeostasis and allostasis.

The process of learning and experimentation enable us to determine the limits of what is possible. If a child places its hand on a hot stove and burn its finger it learns, through the **pain** of the experience and consequent stress stimulus, not to do it again! This same process, of **deterrence**, is responsible for our adherence to the less attractive tasks in our lives e.g. homework: the threat of losing a privilege; parental displeasure; keeping to the law; driving according to the legal limit and procedures; the threat of punishment; working according to the agreed starting and finishing times; the threat of losing your job and income; etc. By contrast we may actively do tasks which bring enjoyment through labour, inventiveness, creativity, sex. These increase the body's natural levels of endorphins – the body's 'pleasure' chemicals.

As psychology and physiology are inter-related, limits of biochemical function are matched by corresponding limits to our behaviour, emotional profile and mental attitude. If exceeded on a long-term basis this can result in phobias, neuroses, vegetative conditions, nightmares, reduced mental capability, etc.

These conclusions lead to a wide range of multi-disciplinary medical approaches such as computational neuroscience, neurobiology, psychoneuroimmunology, neuro-oncology, psychoneuroimmunoendocrinology, health psychology, etc; however the problem for these disciplines is the lack of understanding of the hierarchical nature of the human physiology which involves the 14 identified physiological systems which regulate all aspects of our psychology and physiology.

By introducing specific mathematical models and computing, the researcher I.G.Grakov [75,76] (see chapter 2), has developed a technology which uses these insights in a predictable and understandable format.

Since mind and body are related we are drawn to the conclusion that our mental attitudes, emotional profile, psychological profile and/or behavioural predisposition reflect precisely the levels of biochemical components in our physiology and that the regulation of biochemical components influences our psychoemotional states.

These would affect for example:

(1) Attitudes having a **positive effect** upon our outlook include

Joy, Abstinence/Devotion, Patience, Righteousness, Community, Truth, Goodness, Creativity, Labour and Inventiveness

(2) Attitudes having a **negative effect** upon our outlook include

Ignorance/Obstinacy/Stubborness, Sorrow, Immoderation/lack of self-control, Desire, Injustice/Criticism, Greed, Mendacity/Lies, Envy/Covet, Anger/Resentment, Cunning/Cheat/Sly/Underhand, Hastiness/Impulsiveness, and Guile/Secretiveness

(3) our ability to complete a **decision-making** process from the first element of Intention, through a logical process including the stages: Wish, Will, Faith, Knowledge, Imagination, Implementation, Prioritisation, Ability to Act, Memory, Experience, Supervision, until completion i.e. Effectiveness.

(4) the balance of positive and negative components

All these measures are included in Grakov's psychological profile.

Our psychological profile is the product of our unique biochemistry including the quality of our genes (directly or indirectly) combined with our experiences and hence of our exposure to stress. All these affect our personalities.

We may be good at starting a project or we may be good at finishing a project or we may be good at getting on with a task within a team environment. Some of us may be good at gathering information whilst others may be more disposed to Action whilst some of us may be good at leading a team, being part of a team, communicating, teaching the team or working under management. Those that are successful from an early age may benefit from increasing positive outlook, self-belief and self-esteem.

Grakov's psychological profile uses task performance as well as visual cognition to obtain data. By comparison, other methods of psychometric profiling are based upon colour prioritisation, questions and answers, etc.

Genetic function can directly or indirectly be influenced by stress which affects the production of proteins and conceivably the activity of the proteins [77]. This almost certainly takes place at an epigenetic level.

### 'Is it possible to alter our psychological profile and hence overcome the genetic predisposition which is considered to be irreversible?'

In most cases researchers consider a genetic profile to mean that we will necessarily develop a particular medical condition or behave in a certain manner, only that we are predisposed under the right conditions to develop the medical condition or to behave in a certain manner [78]. If these conditions do not develop, perhaps through their environmental experiences, the person's predisposition to the specified ailment or to their behavioural anomaly can be significantly reduced. Accordingly Nurture is as important as Nurture when considering issues which affect health.

If so, there is clearly a mechanism at play which has the ability, directly or indirectly, to affect the function of our genes. Moreover medical researchers [80] now conclude that our DNA is influenced by how you think and feel.

As an indication that our behaviour has a fundamental biochemical basis [79] consider that there are an estimated 35,000 genes in the human genome of which over 50% are in the brain.

Stress affects the balance of our spirituality and outlook, psychological profile, psychoemotional profile, and our ability to function:

- to value the positive qualities – the need for love, for honour and respect, of aspiration for a better life, to work hard, be good, enjoy life, mix with friends and family, be patient with others, be educated, be well clothed, etc

- and of the negative issues all of which which reduce the quality of our lives  - to lie, steal, commit adultery, murder, covet, and of secretiveness, guile, underhandedness, envy, resentment, frustration, anger, haste, greed, obstinacy, lack of self-control, sorrow, to criticise, cunning, etc

# How these Regulatory Mechanisms Function?

*All functioning systems need to be regulated. The cerebellum is involved in such processing. It used to be considered to be a regulator of active function but is increasingly recognised to have a wider role.*

The human organism does not need certain components of the brain to function. There are examples where, by accident or design, people have had their cerebellum removed and where they have continued to function however their sensory function and longevity have been severely compromised.

The cerebellum contains more neurons than the sum of all other parts of the brain. It acts more speedily than any other brain component processing the information which it receives from other parts of the brain - including an enormous amount of information from the cerebral cortex which is connected to the cerebellum by an estimated 40 million nerve fibres. The optical nerve contains an estimated 1 million nerve fibres which transmit visual data from the retina to the brain i.e. forty times that amount of information can be sent from the cerebral cortex to the cerebellum, including information from the visceral cortex; motor, cognitive and language areas; and even from areas associated with emotional function. The result is that an enormous amount of information is sent to most other regions of the brain by the cerebellum.

**How is the cerebellum able to process this data?** It's structure and its output connections i.e. of the Purkinje cells, bear a remarkable resemblance to the design employed in modern computers.

The cerebellum is a component of the brain which, despite its massive computational capability is not yet fully understood. It is extraordinary to consider that no-one truly understands what is the precise function of the cerebellum. It's [81] function is related to movement, behaviour and sensory function yet its precise role remains a mystery. How can anyone claim to understand the function of the human brain when c50% is effectively excluded from consideration?

If the cerebellum has a processing capability similar to the cerebrum it may be involved in processing most, if not all, data in the cerebrum. It is possible the cerebellum functions as an organ which regulates and controls the limits of our physiological, and therefore of our psychological, function. This would explain the role of the cerebellum in coordinating the brain's acquisition of sensory data, and of the significance of the Purkinje cells which receive inputs from various organs and regions of the body [82].

Correspondingly, if the cerebellum is removed it seems logical to expect that a person's sensory perception would be affected, that their balance and coordination is affected, and their longevity is impaired – and this is what we see in people who have had their cerebellum removed.

Further supportive examples are of savants, associated with reduced interconnection of the two hemispheres of the brain [83], and people with autistic spectrum disorders who can have sensory impairment and yet be hugely talented in processes of calculation and memory.

([84] That there is a systems-based component in autistic-spectrum disorders is indicated by the clinical observations that high fever sometimes alleviates the symptoms, albeit temporarily.).

It appears reasonable to hypothesise that the cerebellum relates the processing of data to our limits of operation (including that of psychology and of physiology). This fits into the latest thinking where it is now suggested that the function of the cerebellum is 'to compensate for its own absence' and that the cerebellum is not responsible for any specific function of the brain and, that it provides a support function for the rest of the brain. This theory, propounded by world-leading neuroscientists, suggests that the cerebellum's function is to provide subtle adjustments regarding the processing of data perhaps involving the precision of data acquisition. This is consistent with the idea that the cerebellum is involved in regulating and processing sensory data from all parts of the body.

A person without a properly functioning cerebellum would lack regulation of their sensory processing and would have impaired sensory function. This would surely be comparable to that of the autistic savant for whom sensory function, connecting them to their environment through a comparison with current and past sensory experiences, is effectively slowed down or stopped. They see the world in 'absolute' terms whereas the vast majority of people see the world in 'relative' terms. For example a savant may give a perfect rendition of a musical piece but without the slight imperfections or intonations which give a musical performance its individual character.

This is consistent with the conclusion that absence of connection between the left and right hemispheres of the brain can result in greater 'linear' thinking and hence of dramatically improved ability to copy, learn, calculate, etc.

Here is an illustration of the fine line which exists between brilliance and malfunction!

The cerebellum in conjunction with our hearing function (involving the cochlea) is involved in the regulation of our movement – but not solely so. The ability to control our balance and physical stability requires massive processing capability and the rapid processing of massive amounts of data which is received from all parts of the body. By comparison the cerebrum does not require such rapid processing of data.

# Do the Systems which Regulate our Physiology, also Regulate our Brain, Psychology, Emotions and Behaviour?

*Is it possible that the physiological systems regulate all aspects of our health and that this is responsible for changes to our mental function which we recognise as cognition, sensory perception, memory, energy, function, behaviour and outlook?*

The brain does not work in a simplistic manner. For example initial studies re Schizophrenia concluded that reduced levels of dopamine were responsible. Like most initial hypotheses this has been shown to be inadequate. The production of the neurotransmitter dopamine is associated with specific components of the brain yet schizophrenia affects most brain's functions. As a result researchers [85] have considered how another neurotransmitter glutamate, also occurring more widely throughout the brain is also associated with schizophrenia and have moved from solely considering the dopamine deficit to include the glutamate deficit. As all aspects of brain function are affected disturbances in the brain's overall function, perhaps involving the stability of the physiological systems, could be responsible. [86,87, 89]

Those who expound such viewpoints [56] recognise the need to move away from the simplistic viewpoint considering single components to consider a systems-based viewpoint which includes networks of components, functions of whole organisms and the interaction of groups of organisms. They now consider that the simplistic consideration of biochemical processes at the molecular or cellular level cannot, by themselves, lead to an understanding of complex brain function (which relate cellular and molecular neuroscience to cognitive neuroscience and computational neuroscience).

Other computational neuroscientists [53] have theorised that the basic function of the brain is essentially due to the connections which exist between brain components and their intrinsic level of activity - which is affected by stress. There is a number of basic observations and precedents which support this theory e.g.

- The **hippocampus** of taxi drivers grows with use. Researchers at UCL using MRI have established that the brain of a taxi driver becomes larger.

- Children trained from an early age to kick a football with both feet, develop an ambidextrous approach. This becomes much harder to learn later in our lives.

- A person born left-handed (in a right-handed world) often develops a degree of ambidexterity. People born left-handed and ambidextrous have up to 11% greater interconnectivity between the left and right hemispheres of the brain [88].

- In dyslexics, the cerebellum is often less developed (cerebellar deficit) although the majority of people with a small cerebellum do not necessarily have dyslexia.

- Damage to the **insula** has been noted to influence a person's addiction to cigarettes

- And of the case of Phineas Gage, a railway worker who suffered a horrific brain injury when an iron bar more than three feet long entered his brain through his cheekbone and exited at the top of his head. He was able to survive this incident and continued to be able to speak, move and his mental abilities appeared to be unimpaired, but whereas before he was hard-working and conscientious he now become impatient, fickle, fond of swearing, etc; illustrating that parts of the brain work together in an inter-connected fashion and influence our mental function.

- There are recorded examples of some people who have had hydroencephalitis as a child, but had survived to adulthood. X-rays revealed that very little of their brain remained and that the hollow central portion was filled with only spinal fluid. For some they have above average intelligence [123-125].

- Some people have damaged particular components of the brain which are associated with specific functions such as memory. Despite these injuries the memories associated with the damaged, or lost, component are still present.

This would be depicted in mathematical terms as follows (see figure 7):

**Figure 7:** Typical illustration of a functional system comprising the inter-relationship of the organs (in this case – the digestive system) with the brain

Sensory Input
from the External Environment

Behavioural
Disposition

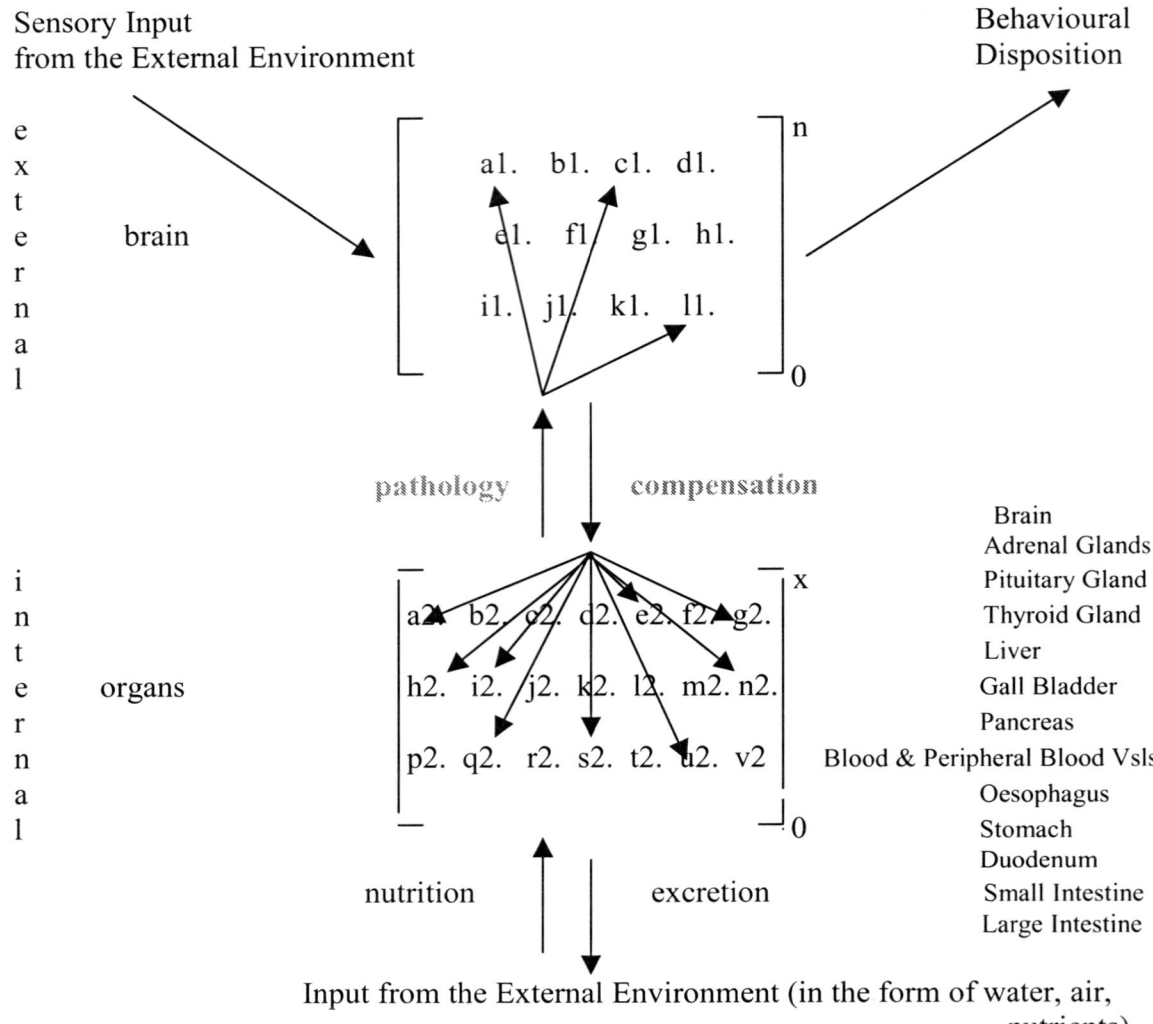

Brain
Adrenal Glands
Pituitary Gland
Thyroid Gland
Liver
Gall Bladder
Pancreas
Blood & Peripheral Blood Vsls
Oesophagus
Stomach
Duodenum
Small Intestine
Large Intestine

Input from the External Environment (in the form of water, air, nutrients)

# The Brain Expands Through Use.

*The brain is an adaptive organ. The more the brain is used; either to acquire facts, process data or to coordinate activity; the more it creates memory associations. The greater this ability to create memory associations, the greater the ability to recall previously acquired information, and also, to form new memories.*

Humans have large brains but are believed to use only a small fraction of the brain's capacity. Much of the brain is apparently obsolete – unless current techniques have not yet been able to observe the subtle mechanisms which use the remaining capacity of the brain – which remains a distinct possibility. The fact that one part of the brain is not used all of the time does not mean that it has no value or use but that its use has not yet been understood. This was true of the prefrontal cortex at one time. No-one knew what was its role so it was considered to be redundant e.g.

"The brain is the only example of evolution providing a species with an organ which it does not know how to use, a luxury organ, which it will take its owner thousands of years to learn to put to proper use – if it ever does." - Arthur Koestler

It can be argued that the human species can develop the use of the brain's full capacity and on occasions does use the apparently redundant areas.

The complex nature of our lives has inhibited our ability to function in a purely rational manner. It is this ability to superimpose our emotional responsibility over our rationality, using all component parts of the brain, which makes us the supreme species.

Many consider that the left brain hemisphere is the most important in brain function. Supporting this point of view researchers consider that the left brain is related to language, mathematics, logic, numbers, sequence, linearity, analysis, song words; whereas the right brain is better at patterns, spatial manipulation, rhythm, images, imagination, daydreaming, tunes. In simple terms, the left brain analyses and rationalises whereas the right brain synthesises.

The reality is that our brain uses all its component parts. The brain and body does not use each organ or component in apparent isolation. That such an explanation, typically reductionist, could suffice to explain the function of the brain, or of our organs, is simplistic and unthinkable.

# The Sensory Function, Complementary Health and the Body's Natural Processes of Compensation.

*Whereas the mechanisms of illness and of pathology are dealt with by drugs where are the mechanisms which maintain our health and which prevent the onset of illness?*

The principles which apply to light and colour, as outlined earlier, appear also relate to sound and tone. (1) Researchers in Spain have been able to relate, empirically, our vocal spectrum to the function of our organs [91], and (2) audiological research has been able to prove, empirically, that the hearing spectrum of some dyslexic children is affected by their health. Conversely the use of music, which has been modified to enhance the depressed elements in their audiological spectrum, is able to bring some improvement to hearing [47], and (3) smell training is also claimed to treat issues such as depression [93].

Such mechanisms fall within those complementary health technologies which are based upon the function of our various senses i.e. upon the receipt of sensory input:

- Colour and light therapy     Colour/Sight

- Audiotherapy, Music     Sound/Hearing

- Massage     Touch

- Aromatherapy     Odour/Smell

- Crystal Voice     Voice/Speech

Elements of these approaches are of course important components of Ayurvedic medicine and other ethnic medicines e.g. Tibetan medicine, Chinese medicine. They contrast with other complementary health systems which involve (1) nutrition, supplementation, and drugs; and (2) the processes which focus upon the body's system of meridians e.g. acupuncture.

Long-term disturbances to our regulatory function [50] result in destabilized functional system and hence of unstable pathology.

This kind of approach can be used to construct models which offer a plausible explanation for the function of almost all therapies including meditation, hypnosis, yoga, and ayurveda; behavioural therapies including sport; the sensory-based therapies including music and sound therapy, reflexology, aromatherapy; of systems which work on the body's meridians e.g. acupuncture; and of herbal remedies, nutrition, and many drugs/medications (see fig 8)

**Figure 8**

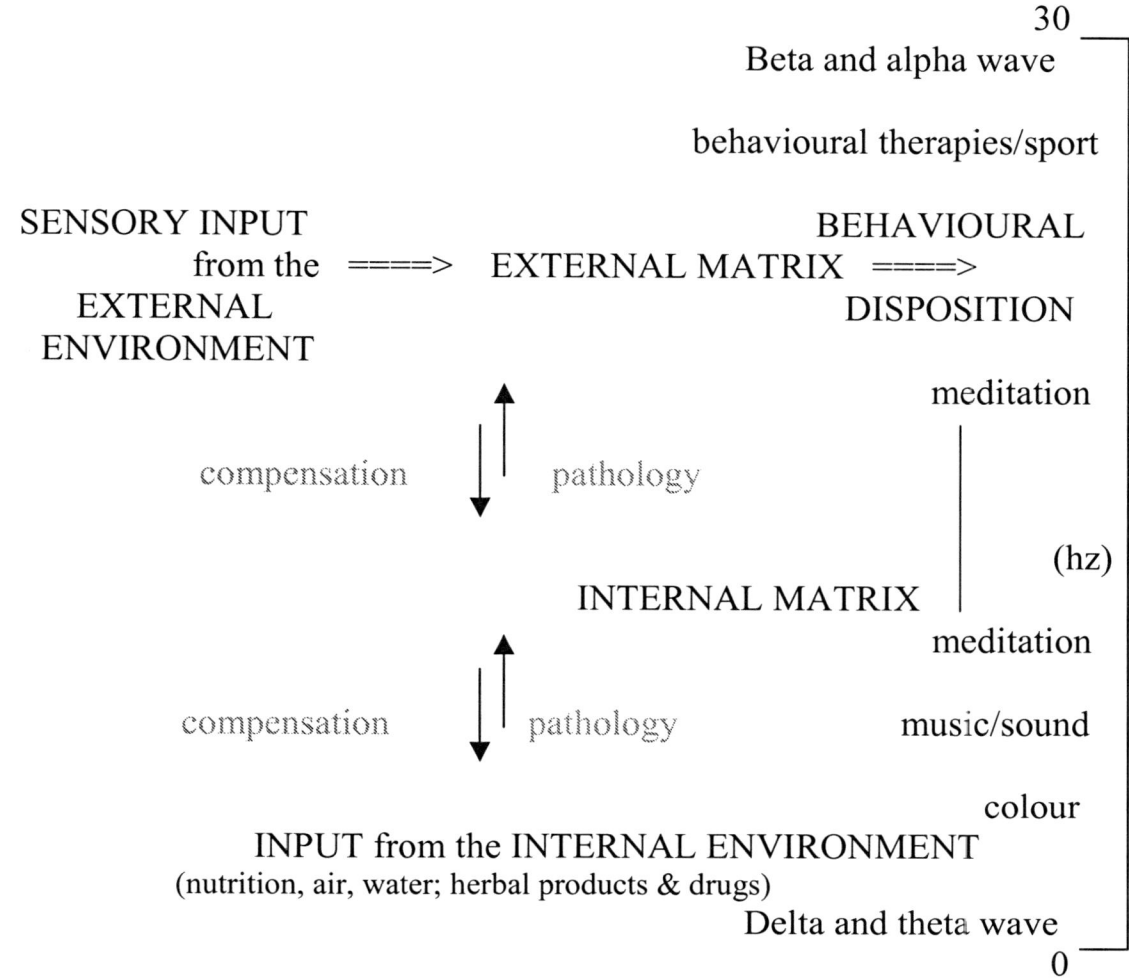

In simple terms our behaviour is regulated by the beta wave which scans at typically 15-30 hz. This rate of scanning is essential for behavioural function however if our health were to be regulated at this frequency and this rate of data input it would be difficult to maintain stability. Our health is fundamentally regulated by the delta wave which scans at typically 1-4 hz which is more appropriate for maintaining the stability of a complex system.

New medical technologies focus upon the means to detect illness and use an understanding of the body's function and physiology to establish new techniques which can be used for diagnosis (MRI scanners, ultrasound, etc) and therapy (radiotherapy, etc). The conventional approach has been to develop invasive techniques based upon the detection and treatment of symptoms, by contrast complementary health technologies offer techniques focussing on the natural processes involved in the regulation of our physiology and hence which treat the cause of the medical condition e.g. the sensory-based approaches.

Other complementary techniques, which can be used to diagnose or treat the symptoms of illness e.g. acupuncture, electroacupuncture; and which use the body's meridians are known to function by suppressing the symptoms of illness e.g. of the pain response. It is worth considering whether this contrasts with an approach involving 'stimulating the natural processes which are responsible for good health and wellbeing'.

The human body interacts with our environment in a multitude of ways. These can be at the biochemical level or structural level in which systems for histological testing or biomedical screening technologies are used to determine the precise levels of biochemicals and hence determine the processes or symptoms of illness. Also used are radiological tests such as MRI, X-rays, Ultrasound, etc.

The body comprises an array of organs and biochemical processes which are all generating and interacting with electrochemical impulses. They can be manifest as electric fields such as the AURA. The interaction of one person's field with another's could have both diagnostic and therapeutic applications. Moreover as the body's biochemistry is based upon our receipt and transmission of DATA it appears plausible consider that this data could be cumulative and could form the basis of the psychological evaluation of a person or indeed of more than one person or groups of persons.

It appears logical to categorise the various health approaches, biomedical or complementary, as follows:

- which are sensory-based and focus on the body's natural compensatory mechanisms i.e. which are responsible for our health and wellbeing.

- which are based on our biochemistry i.e. drug or nutrition-based, and which treat the symptoms of illness

- scanning technologies used to scan our body for physical abnormalities which are based upon fully researched and understood physical parameters

- which are based upon the meridians and work by suppressing the symptoms of illness

- which are based upon inadequately researched parameters for which there is currently an inadequate scientific basis e.g. aura.

The progression of science into obscure phenomena has led to new and more sophisticated technologies. Virtual Scanning, arising from the application of new science and mathematics, now leads to a greater understanding of our sensory perception and cognition. It heralds the introduction into medical practice of a new category of medical device with extraordinary diagnostic and therapeutic capabilities.

# The Negative Effects of Electromagnetic Radiation

*There is now a mass of information concerning the positive and negative effects of electromagnetic radiation [94-96, 118-119].*

The dangers of microwave radiation (i.e. the radiation from cell phones and mobile phone masts): Extensive use of cell phones is clearly associated with damage to the eye and growth of cataracts, and the development of brain tumours [97,98]. Damage to brain cells which initially show up as neurological, reproductive, and cardiac type problems are subsequently manifest as problems such as severe headaches, sleep disturbances, memory loss, learning disabilities, attention deficit disorder, and infertility show up long before cancer. When cancer does appear, it's typically brain tumors, leukemia, and lymphoma.

The danger of microwave radiation is clearly identified by medical researchers [99].

"Some people become ill at power densities of less than 10 nanowatts/cm$^2$. Small children are very sensitive to these emitters, down to field densities of 1 nanowatt/cm$^2$."

Dr. Henry Lai, a well-known bioelectromagnetics researcher at the University of Washington, Seattle, has compiled a 97-page collection of abstracts from studies conducted between 1995 and 2000. The list can be found on the Research page of the EMR Network's web site. As the web site points out, "80% of these studies demonstrate some kind of biological effect." [100].

*The Physiological and Environmental Effects of Non-Ionising Electromagnetic Radiation* is a 34-page report issued in March 2001 by the European Parliament Directorate General for Research, Scientific and Technological Options Assessment (STOA). Written by Dr. Gerard Hyland [101], it pulls no punches in warning of the hazards of microwave radiation.

Recent studies confirm that cell and cordless phone microwave can damage nerves in the scalp, cause headaches and induce extreme fatigue; cause memory loss and mental confusion; precipitate cataracts, retina damage and eye cancer; create burning sensation and rash on the skin; induce ringing in the ears, impair sense of smell; create joint pain, muscle spasms and tremors; cause digestive problems and raise bad cholesterol levels; alter the brain's electrical activity during sleep; open the blood-brain barrier to viruses and toxins; cause blood cells to leak hemoglobin; reduce the number and efficiency of white blood cells; stimulate asthma by producing histamine in mast cells; stress the endocrine system, especially pancreas, thyroid, ovaries, testes; disturb the hormone and immune systems; cause cancerous cells to grow aggressively; promote rapid cell aging.

Other Negative Environmental Effects: It is now proven that living within 500 metres of a main road stunts the lung development of a child.

# Could a Person's Personality Change as a Result of Undergoing an Organ Transplant? Is There a Rational Explanation?

*If mind and body are inter-related as outlined in the earlier text, and body's function is dependent upon the feedback of data to and from an organ, consider whether a person's character may change as a result of undergoing an organ transplant, or blood transfusion.*

A television feature programme [101] reported how, following blood transfusions and organ transplants, people adopted behavioural traits, habits and hobbies which were acquired from the donor. In the absence of a plausible mechanism such issues remain speculative.

It is acknowledged that a person's psychology, psychoemotional profile, character or personal interests can change as a result of a blood transfusion or organ transplant [102] or physical damage to the brain. According to this study of patients who have received transplanted organs, particularly hearts, it is not uncommon for memories, behaviours, preferences and habits associated with the donor to be transferred to the recipient.

Other studies have recounted that a person's memory can be retained or indeed can recover following damage to or removal of the parts of the cerebrum which were considered to have been responsible for specific memories [103]. Memory is more complex. It does not conform to the simplistic assumption that specific parts of the cerebrum are responsible for a specific memory task.

To illustrate how medical research continues to decipher how the brain works - until recently it was assumed that neurotransmitters were to be found in the neural regions i.e. the brain, however recent research has established that neurotransmitters are to be found throughout the body.

If the body functions as a complex biofeedback system with the brain feeding information to the brain and vice versa it is logical to expect that a change of organ would affect personality, emotions, memories, etc.

Could a person's personality and function change as a result of an illness or an induced illness?

A person recovering from a severe illness has less vitality. It takes time for their immune system and energy levels to be replenished, and to recover their natural levels of wellbeing.

In some cases exposure to viruses and bacteria lead to the development of chronic or acute medical conditions thereby affecting the person's wellbeing, mobility and consequently their quality of life [104]. It follows therefore that someone with a chronic condition would experience changes to their personality, behaviour and emotions.

46

# How we Absorb of Data in the Form of Colour.

*Everything that we see is characterised as a shape and as a colour. Can colour also have a therapeutic value?*

Light is amongst the most powerful of therapeutic agents. In hospitals the therapeutic effect of 'light green' is used in heart wards because it is known to reduce heart rate and lower blood pressure. In restaurants 'a rich red' is known to stimulate appetite. In mental hospitals walls were repainted because a cream colour was considered to have a depressive effect.

Light and colour clearly influence our physiology, psychology, emotions and behaviour. The question to be addressed is whether the effect is significant. There are many precedents illustrating the benefits of light-based medicine e.g.

- Photic stimulation and light-based biofeedback technologies have existed since the 1930's [107,108]. Empirical manifestations of the biofeedback approach continue to be researched and have been re-introduced in recent years for treatment of dyslexia.

- In 1903 Nobel Laureate Dr Niels Ryberg Finsen was recognised for his investigative work and clinical application of light therapy.

- 'Diabetic' sailors do not need hypoglycaemic therapy when they are at sea [109] because of increased exposure to light.

- Over 100 medical conditions are known to respond to the positive therapeutic effect of light and colour e.g. [110] Hyperbilirubinema.

- Sunlight stimulates the production of Vitamin D which is necessary for good bone metabolism.

- Light therapy has been scientifically proven to be more effective than Prozac for the treatment of depression.

- There is now a plethora of light-based treatments which are used to treat a variety of ailments e.g. of dermatological conditions [122], pain, memory enhancement, etc.

Exposure to light should not be confused with exposure to strong summer sunlight including infra-red radiation, ultraviolet radiation, x-rays, etc. Over-exposure to ultraviolet radiation is considered to be the main cause of skin cancer. The adverse effect of infra-red radiation results in damage arising from over-heating i.e. blisters, and damage to the epidermis and sub-layers of the skin.

# The Mind-Body Connection

*Your body is a biochemical entity. Anything that influences our psychology must therefore have an influence on our health.*

Stress induces long-term changes to our physiology affecting our health which are manifest as medical conditions, and which subsequently affect our sensory perception and behaviour.

The mind-body relationship is even more precise and predictable than has hitherto been realised. We can hypothesise that the limits of health will be accompanied by limits of behaviour. Short-term changes, arising from short-term exposure to stress, will have little effect upon our health. On the other hand long-term exposure to stress will have a significant effect upon our health.

The resulting pathological conditions are dependent upon a person's

   (1) the genetic profile (i.e. of nature)

   (2) history and experiences (i.e. of nurture)

   (3) age

   (4) weight

   (5) magnitude of the stress event

   (6) length of exposure to the stress event.

In addition the long-term exposure to a stress-effect will have an effect upon the person's behaviour. Moreover we can, therefore, consider the possibility that long-term exposure to a stress-event can result in health and behavioural abnormalities such as RSI (repetitive strain injury), obsessive-compulsive disorders, and perhaps also for phobias, neuroses, etc.

In most cases stress is the result of a visual encounter in which our long-term exposure to the experience, which is beyond the normal limits of behaviour, can shape our thought processes.

In childhood we do not have sufficient memory on which to base independent thought and deduction. Correspondingly, insufficient experience of life in childhood may inhibit adult development and in the most severe cases could result in phobias ranging from fear of height, water, roller-coasters, speed, air travel, etc.

It may also lead to lack of balanced opinions because these are based upon our ability to relate the data which has been made available to us through our experiences, media, books, etc. We just relate together the available data and try to fashion it into an intelligible format.

A major source of stress can be the way advertising creates perceived needs. It influences our opinions and reflects what is desirable in life. In general we relate to such information and our subconscious works it into some kind of intelligible influence.

In advertising, the basic concept is to show the product to the child, illustrate how it brings fun, how their friends want to have it (i.e. to create inclusion), and how to pressurise their parents.

In our teens, childhood memories and experiences are fashioned through imagination to create an identity appropriate to how a person may wish their lives to develop.

A car advert appeals to the raciness of the car and its ability to attract attention from a mate. Beer adverts focus upon the sexiness of the product – in contrast to the reality that beer inhibits the ability of a person's brain and mouth to function in a coordinated manner. Recent advertising even attempts to appeal to the apparent normality of being fat and flabby through drinking beer and how this is normal if you are a football supporter.

For adults, for which associative thinking is increasingly important the car advert relates together the raciness of the car, the attractive wife, and the happy family and promotes the idea that the product is appropriate for the family's complex needs.

In old age, advertising is focussed upon creating an awareness of the product, and thus appeals to the older person's needs. They know what they want, does it do it?

States of mind and body correspond closely enough for the relationship to be predictable. Virtual Scanning highlights this by introducing detailed mathematical models of the connection. This indicates that behavioural changes or abnormalities can be related to precise physiological changes which may, in turn, be related to specific health anomalies.

Further reading about the relationship between mind and body, and of brain wave coherence 111, 112-117.

# References

1. J. Liberman: *Light—Medicine of the Future*, pub, Bear & Co., Vermont, 1991; http://www.egt.bme.hu/!EnglishEducatio/Basic%20Dayl.%20Arch.pdf

2. *Cerebral Cortex*, Vol. 10, No. 8, 772-783, August 2000; Current Biology 13, R10-12, January 8,2003;

3. Dr John Ott: http://www.dickblick.com/vendors/ott-lite/

4. *Psychol Med.* 1998, 28(4):923-33, Effects of fluoxetine versus bright light in the treatment of seasonal affective disorder: Ruhrmann.S, Kasper S, Hawellek.B, Martinez B, Hoflich G, Nickelsen T, Moller HJ:

5. Barrett, D. Preference for Color or Tint and Some Related Personality Data, *Journal of Personality*, pp. 222-232, 15, 1946-47

6. Brainard, G. et al, Effects of Different Wavelengths in Seasonal Affective Disorder, *Journal of Affective Disorders*, pp. 209-216, 20, 1990

7. Cerbus, G. & Nichols, R. Personality Variables and Response to Color, *Psychological Bulletin*, pp. 566-575, 60(6), 1963

8. Cremer, R. et al, Influence of Light on the Hyperbilirubinemia in Infants, *The Lancet*, pp. 1094-1097, 1, 1958

9. Dewan, E. et al. Effects of Photic Stimulation on the Human Menstrual Cycle, *Photochemistry and Photobiology*, pp. 581-585, 27, 1978

10. Erlanger, B., Photoregulation of Biologically Active Macromolecules, *Annual Review of Biochemistry*, pp. 267-283, 45, 1976

11. Erlich, S. & Apuzzo, M. The Pineal Gland, *Journal of Neurosurgery*, pp. 321-341, 63, 1985

12. Evans, B. & Drasdo, N., Tinted Lenses and Related Therapies for Learning Disabilities – a Review, *Opthalmic and Physiological Optics*, pp. 206-217, 11(3), 1991

13. Finsen, N. The Red Light Treatment of Smallpox, *British Medical Journal*, pp. 1412-1414, 7, 1895

14. Fedoseyeva, G. et al, Human Lymphocyte Chromatin Changes Following Irradiation with a He-Ne Laser, *Lasers in the Life Sciences*, pp. 197-205, 2(3), 1988

15. Hamid, P. & Newport, A. Effect of Color on Physical Strength and Mood in Children, *Perceptual and Motor Skills*, pp. 179-185, 69, 1989

16. Hannell, G. et al, Reading Improvement with Tinted Lenses, *Clinical and Experimental Optometry*, pp. 170-176, 72(5), 1989

17.    Hollwich, F. & Dieckhues, B.  The Effect of Natural and Artificial Light via the Eye on the Hormonal and Metabolic Balance of Animal and Man,

18.    *Ophtalmologica*, pp. 188-197, 180, 1980

19.    Lubart, R. et al, Biostimulation of Photosensitized Fibroblasts by Low Incident Levels of Visible Light Energy, *Laser Therapy*, pp. 101-106, 7, 1995

20.    Martin, A. et al, Discrete Cortical Regions Associated with Knowledge of Colour and Knowledge of Action, *Science*, pp. 102-105, 270, 1995

21.    Martinek, K. & Berezin, I.  Artificial Light-Sensitive Enzymatic Systems as Chemical Amplifiers of Weak Light Signals, *Photochemistry and Photobiology*, pp. 637-649, 29, 1979

22.    McDonald, S  Effect of Visible Lightwaves on Arthritis Pain, *International Journal of Biosocial Research*, pp. 49-54, 3(2), 1982

23.    Oren, D. et al, Treatment of Seasonal Affective Disorder with Green Light and Red Light, *American Journal of Psychiatry*, pp. 509-511, 148(4), 1991

24.    Rattemeyer, M. & Popp, F.  Evidence of Photon Emission from DNA in Living Systems, *Naturwissenschaften*, pp. 572-573, 68, 1981

25.    Roberts, J.  Visible Light Induced Changes in the Immune Response through an Eye-Brain Mechanism, *Journal of Photochemistry and Photobiology*, pp. 3-15, 29, 1995

26.    Rochkind, S. et al, Systemic Effects of Low Power Laser Irradiation on the Peripheral and Central Nervous System, *Lasers in Surgery and Medicine*, pp. 174-182, 9, 1989

27.    Rochkind, S. et al, Spinal Chord Response to Laser Treatment of Injured Peripheral Nerve, *Spine*, pp. 6-10, 15, 1990

28.    Rochkind, S. & Ouaknine, G.  New Trend in Neuroscience: Low-Power Laser Effect on Peripheral and Central Nervous System, *Neurobiological Research*, pp. 2-11, 14, 1992

29.    Sato, H. et al, The Effects of Laser Light on Sperm Motility and Velocity in Vitro, *Andrologia*, pp. 23-25, 16(1), 1984

30.    Schaie, W.  On the Relation of Color and Personality, *Journal of Projective Techniques*, pp. 512-524, 30, 1966

31.    Schauss, A.  Tranquilizing Effect of Color Reduces Aggressive Behavior and Potential Violence, *Journal of Orthomolecular Psychiatry*, pp. 218-221, 8(4), 1979

32.    Schauss, A.  The Physiological Effect of Color on the Suppression of Human Aggression, *International Journal of Biosocial Research*, pp. 55-64, 7(2), 1985

33. Sisson, T. Visible Light Therapy of Neonatal Hyperbilirubinemia, *Photochemical and Photobiological Reviews*, pp. 241-268, 1, 1976

34. Tadakuma, T. Possible Application of the Laser in Immunobiology, *Keijo Journal of Medicine*, pp. 180-182, 42(4), 1993

35. Wolfarth, H. & Sam, C. The Effects of Color Psychodynamic Environment Modification upon Psycho-Physical and Behavioral Reactions of Severely Handicapped Children, *International Journal of Biosocial Research*, pp. 10-21, 3(1), 1982

36. Wurtman, R. The Effects of Light on the Human Body, *Scientific American*, pp. 69-77, 233(1), 1975

37. Young, S. et al Macrophage Responsiveness to Light Therapy, *Lasers in Surgery and Medicine*, pp. 497-505, 9, 1989

38. Zelickson, B. et al Clinical and Histological Evaluation of Psoriatic Plaques Treated with a Flashlamp Pulsed Dye Laser, *Journal of American Academy of Dermatology*, pp. 64-68, 35, 1996

39. **http://www.biocybernaut.com/documentation/benefits/agereversal.htm**

40. **http://www.hri.ca/tribune/viewArticle.asp?ID=2650**

41. Sir Michael Rutter, reported in the 'Observer', *Association of Psychological Science:* 19, 8, 28

42. Craik FIM, Salthouse TA. *Handbook of Aging and Cognition*. Hillsdale, NJ: Erlbaum, 1992; Smith GE, Petersen RC, Parisi JE, et al. Definition, course, and outcome of mild cognitive impairment. *Aging Neuropsychol Cogn* 1996;3:141–7.

43. An Interpretation of the Effects of a Single Dose of a Glyconutritional Supplement on the Brain Function of Healthy College Students, Including a Review of Brainwave Function, *Bill H. McAnalley, Roscoe A. Dykman, Kathryn D. Dykman, and John E. Hall:* http://www.glycoscience.com/glycoscience/document_viewer.wm?FILENAME=C011

44. "The adolescent decline of NREM delta, an indicator of brain maturation, is linked to age and sex but not to pubertal stage," Feinberg.I, Higgins.L.M, Khaw.W.K, Campbell.I.G. The *American Physiological Society* & *American Journal of Physiology-Regulatory, Integrative and Comparative Physiology* 291: R1724-1729, 2006

45. Professor Jonathan D. Cohen, Professor of Psychology, Director, Center for the Study of Brain, Mind and Behavior, Princeton University

46. Professor Gary Lynch, Professor of Psychiatry & Human Behaviour, School of Medicine, University of California

47. www.ImmuneSupport.com; Leon Chaitow

48.    comments attributed to Dr Akio Mori; *New Scientist* 11 July 2002

49.    Bullock.T.H et al: *Science* Vol 310, pages 791-793; November 4,2005

50.    http://web.mit.edu/newsoffice/2006/neuron.html; *Cell* July 28, 2006; Nobel laureate Susumu Tonegawa, MIT (a co-author of the study) and Wang.

51.    *New Scientist November 2006*; Action Recognition in the Premotor Cortex: Vittorio Gallese, Luciano Fadiga, Leonardo Fogassi and Giacomo Rizzolatti: published in *Brain*, Vol 119, no2, pages 593-609, April 1996;

52.    A Unifying View of the Basis of Social Cognition. V.Gallese, C.Keysers and G.Rizzolatti in *Trends in Cognitive Sciences*, Vol 8, pages 396-403, 2004.

53.    Paus.T, Director of the Brain and Body Centre, University of Nottingham;

54.    Prof. B. Sahakian, University of Cambridge; extract from article in the Readers Digest 2006.

55.    Syken.J. et al, Harvard Medical School: *Science Express journal* August 2006 (reported in The Times 19th August 2006)

56.    Grakov.I.G: www.mimex.ru

57.    Jung.C.G, http://www.ship.edu/~cgboeree/jung.html

58.    Baldwin; Jung.C.G; Freud.S; Steiner.R; Piaget.J; Lievegoed.B

**59.**    http://ourworld.compuserve.com/homepages/profirst/t.htm

60.    *British Journal of Psychology* November 2006, Irwing.P, Lynn.R,

61.    Craik FIM, Salthouse TA. *Handbook of Aging and Cognition*. Hillsdale, NJ: Erlbaum, 1992.

62.    Smith GE, Petersen RC, Parisi JE, et al. Definition, course, and outcome of mild cognitive impairment. *Aging Neuropsychol Cogn* 1996;3:141–7.

63.    *Experimental Biology and Medicine* 228:800-810 (2003); J.A. Lemon[*], D.R. Boreham[†] and C.D. Rollo[*,‡][*] Departments of Biology and [†]Medical Physics and Applied Radiation Sciences Unit, McMaster University, Hamilton Ontario, Canada L8S 4K1

64.    Borisyuk.R, University of Plymouth, Dept of Computational Neuroscience

65.    comments attributed to Lander.E, MIT

66.    Kandel.E, Nobel Prize for Physiology 2000: *Scientific American Mind* May 2006

67.    Fields.D.R: 'Beyond the Neuron Doctrine': *Scientific American Mind* June/July 2006 p 21–27

68.	Cournot.M.  Toulouse University School of Medicine *Neurology,* October 10 2006.

69.	Dr Steven Narod, University of Toronto *'Breast Cancer Research'*

70.	Merrill F Elias et al, University of Maine professor of psychology, June 2006, *Archives of Neurology*

71.	Mignot.E, Howard Hughes Medical Institute, Stanford University, *Public Library of Science* December 2004.

72.	Indiana University School of Medicine, Dr. Joseph T. Lurito; http://michelemiller.blogs.com/marketing_to_women/2004/02/the_female_brain.html

73.	*The British Journal of Psychiatry* (2002) 181: 22-28 Influence of supplementary vitamins, minerals and essential fatty acids on the antisocial behaviour of young adult prisoners: Gesch C.B, Hammond.S.M, Hampson S, **Eves. A, Crowder M.J.**

74.	comments attributed to Professor Michael Crawford, London's Metropolitan University

75.	*Journal of Alternative & Complementary Medicine 2007 Vol13, no2,* Ewing.G, Ewing.E.N, Hankey.A

76.	*Evidence-based Complementary and Alternative Medicine (eCAM),* September 2006: Hankey.A, Ewing.E

77.	comments attributed to Crick.F, Nobel Prize for Medicine 1962

78.	comments attributed to Lander.E, MIT

79.	systemic memory hypothesis for science and society. In KH Pribram (ed.). *Brain and Values: Is a Biological Science of Values Possible?* Hillsdale, NJ: Lawrence Erlbaum Associates, 1998.

80.	*It's the Thought that Counts,* Hamilton D.R. Dr, pub. Hay House; *The Biology of Belief,* Lipton B.

81.	*'The Treasure at the Bottom of the Brain',* Henrietta C. Leiner and Alan L. Leiner, pub., Channing House

82.	*Scientific American* 2003, 289: 50-57, Bower, J.M. and Parsons, L.; 'Rethinking the Lesser Brain'

83.	http://www.ninds.nih.gov/disorders/agenesis/agenesis.htm

84.	*New Scientist* November 2006; Ramachandrayan V.S., Oberman. L.M;

85. Autonomic Responses of Autistic Children to People and Objects. Hirstein.W, Iversen.P and Ramachandran. V.S in *Proceedings of the Royal Society of London B*, Vol 268, pages 1883-1888, 2001;

86. EEG Evidence for Mirror Neuron Dysfunction in Autistic Spectrum Disorders; Oberman.L.M, Hubbard. E.M, McCleery.J.P, Altschuler.E.L, Pineda.J.A, Ramachandran. V.S, in *Cognitive Brain Research* Vol 24, pages 190-198, 2005

87. *Scientific American*, January 2004, Daniel C.Javitt, Joseph T Coyle

88. *Science*, Vol 229, Issue 4714, 665-668; 1985 American Association for the Advancement of Science

89. *Science*, 26 January 2007, Bechara.A

90. Lekander.M, Director, Department of Clinical Neuroscience, Section of Psychology, Karolinska Institute

91. Biosonics, Gonzalez-Sterling.M, http://www.biosonic.org/ManualEng/ANALYSIS.html

92. Alvin, J. and Warwick, A. (1991) '*Music therapy for the autistic child*'. 2nd ed. Oxford: Oxford University Press

93. *Scientific American Mind*, Vol 17; 5: 62-65, Van Bothmer. E;

94. *The Lancet*, 2004; 363: 345-51

95. *J.Nat Can Inst*, 2005; 97: 1035-43

96. *Radiology*, 2004; 232: 735-8;

97. *American Journal of Epidemiology*, March 15 issue 2006

98. *British Medical Journal*, doi:10.1136/bmj.38720.687975.55 (published 20 January 2006

99. September 2000 newsletter of the Cellular Phone Taskforce, *No Place To Hide;* studies presented at the June 2000 European Parliament meeting on mobile phones and health; comments attributed to Dr. Lebrecht von Klitzing, Medical University of Lubeck, Germany

100. Dr. Henry Lai, bioelectromagnetics researcher, University of Washington, Seattle

101. *The Physiological and Environmental Effects of Non-Ionising Electromagnetic Radiation*, report issued in March 2001 by the European Parliament Directorate General for Research, Scientific and Technological Options Assessment (STOA). Dr. Gerard Hyland

102. *Nexus Magazine*, Volume 12, Number 3 (April - May 2005) Organ Transplants and Cellular Memories

103. FDA web site

104. *The Lancet* 340, 81 – 82, Detection of Chlamydia trachomatis DNA in joints of reactive arthritis patients by polymerase chain reaction

105. *British Medical Journal,* 2006; 333: 912-5

106. *Archives of Internal Medicine* November 2006

107. *Journal of Neurotherapy:* http://www.snr-jnt.org/JournalNT/JNT(2-2)2.html

108. PMS, EEG, and Photic Stimulation: Noton.D

109. Longo.L, University of Siena; Laser therapy for the treatment of diabetes; *Private Hospital Healthcare Europe 2006.*

110. 'Light, Medicine of the Future', Liberman.J, publisher Bear & Company

111. Dr David.R.Hamilton: *'It's the thought that Counts'*, publisher Hay House

112. Travis, F.T., Tecce, J., Arenander, A., Wallace, R.K. (2002). Patterns of EEG Coherence, Power, and Contingent Negative Variation Characterize the Integration of Transcendental and Waking States. *Biological Psychology,* 61, 293-319.

113. Travis, F.T. (2001). Autonomic and EEG patterns distinguish transcending from other experiences during Transcendental Meditation practice. *International Journal of Psychophysiology*, 42, 1-9.

114. Travis, F.T., (1996). Invincible Athletics program: Aerobic exercise and performance without strain. *International Journal of Neuroscience*, 85: 301–308

115. Feinberg I, March J., Flach K., Maloney T., Chern W-J., Travis F.T. (1989). Late maturational decline in 0–3 Hz EEG amplitude during sleep: A reflection of synaptic elimination? *Society for Neuroscience Abstracts*, 15(1): 244.

116. Gaylord C., Orme-Johnson D.W., and Travis F.T. (1989). The effects of the Transcendental Meditation technique and progressive muscle relaxation on EEG coherence, stress reactivity, and mental health in black adults. *International Journal of Neuroscience*, 46: 77–86.

117. *J Behav Med*, 1998; 21; 581-99 Meditation can reduce anxiety and panic attacks

118. *Journal of the American Medical Association*, 2004; 292: 1669

119. *British Medical Journal*, 2004; 329: 849-51, Picano E.

120. 'Nutrition, Stress and the Visual Pathway', *2nd Annual South Eastern Conference,* Atlanta 1981, Morgan.R.B.

121. Felleman.D, *Nature* January 2003

122. Photorejuvenation with intense pulsed light: results of a multi-center study, Journal of Dermatology, Jan-Feb 2004, Sadick.N.S, Weiss.R, Kilmer.S, Bitter.P

123. http://www.flatrock.org.nz/topics/science/is_the_brain_really_necessary.htm

124. http://www.alternativescience.com/no_brainer.htm

125. *Developmental Medicine and Child Neurology* 7: 628–33, Lorber J. (1965)

126. http://www.subliminalworld.org/flickers.htm

127. Hogl.B; http://www.aasmnet.org/jcsm/AcceptedPapers/PLMDisturbedSleep.pdf

128. http://www.colour-experience.org/matching/matcol_psych_tests/matcol_psych_test5.htm

# Chapter 2

# What is Virtual Scanning?

by

Elena Ewing (Dr)

# The Test Procedure and Report

Virtual Scanning is a cognitive type technology, a software programme, which is conducted on a computer

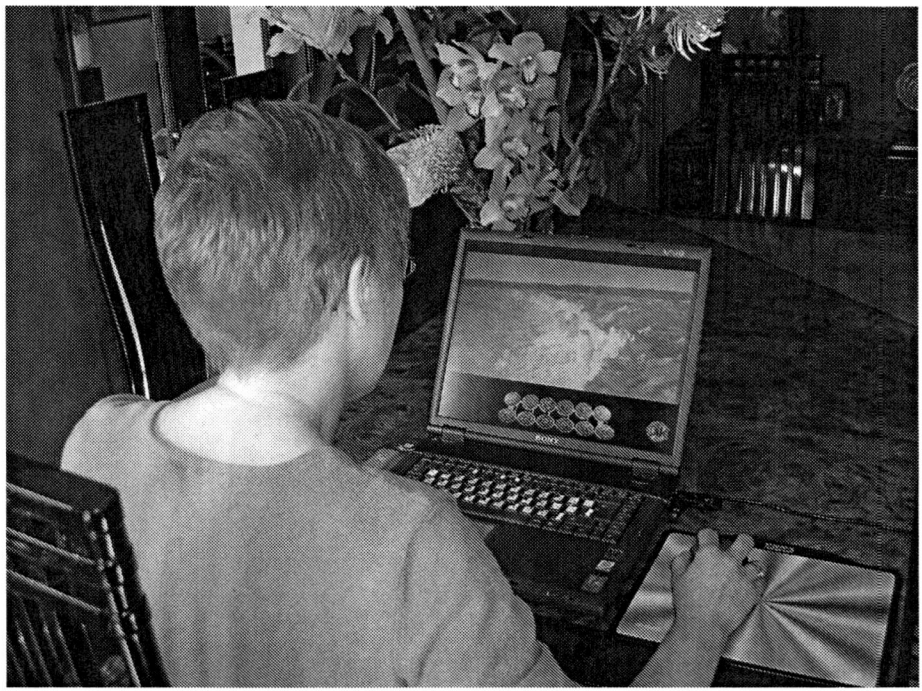

Following a process of registration which involves gaining patient authorization, e.g. as required under the data protection regulations, the patient consultation commences.

Firstly, the patient is required to register their personal details in the programme which includes their weight, age and sex.

The patient is given a picture to study for a period of 15 seconds during which they are required to study and memorise the content of the picture (picture 1) and in particular the colours which are displayed. At the end of the 15 seconds the picture is over-wiped by a colour filter (see picture 2) and the task of the patient is to use the 'mouse' to select colours from the colour palette and hence to increase or decrease the colours in order to recover the original picture (see picture 3). There is no right way or wrong way to complete the task – just the patient's own inimitable style and efforts. Each movement, thought process, delay, rate of movement, memory and style of recovering the colours is a unique blueprint which is a simulation of the patient's neural processing.

1

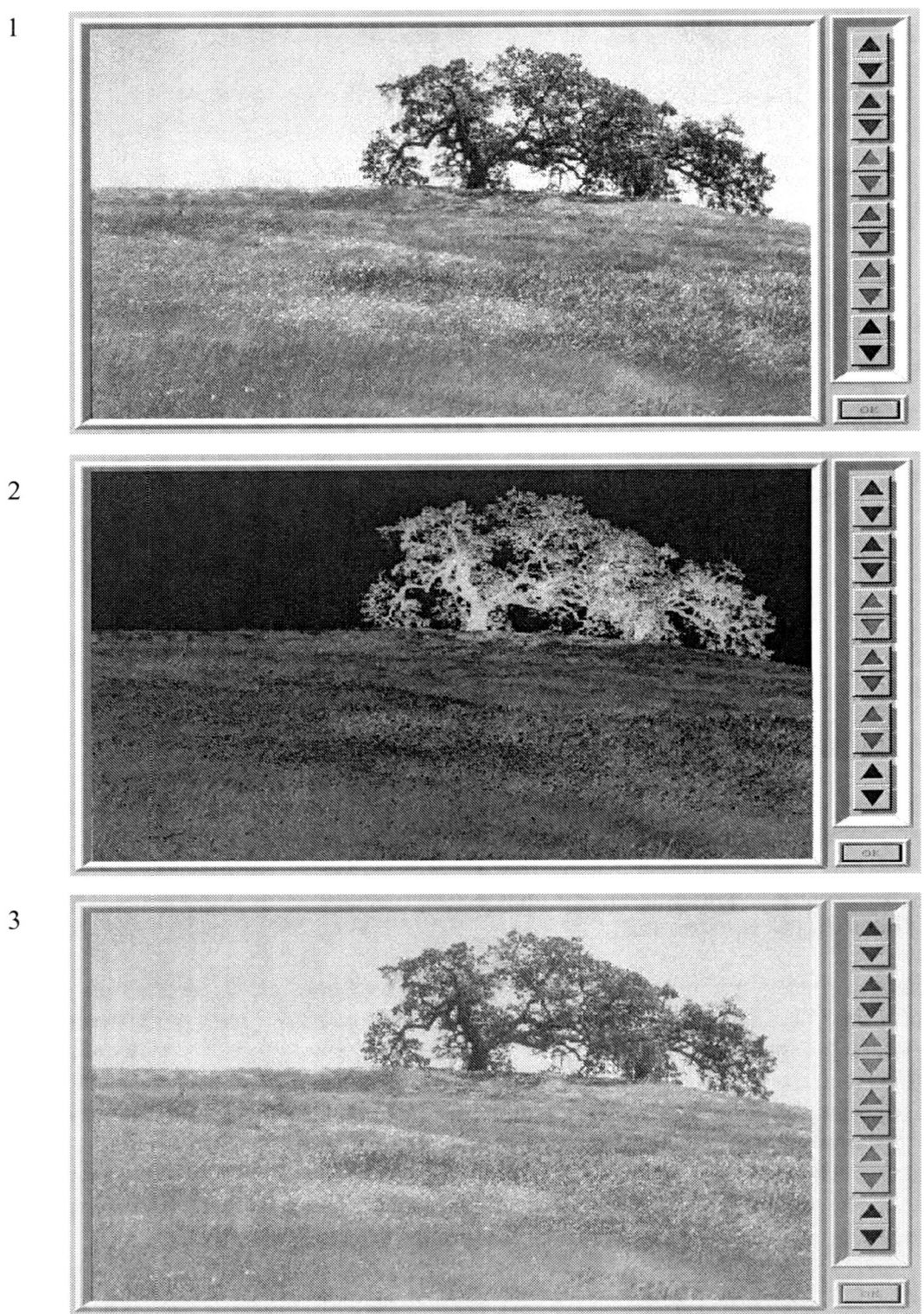

2

3

Upon completion of the task i.e. the patient is not able to make any further adjustments
and has completed the task which usually takes 1-2 minutes for each picture, the program

moves onto the next picture. This continues until the program has sufficient data for processing – usually 3-5 pictures.

The pictures – which in version 7 is now a short video – comprise an entertaining and beautifully presented sequence in which are featured e.g. polar bears, seals, penguins, dolphins, ducks, geese and beautiful landscapes comprising volcanos, pacific islands, geological formations, rivers, geysers, etc.

At the completion of the test the data is sent for processing by the remote server and the processed data is returned after a pause of typically 10 minutes.

The information is presented in a number of reports:  see figs 1-13; which may be discussed with the patient at a level which is appropriate for each situation.  If anything significant and of concern is noted the patient is advised to contact their GP.

Upon receipt of data from the remote server after typically 10 minutes the appropriate therapy is selected and again sent for processing by the remote server.

Upon receipt of the therapy from the remote server the practitioner copies or 'burns' the treatment onto a CD which is given to the patient who installs the therapy on their home computer.

The correctional therapy involves sitting in front of the computer and studying the contents of the computer screen for typically two sessions per day – one in the morning and the second in the early evening – for typically 20 minutes per session.

The therapy is experienced as a series of colours – typically 3-5 minutes of one colour which is presented as a shape and which flashes on and off typically 1-4 times per second.

A typical session would, for example, be 3-5 minutes of a pink triangle which is presented at 2.7 times per second, a further 3-5 minutes of a blue circle which is presented at 3.5 times per second, and a further 10 minutes of a pink square which is presented at 2.1 times per second.

Each therapy is unique for each patient and for their precise physical parameters and medical conditions.

Virtual Scanning version 4 (1998-2002)

# Figure 1

In version 4 of the technology, the results are presented as follows:

## 1.    Brain Functions

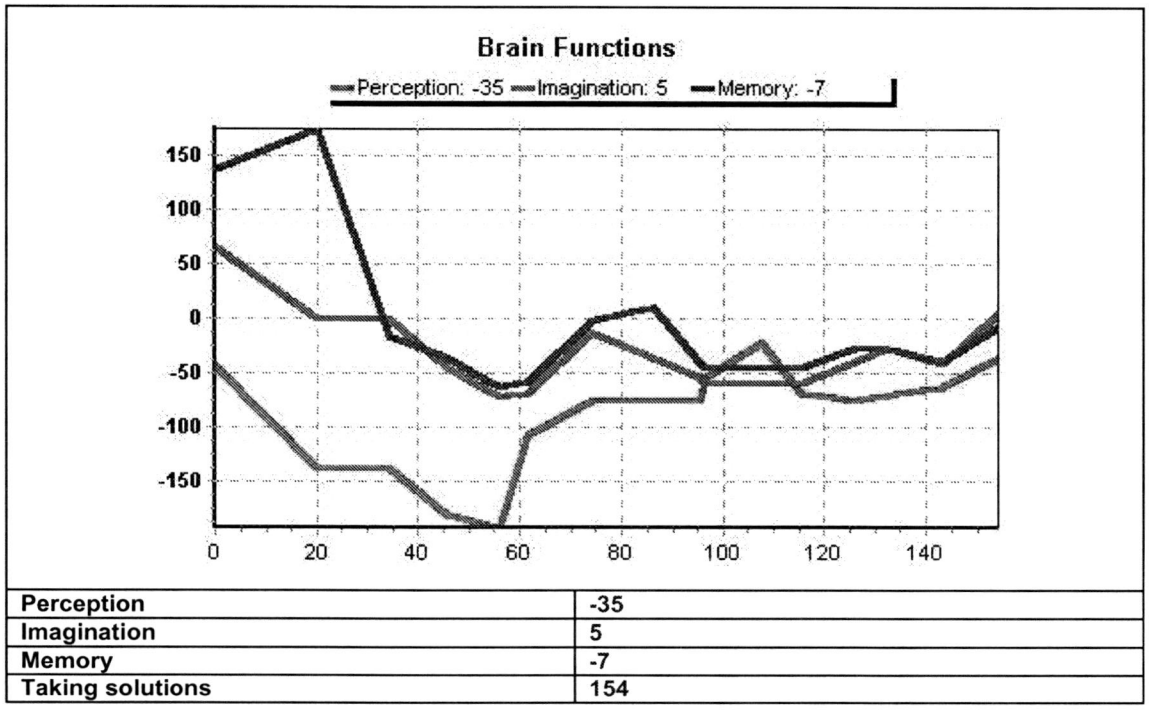

| Perception | -35 |
|---|---|
| Imagination | 5 |
| Memory | -7 |
| Taking solutions | 154 |

## 2. Detailed report of organs

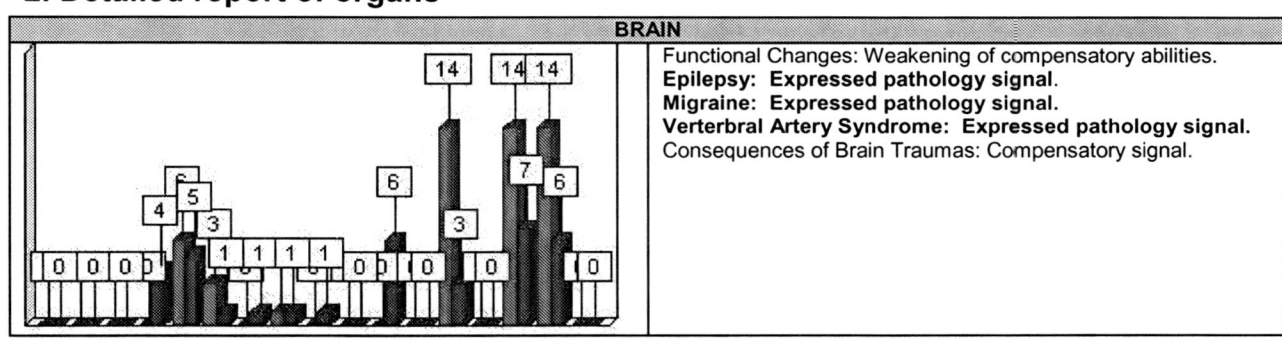

**BRAIN**

Functional Changes: Weakening of compensatory abilities.
**Epilepsy: Expressed pathology signal.**
**Migraine: Expressed pathology signal.**
**Verterbral Artery Syndrome: Expressed pathology signal.**
Consequences of Brain Traumas: Compensatory signal.

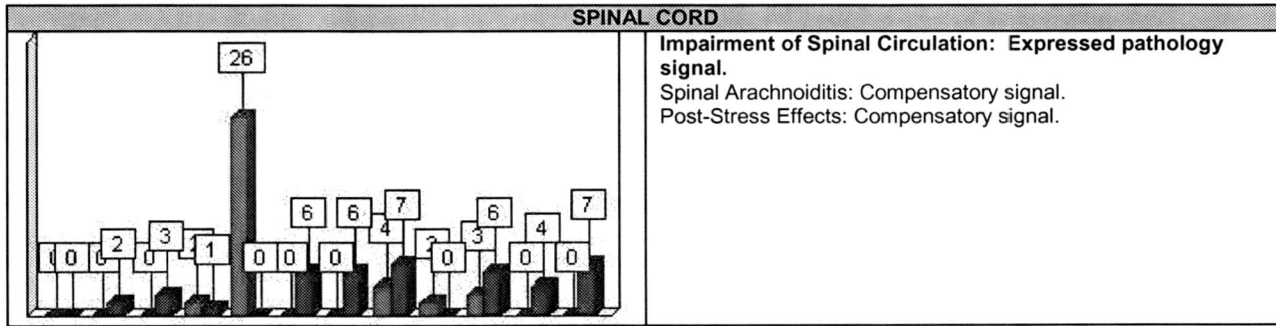

**SPINAL CORD**

**Impairment of Spinal Circulation: Expressed pathology signal.**
Spinal Arachnoiditis: Compensatory signal.
Post-Stress Effects: Compensatory signal.

## PERIPHERAL NERVOUS SYSTEM

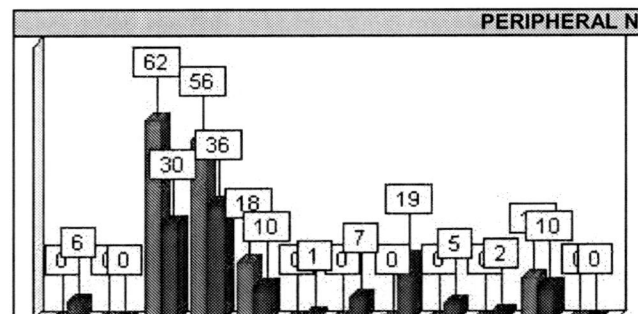

Chronic Fatigue: Expressed pathology signal.
**Spinal Osteochondrosis with Neurological Effects: Weakening of compensatory abilities.**
Allergic Process: Weakening of compensatory abilities.
Hereditary-Degenerative Process: Weakening of compensatory abilities.
Intoxication Effects: Compensatory signal.
Polyneuropathy: Expressed compensatory signal.

## EAR

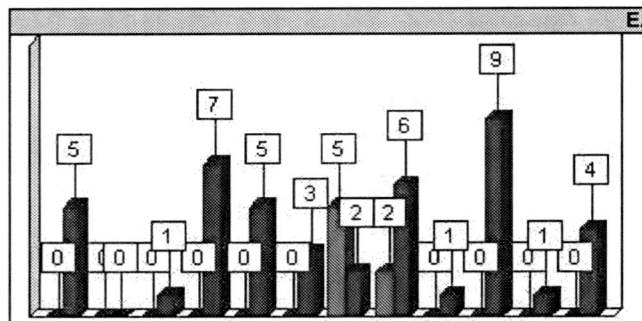

Degenerative Process: Compensatory signal.
Chronic Fatigue: Compensatory signal.

## NOSE

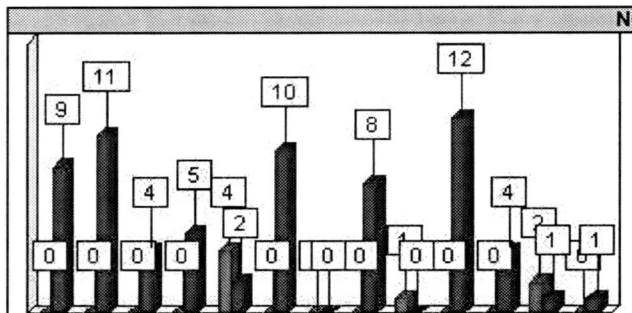

Tension of compensatory abilities.

## PITUITARY GLAND

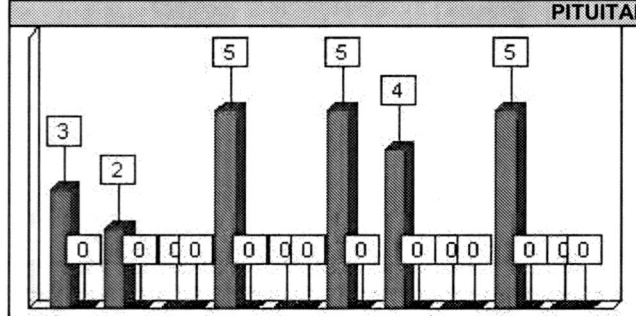

No changes detected.

64

## THYROID GLAND

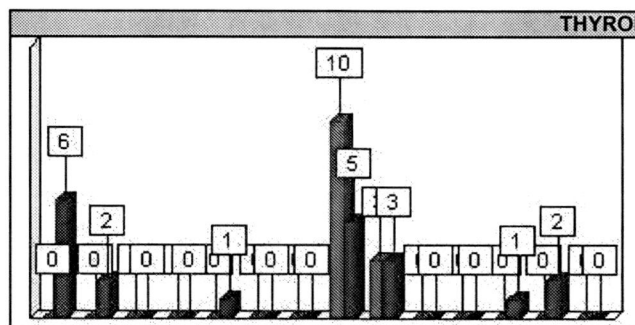

Allergic Process:  Pathology signal.
Abnormalities of Development: Compensatory signal.

## ADRENAL GLANDS

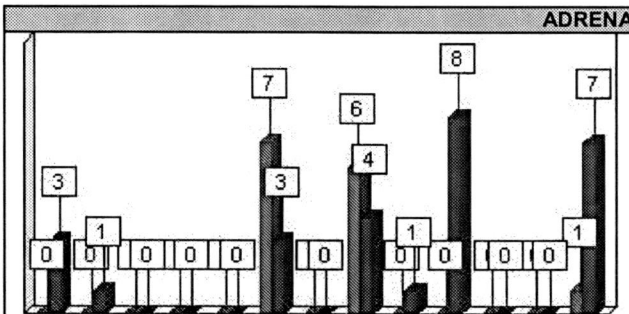

Allergic Process:  Pathology signal.
Cushing Syndrome: Compensatory signal.
Functional Changes: Compensatory signal.

## OVARIES

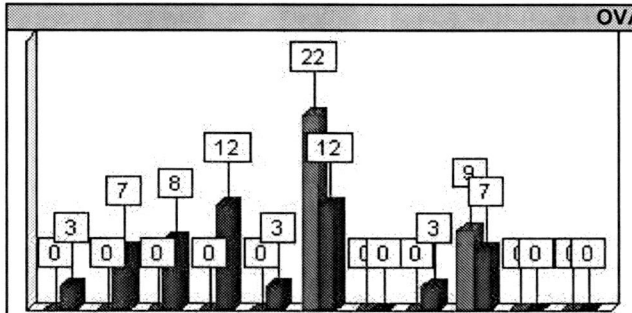

Degenerative Process: Weakening of compensatory abilities.
Allergic Process: Weakening of compensatory abilities.
Post-Stress Effects: Compensatory signal.
Ovarian Cyst: Compensatory signal.

## MAMMARY GLAND

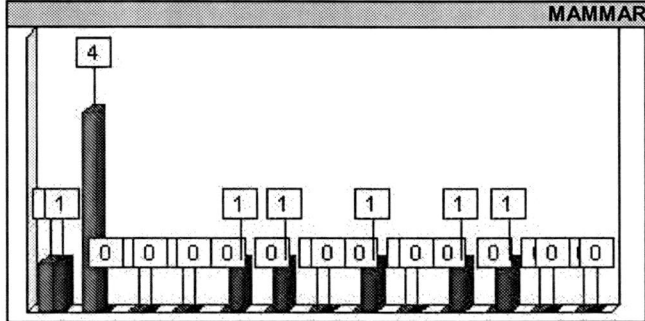

No changes detected.

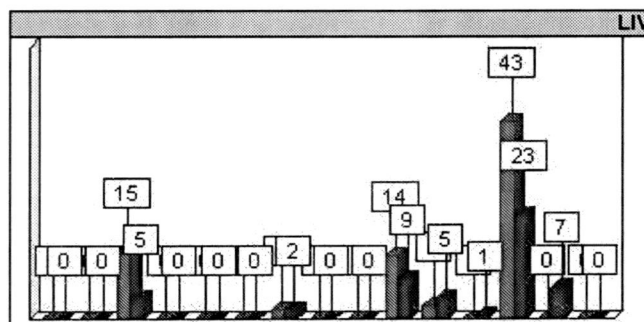

**LIVER**

Allergic Process: Expressed pathology signal.
Disruption of Bilirubin Metabolism: Weakening of compensatory abilities.
Liver Insufficiency: Weakening of compensatory abilities.
Neoplasm: Compensatory signal.

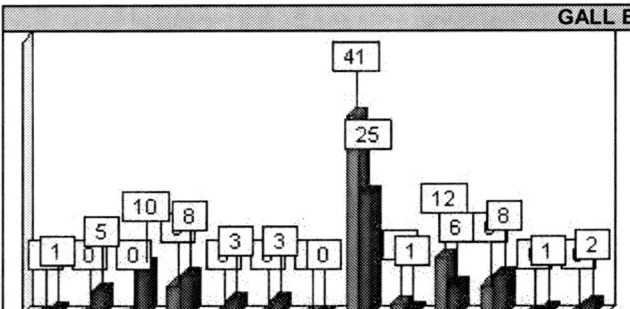

**GALL BLADDER**

Dyskinesia of Biliary Ducts and Gall Bladder: Weakening of compensatory abilities.
Chronic Fatigue: Pathology signal.
Post-Stress Effects: Compensatory signal.
Tissue Growth: Compensatory signal.
Cholangitis: Compensatory signal.

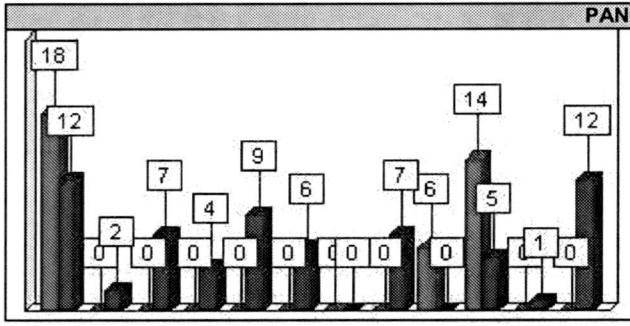

**PANCREAS**

Chronic Fatigue: Weakening of compensatory abilities.
Pathology of Islands of Langerhans: Expressed pathology signal.
Post-Stress Effects: Compensatory signal.
Age-Related Changes: Compensatory signal.
Functional Changes: Compensatory signal.
Abnormalities of Development: Compensatory signal.

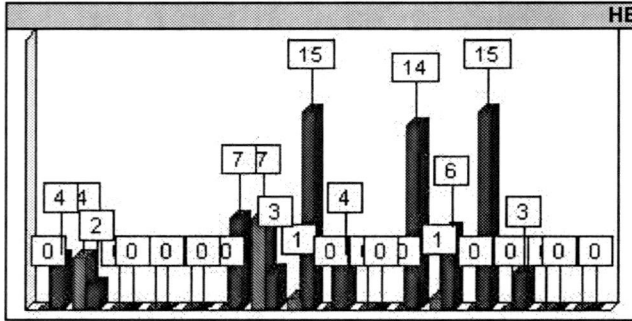

**HEART**

Chronic Fatigue: Pathology signal.
Cardiosclerosis: Compensatory signal.
Myocardial Dystrophy: Expressed compensatory signal.
Intoxication Effects: Expressed compensatory signal.
Cardiac Insufficiency: Compensatory signal.
Cardiac Myopathy: Expressed compensatory signal.

66

## BLOOD AND PERIPHERAL BLOOD VESSELS

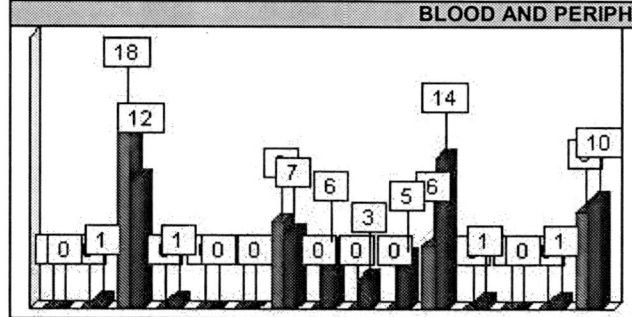

**Leukopenia: Weakening of compensatory abilities.**
**Hemorrhagic Vasculitis: Weakening of compensatory abilities.**
**Idiopathic Hypotension: Expressed compensatory signal.**
Post-Stress Effects: Compensatory signal.
Neoplasm: Compensatory signal.

## SPLEEN

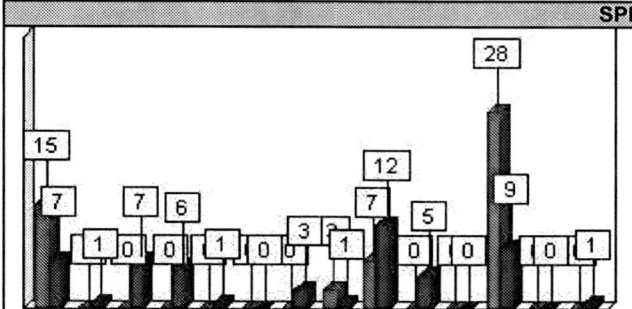

Chronic Fatigue:  Expressed pathology signal.
Hyposplenism: Compensatory signal.
Chronic Staying Splenomegaly:  Expressed pathology signal.
Splenomegaly: Compensatory signal.
Functional Changes: Compensatory signal.

## LUNGS AND BRONCHI

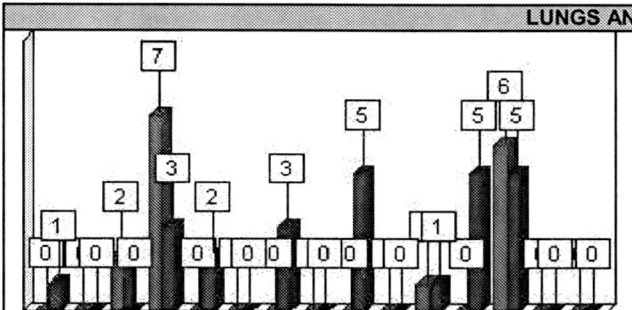

Bronchiectatic disease:  Pathology signal.
Post-Stress Effects: Weakening of compensatory abilities.

## SKIN

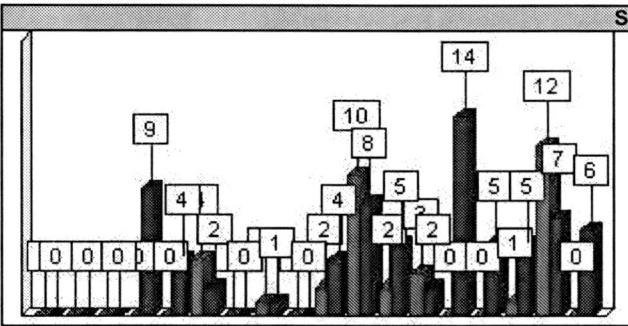

Eczema: Weakening of compensatory abilities.
Herpes: Weakening of compensatory abilities.
Neoplasm: Expressed compensatory signal.
Age-Related Changes: Compensatory signal.
Degenerative Process: Expressed compensatory signal.
Erythema: Compensatory signal.
Post-Stress Effects: Compensatory signal.
Intoxication Effects: Compensatory signal.

67

## OESOPHAGUS

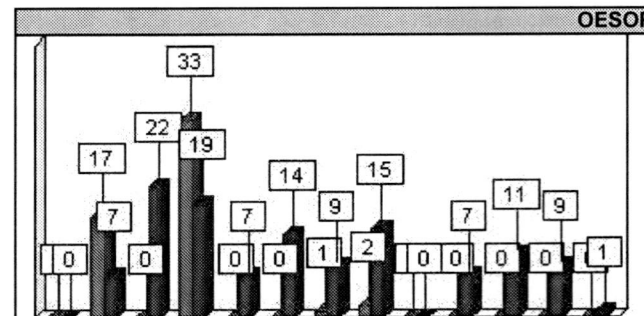

Degenerative Process: Expressed pathology signal.
Chronic Fatigue: Weakening of compensatory abilities.
Tension of compensatory abilities.

## STOMACH

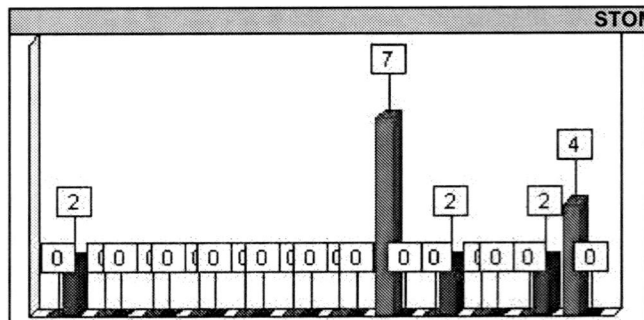

Ulcerative Disease: Pathology signal.

## DUODENUM

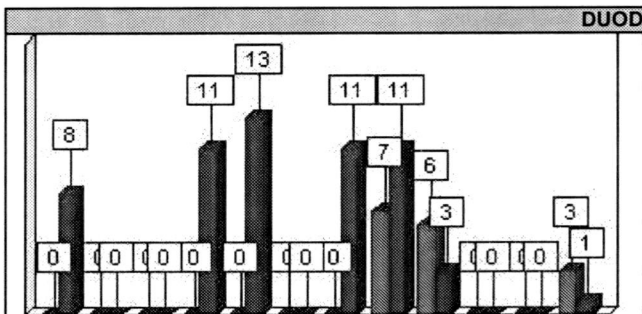

Allergic Process: Compensatory signal.
Neoplasm: Compensatory signal.
Duodenitis: Compensatory signal.
Intoxication Effects: Expressed compensatory signal.
Ulcerative Disease: Compensatory signal.

## SMALL INTESTINE

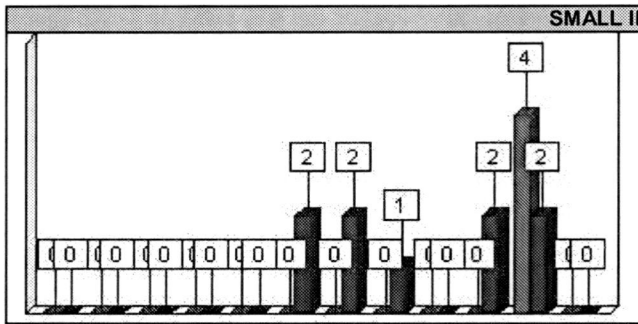

No changes detected.

## LARGE INTESTINE

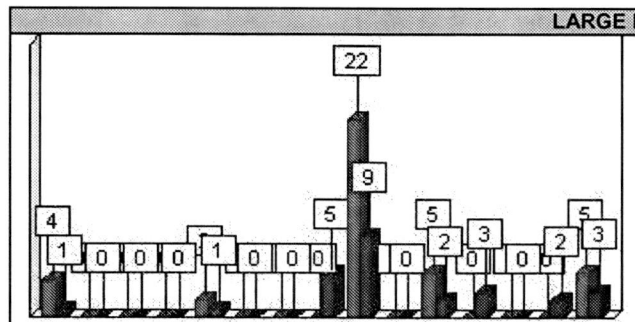

Degenerative Process: Expressed pathology signal.

## KIDNEYS

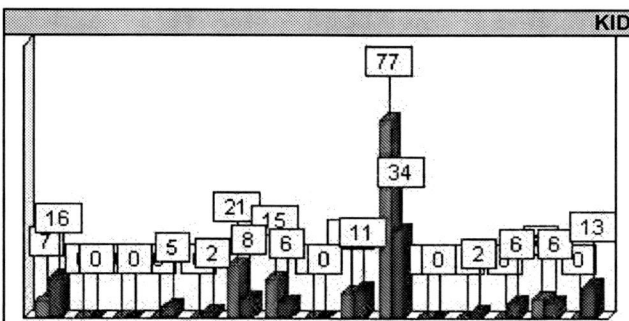

General weakening of compensatory abilities.
Glomerulonephritis: Expressed compensatory signal.
General weakening of compensatory abilities. Tissue Growth:
Compensatory signal.
Urolithiasis: Compensatory signal.
Functional Changes: Expressed compensatory signal.

## URINARY BLADDER

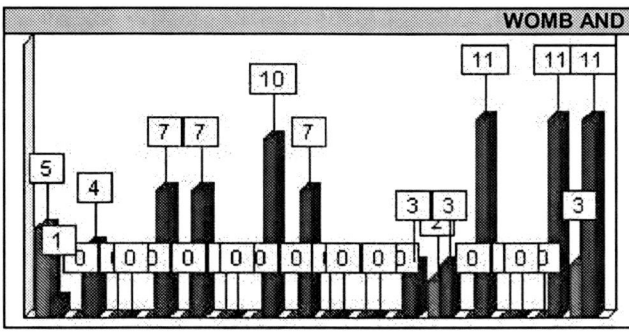

Chronic Fatigue: Pathology signal.
Age-Related Changes: Compensatory signal.

## WOMB AND APPENDAGES

Allergic Process: Pathology signal.
Tension of compensatory abilities.

## SKELETAL AND MUSCULAR SYSTEM

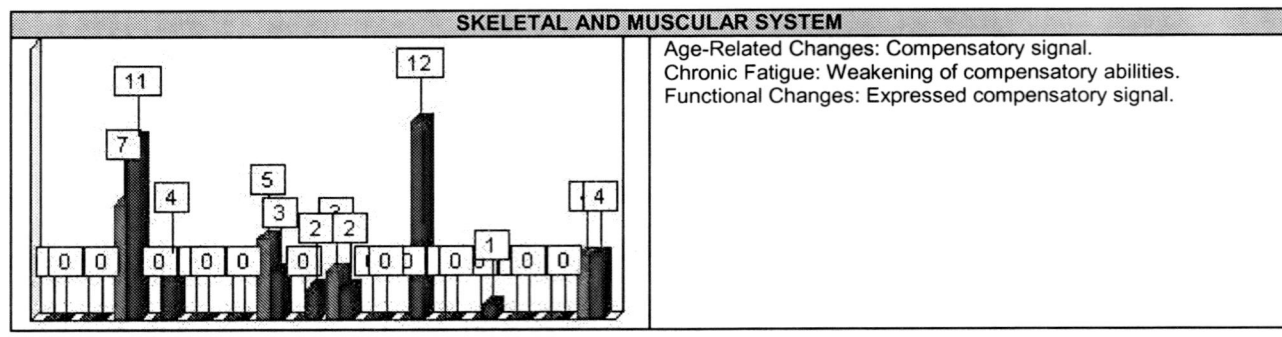

Age-Related Changes: Compensatory signal.
Chronic Fatigue: Weakening of compensatory abilities.
Functional Changes: Expressed compensatory signal.

# Virtual Scanning version 7 (2002-    )

In version 7G the results are presented in figures 2-13 as follows:

## Figure 2/Report1

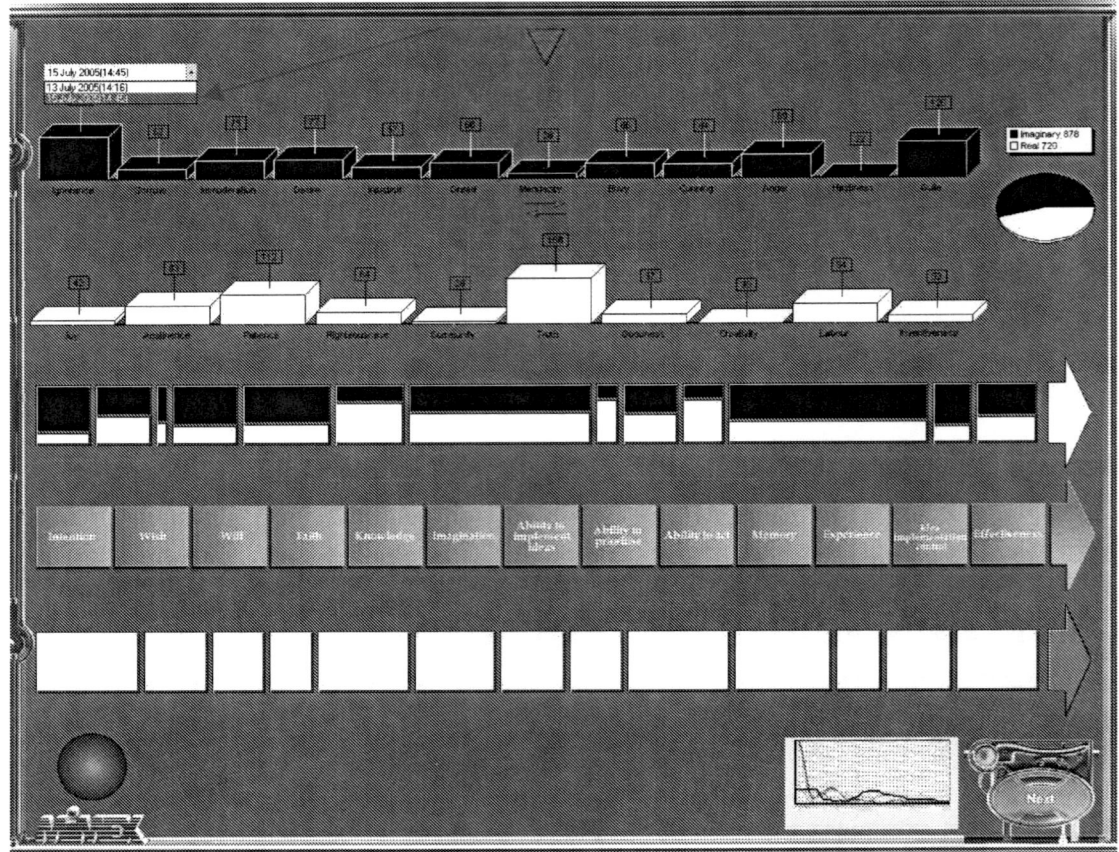

**The results of the psychological profile are expressed in the following terms**:

1. (line 2: in white) The positive psycho-emotional traits which are expressed as Joy, Abstinence (Devotion), Patience, Righteousness, Community, Truth, Goodness, Creativity, Labour and Inventiveness.

2. (line 1: in black) The negative psycho-emotional traits which are expressed as Ignorance (Obstinacy/Stubborness), Sorrow, Immoderation, Desire, Injustice, Greed, Mendacity (to lie), Envy, Cunning, Anger (Resentment), Hastiness, and Guile (Secretiveness).

3. (see pie chart) The balance of positive and negative aspects and the scale of the positive and negative aspects.

4.  (see line 3) The individual balance of the 14 positive and negative factors (see black and white flow chart

5.  (see line 4) The influence of the positive and/or negative factors upon the decision-making process which comprises 14 components:

    Intention, Wish, Will, Faith, Knowledge, Imagination, Implementation, Prioritisation, Ability to Act, Memory, Experience, Monitoring and Supervision of an idea, Effectiveness

6.  (see graph line 6) The balance of neurological issues expressed as perception, imagination, associative thinking, and speed of decision-making.

7.  (see line 5) The 14 functional systems of the body which are reported in sequence from the most stable (left) to the most destabilized (right) – (see below)

## Table 1: List of Physiological or Functional Systems

| | |
|---|---|
| (1) Blood Cell Content | (2) Circulating Blood Volume |
| (3) pH Level | (4) Osmotic Pressure in the Body |
| (5) Blood glucose | (6) Blood pressure |
| (7) Breathing Level | (8) Digestion |
| (9) Body temperature | (10) Excretion |
| (11) Sexual Function | (12) Bodily Posture |
| (13) Sleeping Patterns | (14) Locomotion, Communication and Manipulation |

**Figure 3/Report 2:**

## Summary of the most destabilized Systems and Organs

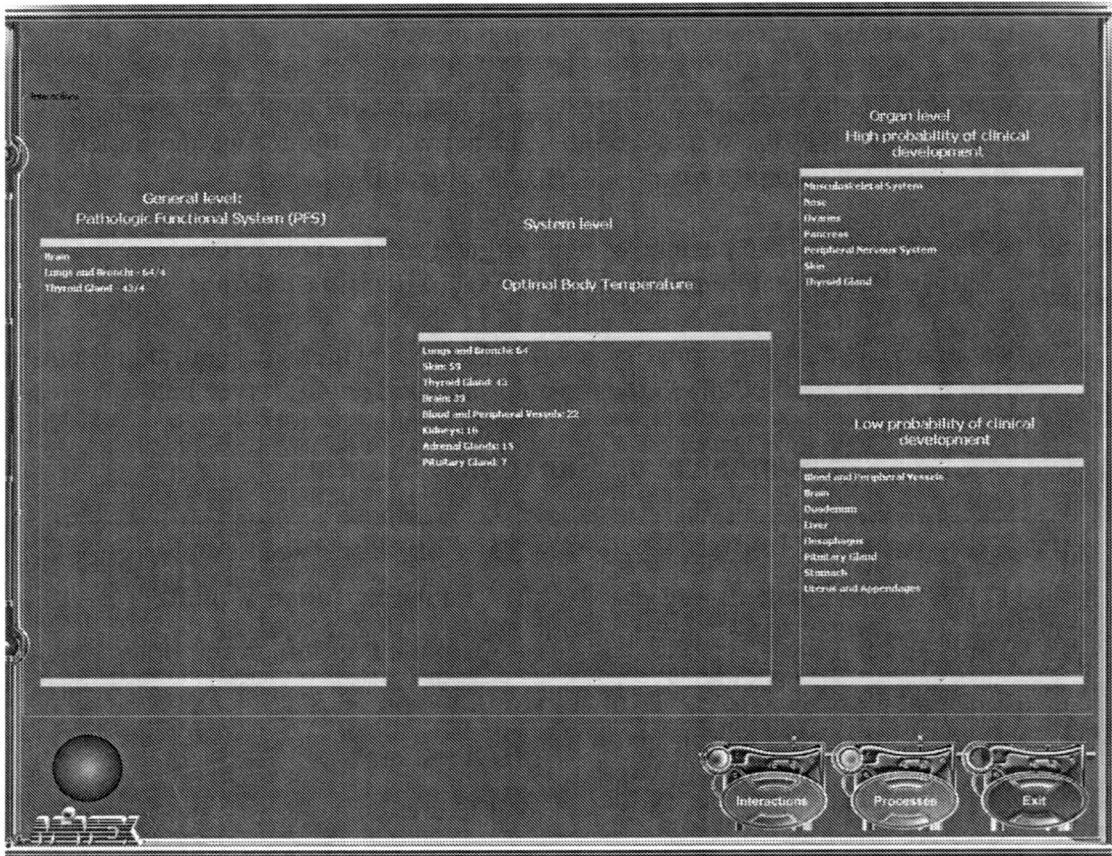

From this report we are able to identify the specific pathological functional systems which exist at the GENERAL Level and which, in this case, affect the Brain, Lungs and Bronchii, and Thyroid Gland of the lady patient.

At the SYSTEM level we can identify that the most affected system is that which maintains 'optimal body temperature' and that the most affected organs in this system as Lungs and Bronchii, Skin, Thyroid Gland and Brain. Other organs listed, but which have lesser indications, include Blood & Peripheral Blood Vessels, Kidneys, Adrenal Gland and Pituitary Gland

The organs listed which have greatest risk of clinical development include: Musculoskeletal System, Nose, Ovaries, Pancreas, Peripheral Nervous System, Skin and Thyroid Gland.

# Figure 4/Tables 2 & 3

## TABLE 2  REGULATORY SYSTEMS
for which Virtual Scanning identifies quality of function
(named for the physiological factors for which they maintain optimal functional levels)

(1) Blood Cell Content

(2) Circulating Blood Volume

(3) pH Level

(4) Osmotic Pressure in the Body

(5) Blood glucose

(6) Blood pressure

(7) Breathing Level

(8) Digestion

(9) Body temperature

(10) Excretion

(11) Sexual Function

(12) Bodily Posture

(13) Sleeping Patterns

(14) Locomotion, Communication and Manipulation

## TABLE 3  ORGANS
for which Virtual Scanning yields scales of pathology / compensation
(note the six organs 24 – 29 in three pairs of alternatives for each sex)

(1) Brain

(2) Spinal Cord

(3) Peripheral Nervous System

(4) Ear

(5) Nose

(6) Pituitary

(7) Thyroid

(8) Adrenals

(9) Liver

(10) Gall Bladder

(11) Pancreas

(12) Heart

(13) Blood and Peripheral Blood Vessels

(14) Spleen

(15) Lungs and Bronchi

(16) Skin

(17) Oesophagus

(18) Stomach

(19) Duodenum

(20) Small Intestine

(21) Colon

(22) Kidneys

(23) Urinary Bladder

(24/25) Penis / Uterus

(26/27) Testicles / Ovaries

(28/29) Prostate / Mammary Glands

(30) Muscular Skeletal System

## Figure 5/Report 3 (a):

## Summary of the most Prevalent Conditions for each Organ

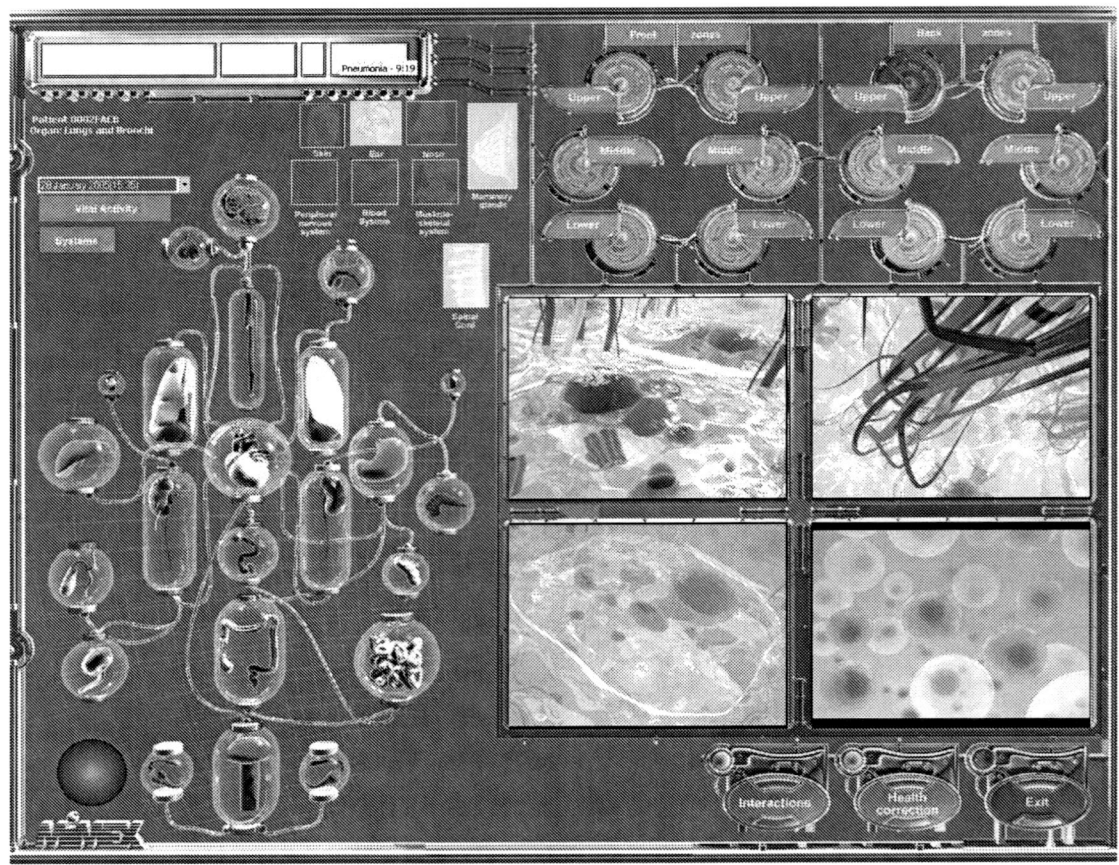

From this report we can assess the extent of the medical indications which affect each organ. In this example we are able to look at the Lungs and Bronchii of the patient and can establish that the major indications of concern are

**Pneumonia 9/19**
Bronchiectatic Disease 4/5
Post natal growth abnormalities 20/7
Bronchial asthma 51/11

As each medical condition can be assessed in terms of the balance (C/P) of firstly, their compensatory signal (C) and secondly, of their pathology signal (P) we can note that of the listed conditions Pneumonia has greater pathology whilst Bronchial Asthma is highly compensated. If the medical condition is above 10 units pathology it will be diagnosed at the symptomatic level and this proved to be the case with this patient.

We are also able to review the patient's morphology and can establish that this patient has at the back, left, upper region of the lungs increased blood flow to and from this part of the lung and significantly increased cell differentiation which should be subject to further investigation by conventional diagnostic scanning technologies.

## Figure 6/Report 3(b):

### Summary of the most prevalent Medical Conditions for all organs:

Each medical condition is prioritized according to scale and importance i.e. acute conditions are manifest as the red signals, chronic conditions are manifest as the yellow signals and emerging conditions are manifest as the green signals.

**Figure 7/Table 4:**

## Pathology Reported for each Organ

The following list is indicative of the medical conditions which can be diagnosed.

**1.      General Measures Reported for Each Organ**

Reports for all organs evaluate:

Intoxication Effects, Degenerative Process, Chronic Fatigue, Tissue Growth, Age-related Changes, Functional Changes, Abnormalities of Development, Allergic Process, Neoplasm (growth of new cells), and Post-stress Effects

**2.      Specific Medical Conditions Reported for Each Organ**

### 1. BRAIN (18)
Epilepsy,  Migraine, Encephalitis, Vertebral Artery Syndrome, Arachnoiditis, Encephalopathy,  Impairment of Cerebral Circulation, Consequences of Brain Traumas

### 2. SPINAL CORD (13):
Myelitis, Spinal Arachnoiditis,  Impairment of Spinal Circulation,

### 3. PERIPHERAL NERVOUS SYSTEM (15):
Neuritis, Ganglioradiculitis, Polyneuropathy, Radiculitis,

### 4. EAR (15)
Otogenous Labyrynthitis, Cochlear Neuritis, Chronic Otitis, Inflammation of External Ear, Inflammation of Middle Ear,

### 5. NOSE (13)
Maxillary Sinusitis, Rhinitis, Frontitis,

### 7. THYROID GLAND (13)
Hypoparathyrosis, Thyroiditis, Hypothyrosis,

### 8. ADRENAL GLAND (13)
Insufficiency of Adrenal Cortex, Crohn's Syndrome, Cushings Syndrome,

### 9. LIVER (14)
Portal Hypertension, Liver Insufficiency, Cirrhosis, Hepatitis

### 10. GALL BLADDER (14)
Cholecystitis, Cholelithiasis, Cholangitis, Dyskinesia of Biliary Ducts & Gall Bladder

### 11. PANCREAS (13)
Sclerotic Pancreatitis, Pancreatitis, Pathology of Islands of Langerhans

## 12. HEART (19)

Myocarditis, Cardiosclerosis, Ischaemic Heart Disease, Cardiac Insufficiency, Cardiac Myopathy, Angina Pectoris, Cardiac Infarction, Myocardial Dystrophy, Impairment of Rhythm and Conduction

## 13. BLOOD & PERIPHERAL BLOOD VESSELS (17)

Haemorrhagic Diathesis, Anaemia, Haemorrhagic Vasculitis, Leukopenia, Idiopathic Hypotension,, Hypertonia, Phlebitis and Thrombophlebitis

## 14. SPLEEN (13)

Hyposplenism, Hypersplenism, Splenomegaly

## 15. LUNGS & BRONCHI (16)

Chronic Breathing Insufficiency, Pleurisy, Pneumonia, Bronchitis, Bronchal Asthma, Bronchiectatic Disease

## 16. SKIN (18)

Urticaria, Psoriasis, Herpes, Erythema, Eczema, Dermatitis, Lichen Planus, Neurodermatitis, Dermatomyositis

## 17. OESOPHAGUS (13)

Diverticulum, Neurosis of Oesophagus, Oesophagitis

## 18. STOMACH (12)

Ulcerative Disease, Gastritis

## 19. DUODENUM (12)

Dyskinesia, Duodenitis, Ulcerative Disease

## 20. SMALL INTESTINE (12)

Dyskinesia, Enteritis, Diverticulum

## 21. LARGE INTESTINE(12)

Diverticulum, Colitis, Proctitis, Haemorrhoids, Sigmoiditis

## 22. KIDNEYS (14)

Renal Insufficiency, Pyelonephritis, Urolithiasis, Glomerulonephritis

## 23. URINARY BLADDER (14)

Urethral Infections, Urinary Bladder Polyposis, Urolithiasis, Cystitis

## 25. UTERUS (15)

Kraurosis, Uterine Myoma, Salpingitis, Cervical Erosion, Endometritis

## 27. OVARIES (11)

Ovarian Cyst,

## 28. PROSTATE GLAND (12)

Calculous Prostatitis, Prostatitis,

## 29. MAMMARY GLANDS (12)
Mammary Gland Cyst, Mastitis, Mastopathy,

## 30. MUSCULAR SKELETAL SYSTEM (17)
Arthrosis. Polyarthritis, Arthritis, Osteochondrosis, Osteoporosis, Radiculitis, Myositis

## For Nos 6. PITUITARY GLAND (10); 24. PENIS (10); & 26. TESTICLES (10)
No specific medical indications were reported

# Figure 8/Report 4:

## Summary of the proposed Treatment Options

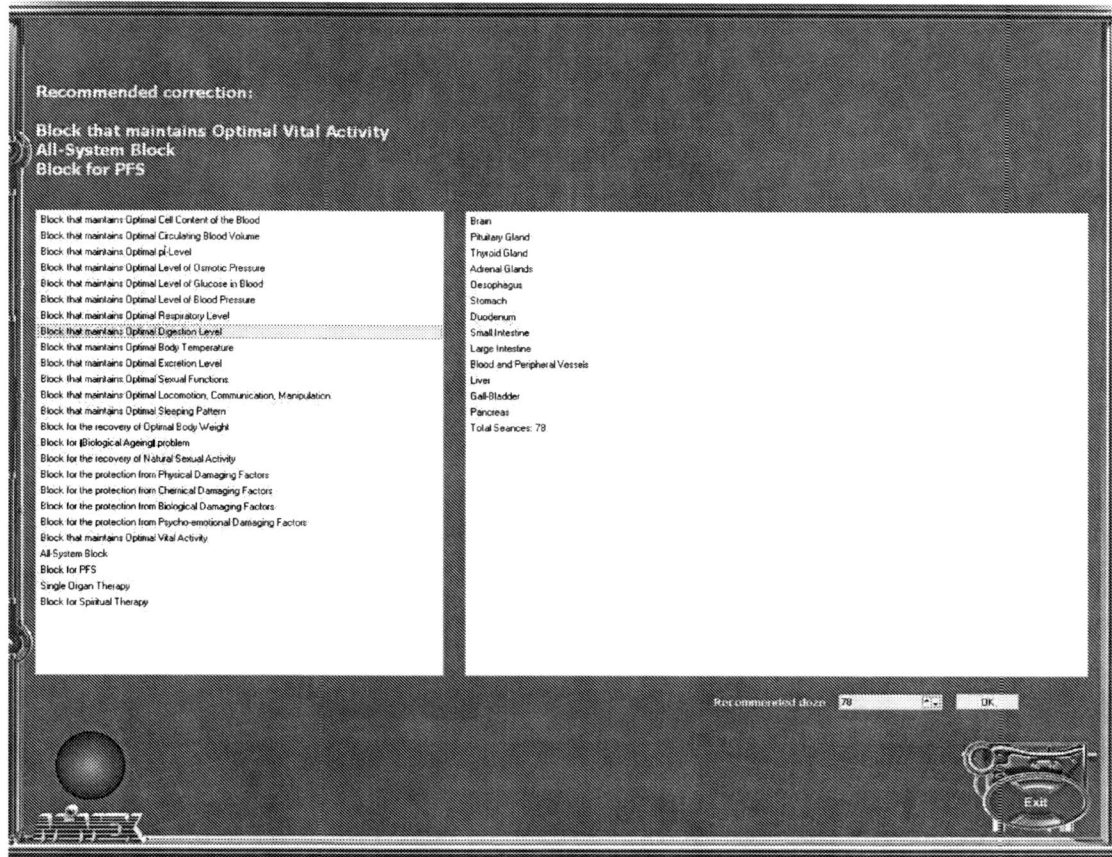

The correctional therapy can be targeted upon specific features e.g.

- the specific functional system of concern

- the specific organ of concern

- to prevent premature biological aging

- to maintain optimum body weight

- to focus upon specific issues which have been responsible for damage i.e. physical, chemical or biological factors

- to focus upon the wellbeing, emotional and/or spiritual needs of the person

**Figure 9/Report 6(a):**

## Summary of the Psychology of the Group

The following example illustrates the ability to diagnose the psychology of the group. In this case the group comprised

Patient 00B7373C – Male, 100 kg, 04.12.60 DOB (Father)
Patient 00C26CAE – Female, 63 kg, 05.10.62 DOB (Mother)
Patient 00CD4AE8 – Male, 63 kg, 21.08.84 DOB (Son)
Patient 00A9ECC5 – Male, 77 kg, 15.03.86 DOB (Son)

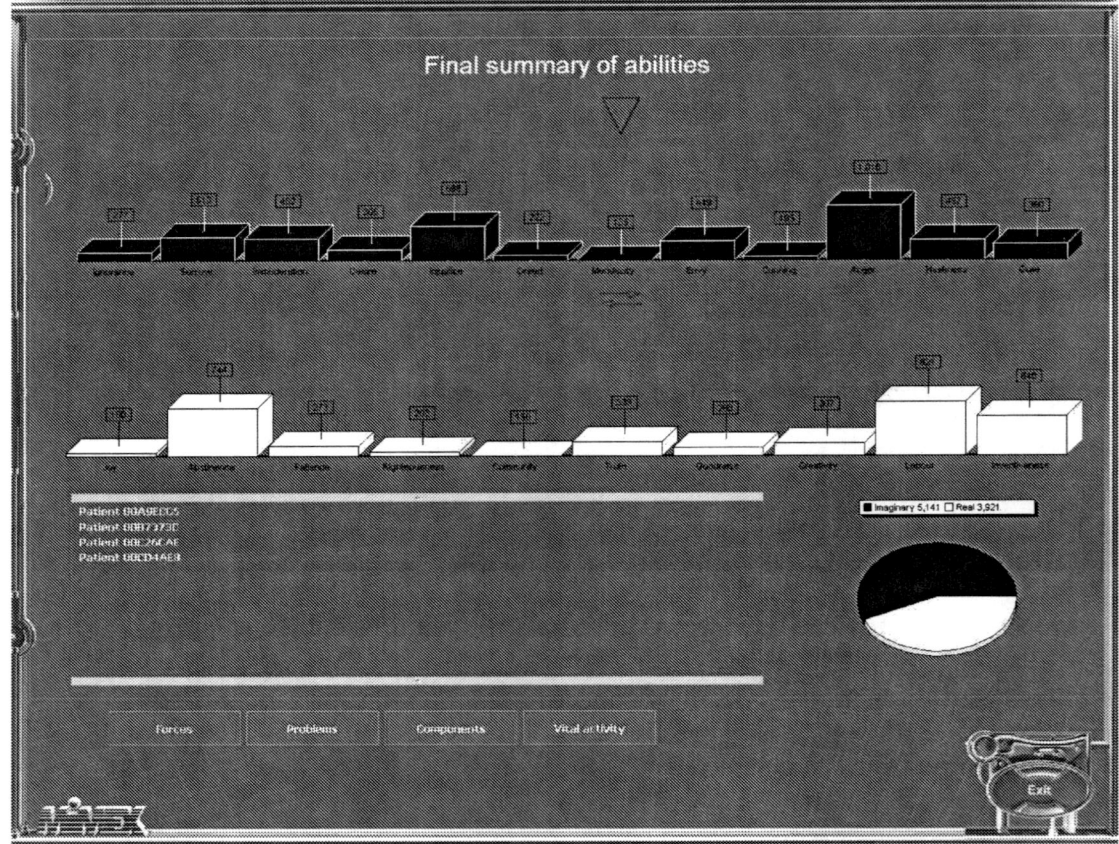

The psychology of the group, in which the negative components outweighed the positive components, was dominated by issues such as Anger, Labour, Inventiveness, Abstinence and Injustice.

**Figure 10/Report 6(b):**

## Problem Creator and Problem Solver

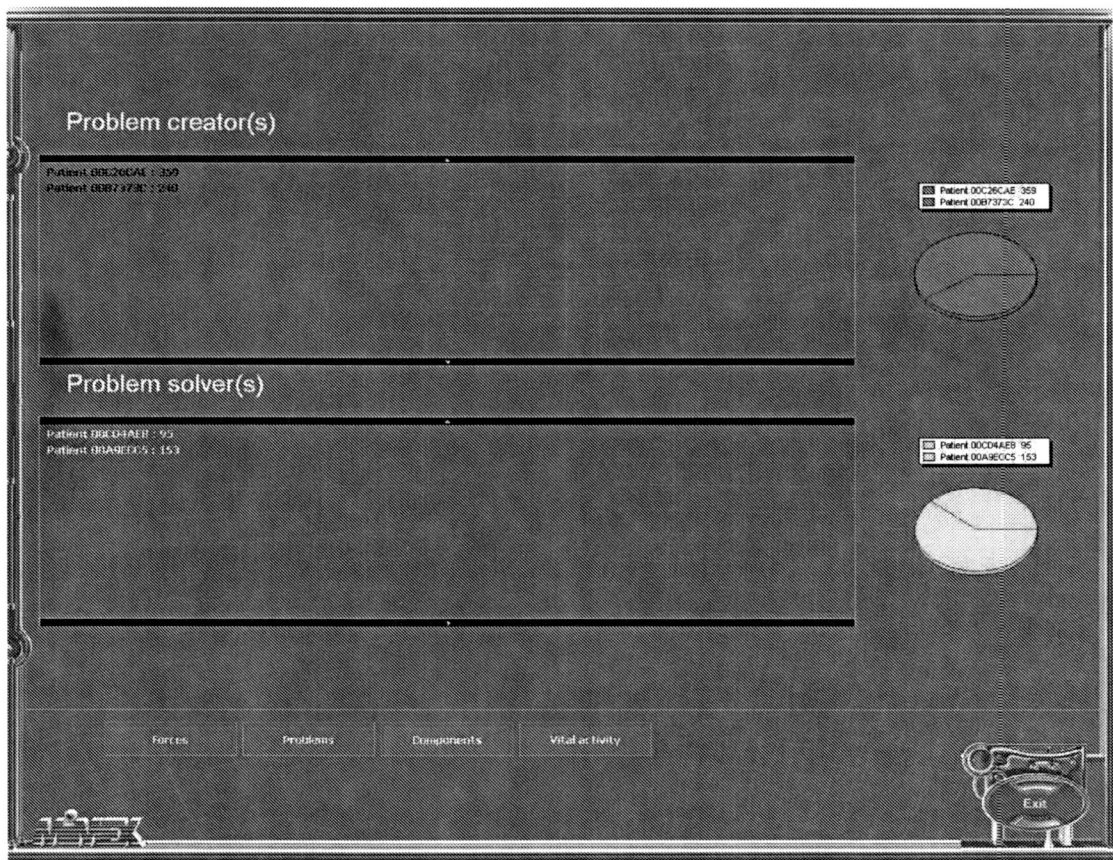

Both parents were identified as the problem creators whilst both boys were identified as the problem solvers.

## Figure 11/Report 6(c):

## Components of the Forces

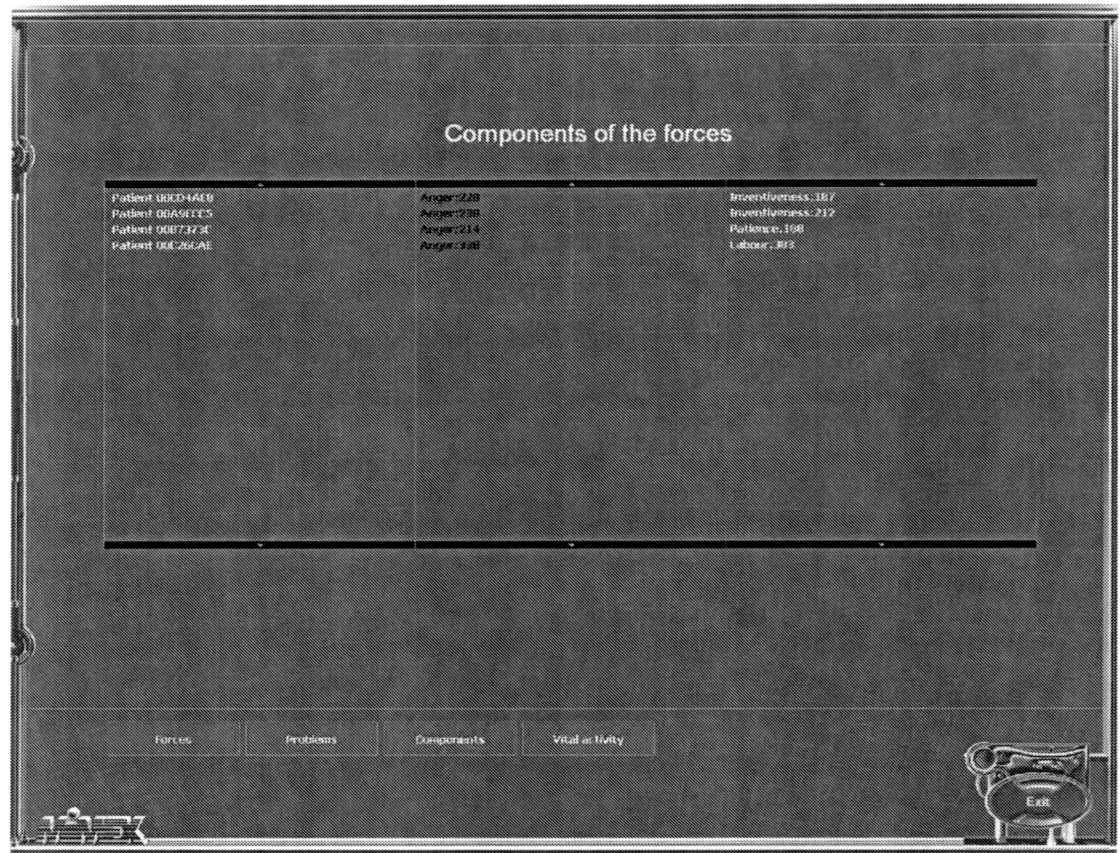

The Anger felt by all four family members was being counterbalanced by the Inventiveness of the teenage boys, the patience of the father and the labour of the mother.

# Figure 12/Report 6(d):

## Vital Activity of the Group and its Components

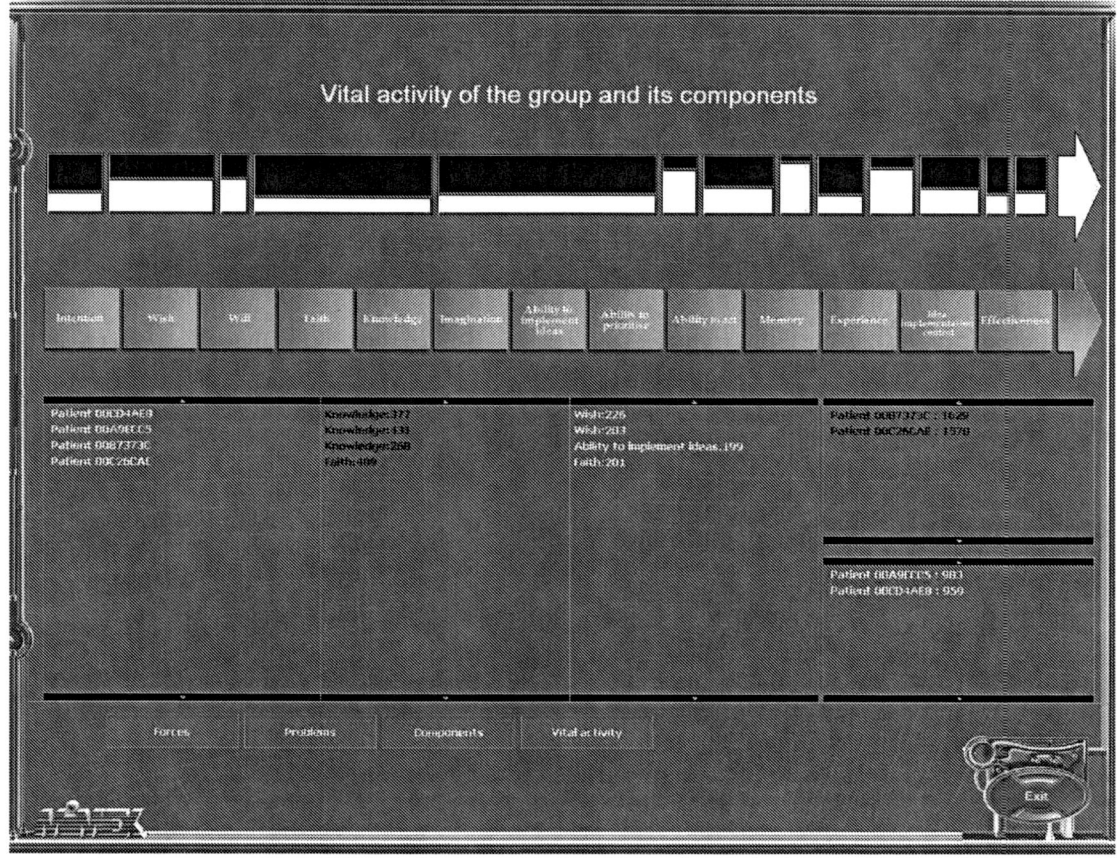

## Figure 13/Report 6(e):

### Ratio of Success

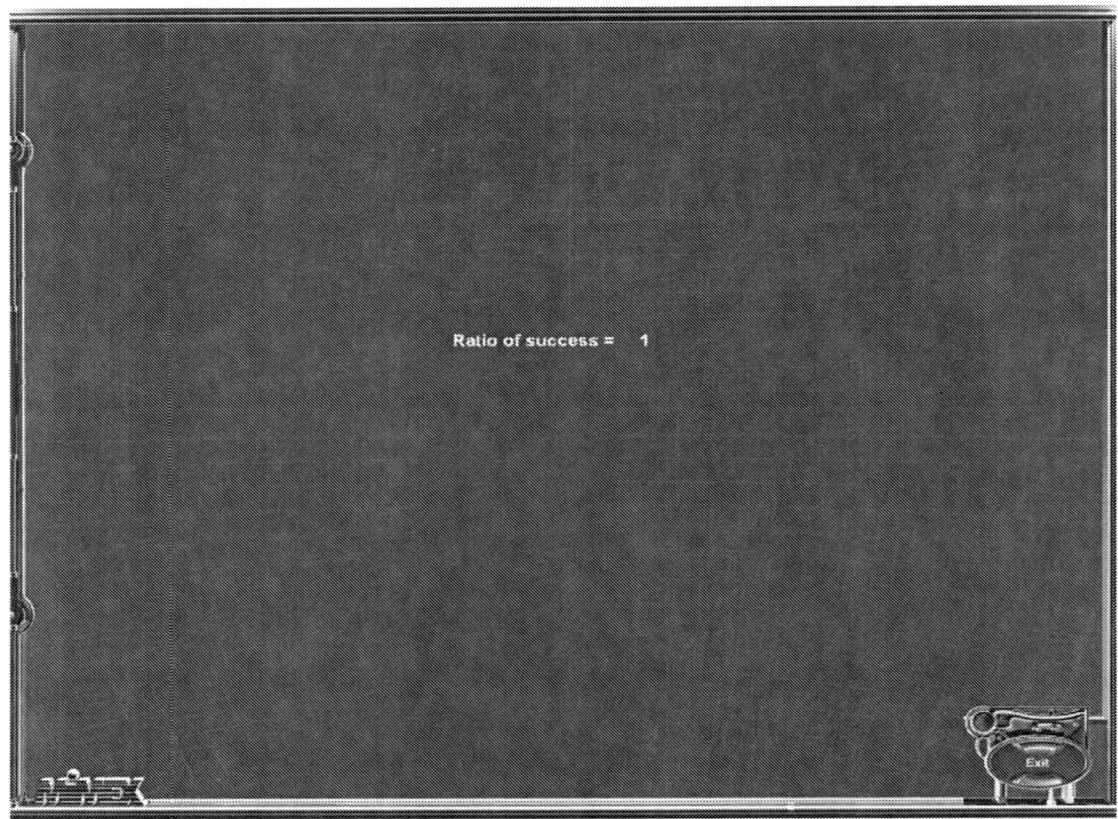

If the ratio of success is reported as 1 this indicates that the group is performing at a satisfactory level whereas if the results were at 0.5 this would indicate that the group was performing at an unsatisfactory level.

If for example a group of two person, perhaps a small company (husband and wife) with a result of 1.0 were to be augmented by a third person the group would be seeking to recruit an employee with attributes which would maintain this level of efficiency of the group or improve the level of efficiency of the group (1.3)

If for example a small team was working at a level of 0.75 it would be worth looking at the profiles of each person to identify specific factors which are affecting his/her ability to contribute to the efficiency of the team. If a health or psychological problem were identified this could lead to remedial therapy. If a problem was identified between team members it may be decided to reorganize the team, perhaps involving swapping team members, changing responsibilities, changing schedules, or recruiting new employees; to overcome the problem and improve the efficiency of the team(s).

# Discussion of Results

Description of the Group: The mother, a highly motivated and achievement oriented lady of 43 years chose to move from the Ural region of Russia to live in Moscow and to look after her elder son who had chosen to attend University. She was seeking to live as an independent lady free from the constraints of her marriage. She has become a very successful, ruthless, commercial manager in the telecommunications business. Her sole focus is that of achievement and of providing for her children.

There are two very pleasant, good-looking sons, aged 17 and 19 years, who are highly intelligent achievers and who are both at university in Moscow. They love both of their parents equally and seek to maintain the harmony of the family relationship whilst understanding fully that their mother seeks to be free from their father. Both sons are achievers, and are achieving good grades at University, although the younger son's performance appears to be affected by the family stresses to a greater extent than the older son.

The father, aged 45 years, is also highly intelligent and works at the level of Technical Director in the development and manufacture of electrical equipment. He is highly respected and sought-after in his profession and is a calm, knowledgeable, capable, intelligent, rational and efficient manager.

## Assessing the Group's Psycho-emotional Profile

Using Virtual Scanning we are able to assess the psycho-emotional profile of each person and of the sum of the group's abilities.

We identify that the father and mother are the 'Problem Creators' whilst the two sons are the 'Problem Solvers'. The two sons have the 'inventiveness' to overcome the problems of their parents very difficult relationship and of an underlying level of 'anger' (which may be better described as frustration or resentment). The group's activity is dominated by labour, inventiveness and abstinence i.e. of working to have a better future but of the negative emotions which are the cause or effect of this programme.

The parents psycho-emotional profile comprise 'Patience' (the father) and 'Labour' (the mother) and also of an underlying level of 'anger' (and/or resentment). The 'vital activity of the group and its components' is dominated by negative components although this does not affect the ability of the group to initiate and complete a course of action.

The 'ratio of success' of the group is 1.0 which, surprisingly, is just the average level and which is not affected by the tension in the household.

# Virtual Scanning version 4

# Psychological Profile

The earlier versions of this technology (version 4) were developed as two different programmes with differing outcomes for the same test procedure i.e. as the psychological profile and the health profile. Whilst the health report was described earlier the psychological report was excluded and is now discussed within this text.

This first version of the technology tests the patient's ability to complete the test under normal conditions and then under pressure (i.e. to complete the test as quickly as possible). The mathematics of the programme were able to differentiate the person's results and hence to comment upon whether the patient performed well under pressure.

In the example (figures 14 -17) the patient was noted to be pre-disposed to action rather than gathering information.

Figures 18-21 enable us to have an understanding of the person's psychological profile. The red and blue bars of the psychological profile are considered to represent the rational and emotional aspects of each trait.

## Figure 14

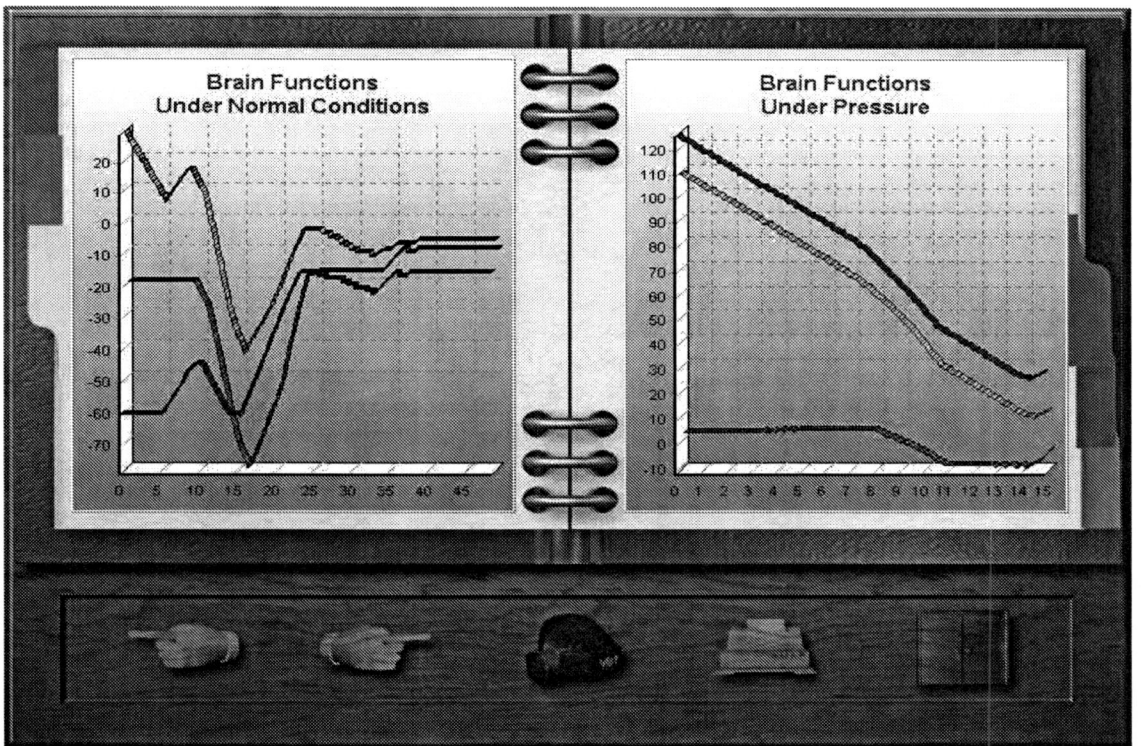

# Figure 15

1. CARBOHYDRATE EXCHANGE
2. BLOOD AND PERIPHERAL VESSELS
3. PROTEIN EXCHANGE

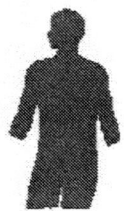

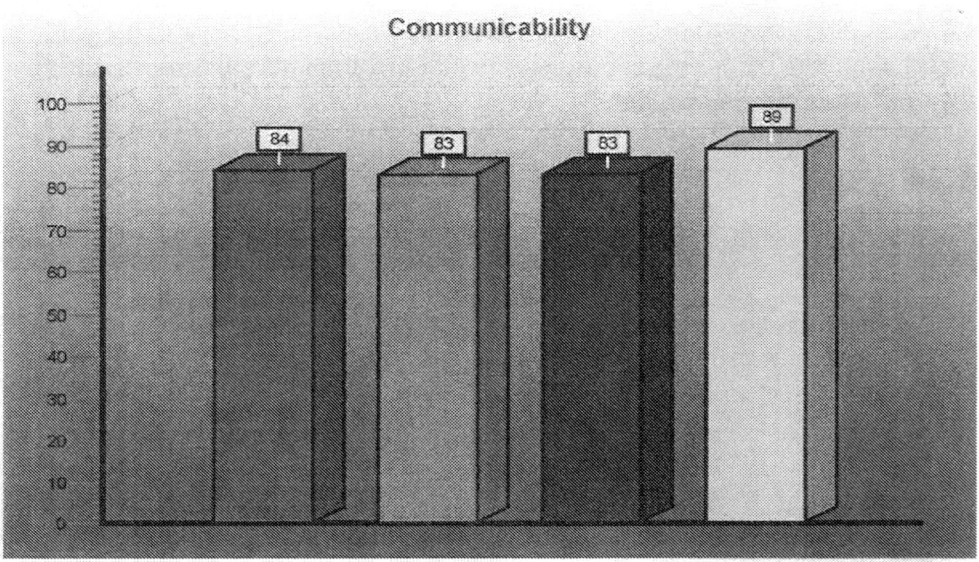

Ability to work under management 84
Ability to communicate with other people 83
Ability to teach/train 83
Ability to manage others 89

## Information to action

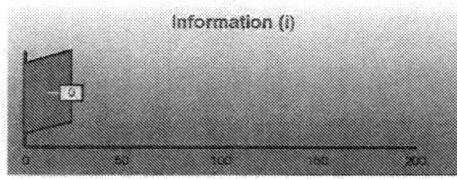

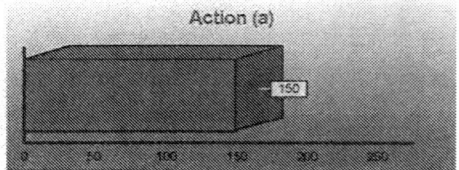

Preference to action

# Figures 16 & 17

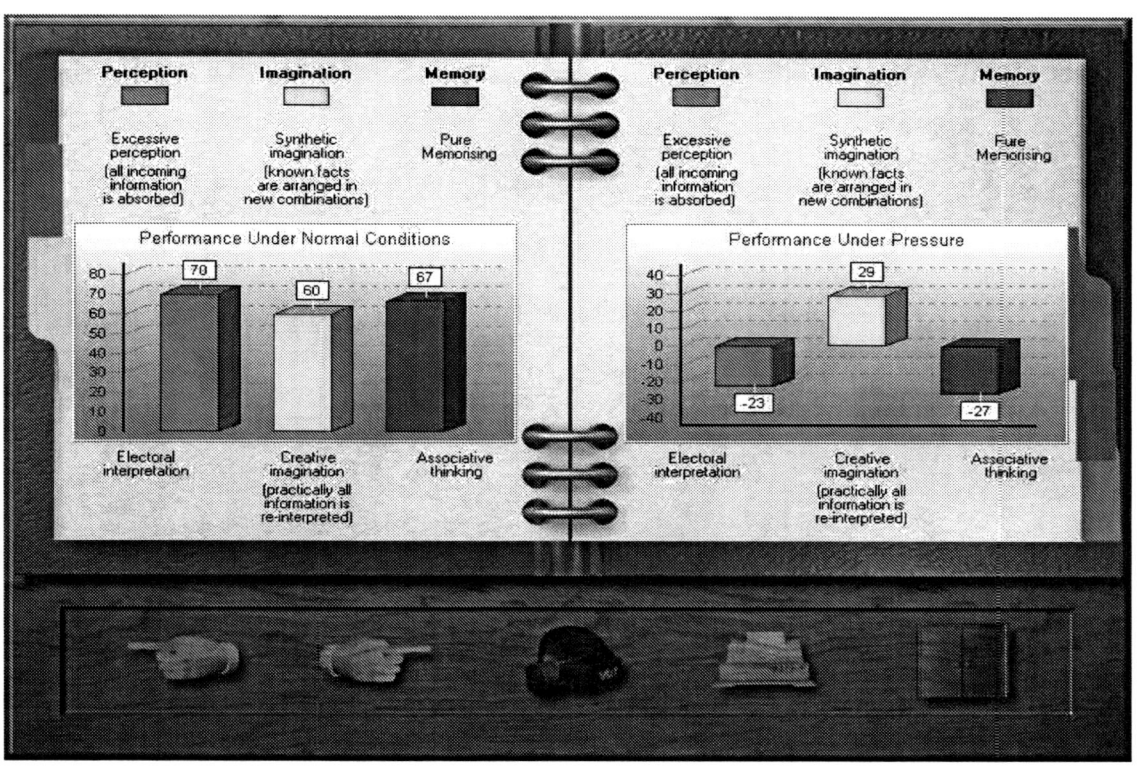

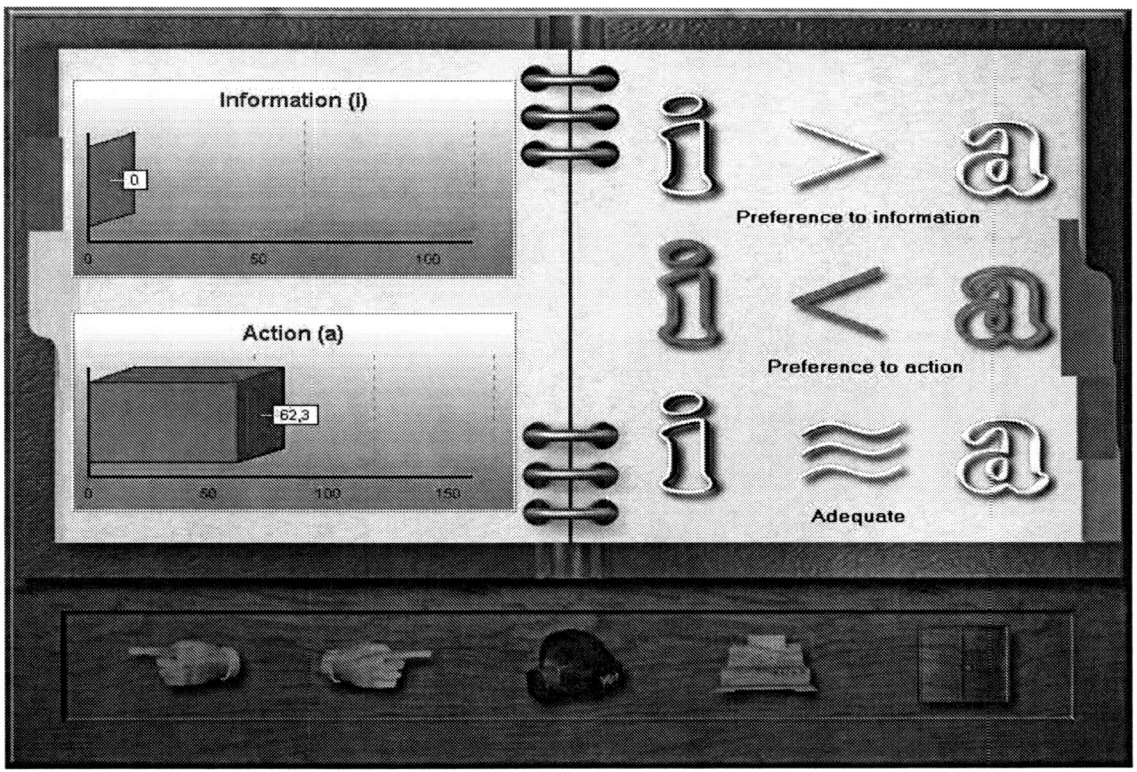

## Figures 18 & 19

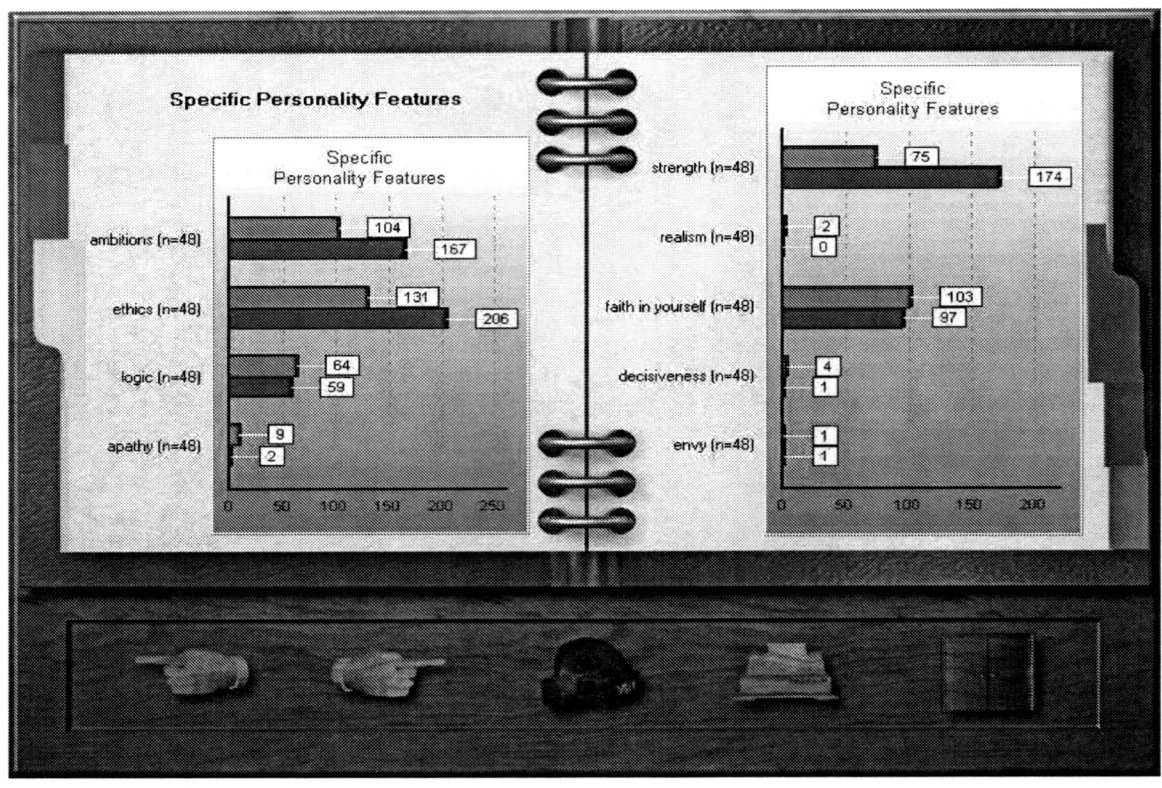

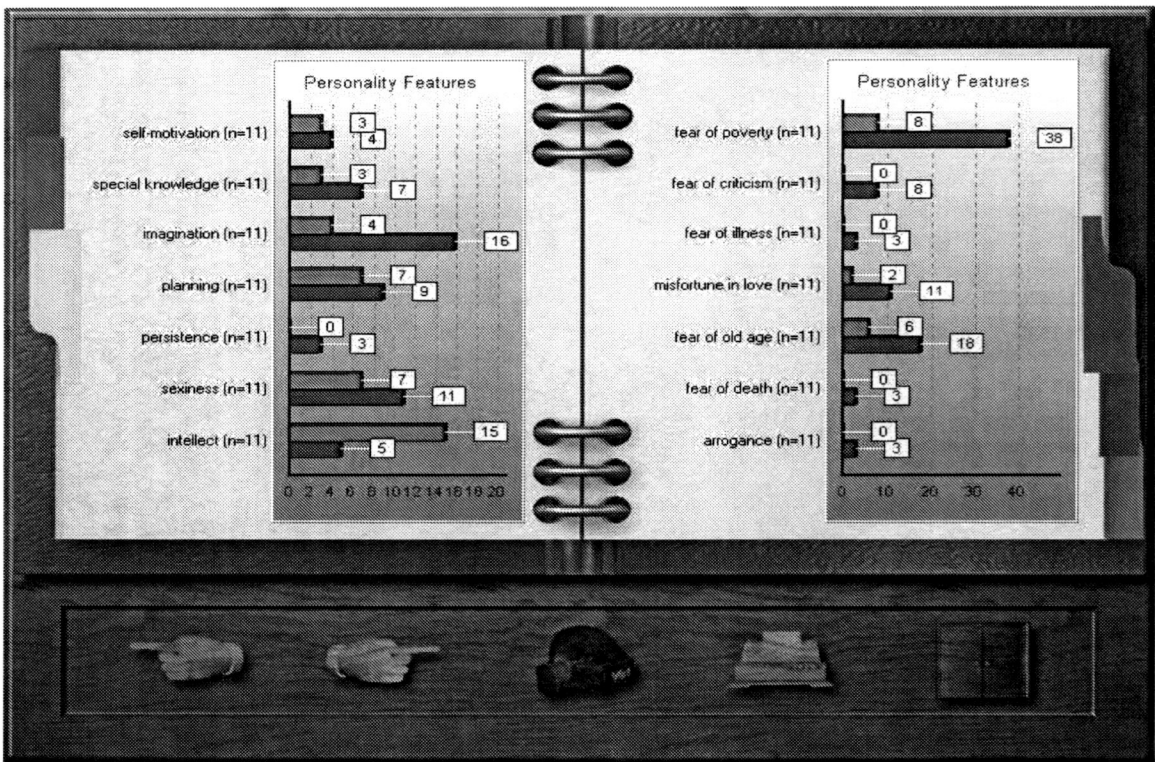

# Figures 20 & 21

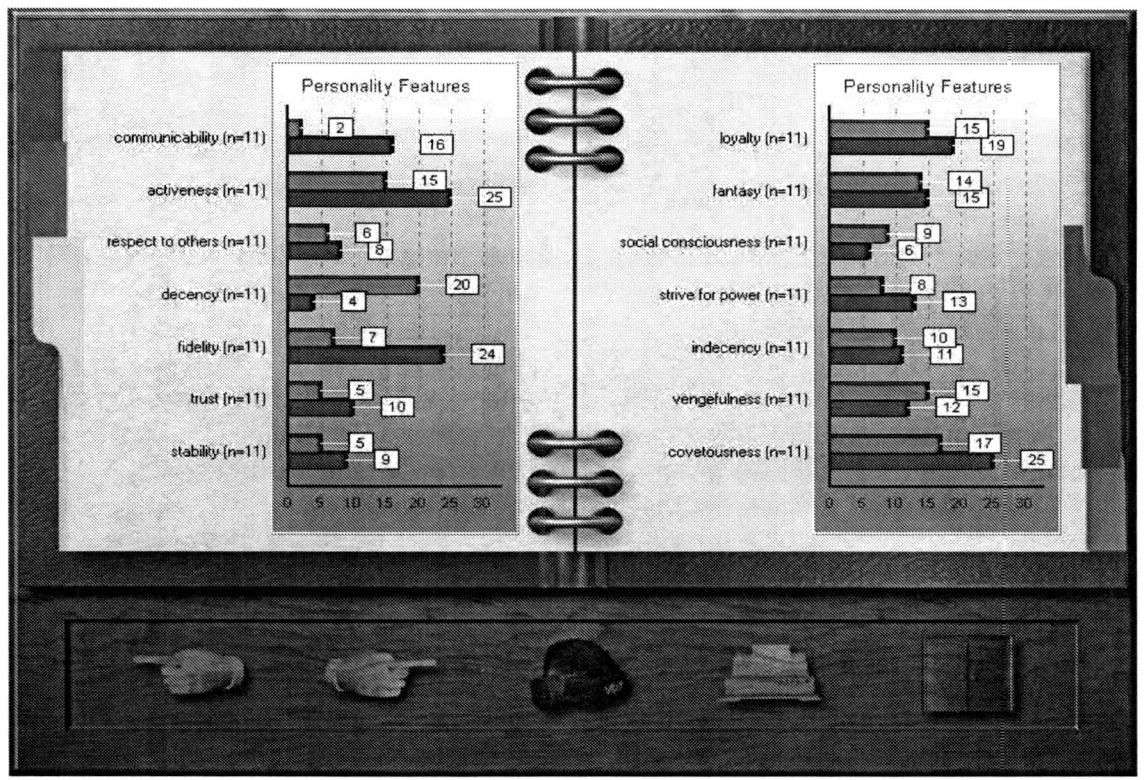

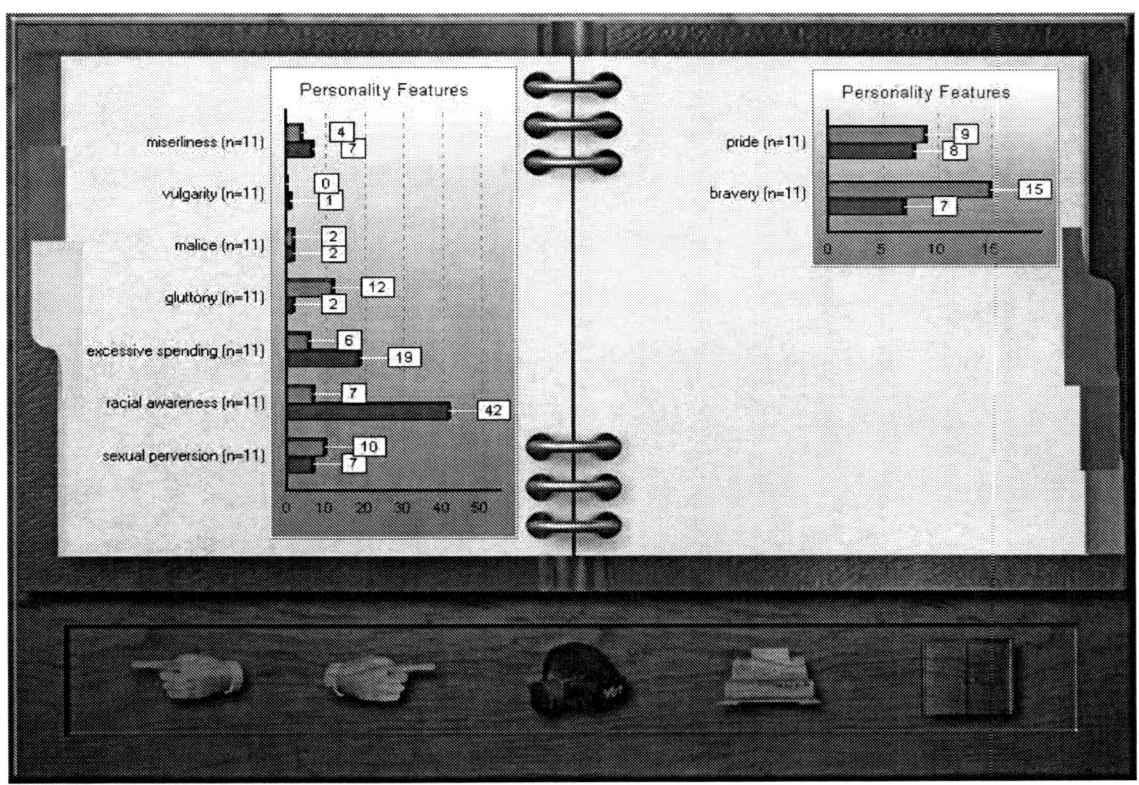

# Patient Summary

The person is predisposed to action and not to gathering information and they do not work well under pressure.

They are highly ambitious, highly ethical, have high inner strength, are above-average in logical thought and have a high level of self-confidence. By contrast they are not in the slightest bit apathetic, have little realism, are indecisive and are not envious.

Specific Personality traits include a lack of persistence and of self-motivation; fear of criticism, illness and death; that they are loyal, vengeful, covetousness; not vulgar or miserly, and have little malice.

Each report is able to comment upon the extent of their particular personality trait e.g. (1) that the person has a high level of rationality (15) to bravery but on the emotional level has a below average level (7). Similarly with decency the person has an above average level (20) rationally and is below average (4) on the emotional level.

# Chapter 3

# How does VIRTUAL SCANNING work?

by

Graham Ewing

# Why do we get ill?

*What is it that overcomes our body's natural stability and makes it prone to the development of pathologies?*

The conventional medical viewpoint is that we get ill for some reason and that stress makes these illnesses worse. By contrast the complementary health view is that stress is the fundamental cause for illness [1] and lowers the immune system. This leaves the person vulnerable to the onset of pathologies and hence of the establishment of the unnatural pathological processes in the body.

A stress effect is anything which affects our body's function e.g. anxiety, violence or the threat of harm; of underperformance in school, sport or at work; social stresses, death of a close relative, divorce; excessive heat or cold; exposure to subtle radiation; bacterial or viral infection; reduced amounts of sleep; disturbed diet or dietary overindulgence; etc.

Stress is any effect, the influence of any phenomena, which is beyond the body's natural tolerance limits and which affects the regulation of the body's systems, organs and of the levels of biochemicals associated with body's stability i.e. of homeostasis.

Long-term exposure to stress or exposure to high levels of stress inhibits the body's natural processes of compensation. The mechanisms which regulate our health are weakened and the processes of pathology become established. These biochemical changes subsequently affect our sensory perception, cognition, and behaviour.

While there is not yet an accepted mechanism for the development of pathology it appears that Russian medical science has for many years been more advanced in their understanding of specific aspects of pathophysiology than western medicine [142]. Researchers such as [2] Anokhin , Gorizontov [147], Medvedev [149], Sudakov [156], and others have contributed to a robust theory which defines the PATHOLOGICAL FUNCTIONAL SYSTEMS which are responsible for the development of pathology and of illness. These have been used in the development of Virtual Scanning technology and other medical devices [160].

They consider that stress, defined in its broadest terms – affecting organ and cell function - is the fundamental cause of illness (see figure 1). By contrast the conventional outlook considers that the adverse influences of stress make a medical condition worse but are not considered to be the fundamental cause of illness.

This is represented as follows:

# Figure 1

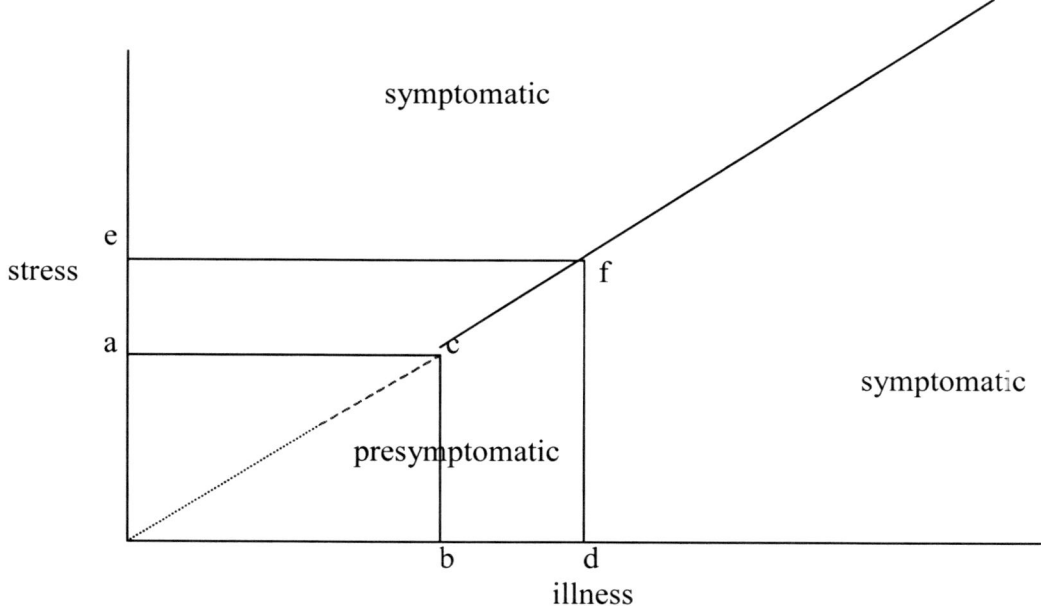

i.e. the conventional model commences at point c whereas the Russian model extrapolates the data back to zero. Points e, f and d indicates how the pathophysiological process would progress from the pre-symptomatic level to the symptomatic.

Data received from the external environment, perceived in the form of others' behaviour, is experienced through the effect of light and other senses on our physiology. This enables us to define our stability and to define the threats which affect our existence.

All extreme experiences create short-term exposure to stress however it is the long-term exposure to stress, or the magnitude of the exposure, which overrides the body's natural stability 3. This depresses the normal levels of immunochemicals thereby enabling the development of the pathological functional systems and of the development of medical conditions.

Our neural functions - of perception, imagination, memory and associative thinking, and of decision-making - are affected by the development of pathological functional systems. These can be measured and related to our psychology and to our physiology.

In particular our perception of light and colour changes according to the influence of our autonomic nervous system 5,6, and the levels of biochemicals in our physiology. The ability to use autonomic information flow (AIF) in medical diagnosis 162 has been demonstrated in patients with heart failure and complex medical conditions.

These neural functions, which can be measured and related to the physiology of the person, are unique to each person at any point in time, i.e

- cognitive response is related to health;

- visual perception and cognition are related to the levels of components in blood (of proteins, neurotransmitters, etc);
- levels of specific biochemical components reflect the nature and magnitude of the medical condition;
- colour perception is defined by our experiences [4];

- colour perception is influenced by the levels of photopsins in the retina [136];

therefore by using a colour-based cognitive test procedure, which measures the cognitive parameters, the results can be related to psychology and health. Due to the complexity of the process, mathematical modelling and computing are used to process the data into an intelligible format.

The components in our blood absorb and transmit light of different colours and that this is, directly or indirectly, dependent upon the interaction between proteins, neurotransmitters, etc; which affect our perception of colour.

[7] According to Neurochemist Dr Candace Pert:

**"There's a revolution going on. There used to be two systems of knowledge: hard science of chemistry, physics, biophysics -- on the one hand, and, on the other, a system of knowledge that included ethology, psychology and psychiatry. And now it's as if a lightning bolt had connected the two. It's all one system -neuroscience. The present era in neuroscience is comparable to the time when Louis Pasteur first found out that germs cause disease."**

[8] According to David Krech, University of California at Berkeley psychologist, who predicted almost twenty-five years ago:

**"I foresee the day when we shall have the means, and therefore, inevitably, the temptation to manipulate the behavior and intellectual functioning of all people through environmental and biochemical manipulation of the brain."**

# What evidence is there to relate our cognition to our psychology?

*There is a surprising number of precedents which enable us to illustrates how our cognition is related to our psychology.*

There are established psychometric profiling technologies such as the Colormetrics [9] approach which is based upon the prioritisation of shapes and colours. Other methods use written questionnaires. Typical commercial techniques include the Occupational Personality Questionnaire (OPQ), Watson-Glaser Critical Thinking Appraisal, 16PF, Myers-Briggs Type Indicator (MBI), Innovation Potential Indicator (IPI). The MBI and IPI approaches claim to identify the cumulativeness of the profiles for groups of people.

There are two types of psychometric tests: aptitude tests, which assess your abilities; and personality questionnaires, which help to build up a profile of your characteristics and personality. Virtual Scanning offers an approach which covers all aspects of the person's specific personality and aptitude. Unlike the word-based approach - because Virtual Scanning uses cognitive response - it is not possible to cheat the test.

The Luscher [133] colour test measures a person's psychophysical state, his or her ability to withstand stress, to perform, and to communicate. It is claimed that the Luscher test uncovers the cause of psychological stress, which can lead to physical symptoms.

**Consider for a moment what is cognition?**

Our cognitive abilities are a function of our biochemical interaction with our environment. This involves how we receive data, how we process data, and how we behave? This involves sense perception (of vision, hearing, smell, touch and taste), memory and movement. It must therefore be related to the health of the systems, organs and cells which regulate our receipt and processing of data.

**There are many precedents which illustrate how our cognition is subjectively associated with our health e.g.**

- If we are ill, perhaps with influenza, our cognitive abilities are severely affected; if we have a heart condition we are hardly likely to consider running 100 metres; and if we are stressed out it becomes difficult to concentrate or to memorise. Every medical condition affects our cognition in some way.

- Research [13] has illustrated that being forgetful is indicative of poor heart function and that those with poor memories and slower reaction times are more likely to die from a heart attack.

**and how drugs affect our colour perception e.g.**

- W.Paulus [10] reports in the International Color Vision Society 1999 symposium upon the 'Effects of Medication on Colour Vision' and in particular that anti-epileptic and dopaminergic drugs influence colour perception.

- Viagra [11] affects colour perception, mild and temporary visual changes (blue/green color perception changes, light perception changes, and blurred vision) and can cause increased sensitivity to light or blurred vision. It inhibits the function of the enzyme PDE6 which is involved in transduction in the retina and hence affects colour perception.

- Other drugs which influence colour perception include:

  1.    sulpha drugs and antibiotics are associated with a misperception of yellow;

  2.    the anticonvulsant drug Triodone can cause the complete disappearance of some colours;

  3.    and oral contraceptives cause a blue-yellow perception deficit.

  4.    Other drugs which have known effects upon colour perception include: ethambutol, vigabatrin, voriconazole, pregabalin, quinine, carbamazepine, midazolam, ecstacy, lsd, etc.

- This induced colour perception deficit is often referred to as a drug-induced **dyschromatopia**.

**and how our medical condition is associated with visual perception deficits e.g.**

- Further research of available literature identifies visual perception deficits in those with autism, parkinsonism, alzheimer's disease [12], schizophrenia and in the elderly [14].

- Some medical conditions are associated with colour perception deficits eg. blue colour deficiency is associated with liver disease and diabetes; a green colour deficiency is associated with heart conditions [16]

Those with a Red-green deficiency (**deuteranopia**) is the most frequently diagnosed deficiency. Those with this condition cannot distinguish certain shades of red and green. Blue deficiency (**protanopia**) is relatively rare. Blue and yellow are not distinguished by those with this condition, and may be seen as white or grey. Total colour blindness (**achromatopsia**) is extremely rare. In this condition, no colours can be detected and the world is viewed in shades of black, white and grey. People with this condition have poor sight and are extremely sensitive to light.

Our visual perception is therefore associated, directly or indirectly, with the mechanisms which regulate our biochemistry. Changes to the physiological systems induced by illness or by drug substances, influence our perception of colour therefore by assessing the cognitive deficit it is possible to make an evaluation of a person's health.

Changes to the levels of proteins and of protein-substrates in the body affect the release of biophotons and hence the intensity and colour of the light released.

Research now questions the conventional explanation for sight and visual perception which is based upon the number and type of colour-sensitive cones, and the role of photopsins in the retina [136, 137]. The number of colour-sensitive cones in the retina differs by up to 40 times, yet we perceive colours in the same way. This suggests that our colour perception is influenced more by our brains than our eyes i.e. that our visual perception is affected by other factors.

# Grakov's Work

*Dr I.G.Grakov, medical researcher University of Krasnoyarksk, in 1985 initiated the programme which developed the first commercial version Virtual Scanner* 171-175 *by 1998.*

Grakov has built upon the work of Anokhin, Bekhtereva, Sudakov, et al; which define the mechanisms for the maintenance of the body's regulation and stability. Stress is considered to be the main culprit and depresses cognitive function, the immune system, the production of proteins and/or neurotransmitters, etc 157-159; and is related to the function of the short-term and long-term memory(s).

The sensitivity of the stress mechanism is related to the current health, weight and age of the person. For example a young person with good health would be less affected by issues which could induce stress (see figure 4) whereas an older person is much more susceptible to stress.

Long-term exposure to stress effects, which exceed the natural tolerance limits, create the conditions which result in the development of the pathological functional systems which we ultimately observe as the symptoms of illness. (see figure 2 – process of regulation (1)). Over a period the brain recognises the errant stress-related condition as the stable state rather than the long-term memory i.e. the short-term memory replaces the long-term memory (see figures 3 – process of regulation (2)).

Stress affects all aspects of our physical performance. It affects our sexual performance, our physical performance (including the speed, duration and extent of energy expenditure) and it also affects the function of our senses. It inhibits blood flow to the brain, spinal chord, organs, muscles and the senses.

The belief that the anatomical and biochemical models of our physiology are the sole models upon which credible new technologies, medications or therapies can be based is therefore a fundamentally wrong assumption.

This approach fails to consider that the biochemical model includes biophysical concepts which are regulated by the autonomic nervous system including: the pressure and flow of blood through the blood vessels and the pumping of liquids by the heart; of bio-electrical influences which influence the function of the heart, the communication between cells; of bio-mechanical systems which effect our motion, posture, etc.

There are theoretical concepts based upon the function of the autonomic nervous system which could, in principle, be a more precise method of determining the health of the patient than the conventional biochemical approach. These involve the sensory processes e.g. (1) vision: which affects our perception of light and colour; (2) hearing: which affects our perception of sound and is involved in the regulation of balance; and (3) smell, taste and touch. Changes to our sensory spectrum induced by external stress influences will therefore affect our physiology and vice-versa.

Virtual Scanning illustrates how stress induces changes in the autonomic nervous system and hence affects our health. This is reflected in our cognition and colour perception.

(Similarly Berard.G [165] and others have illustrated that the hearing spectrum [164, 165, 167-169] and the vocal spectrum can be affected by changes to our health. No doubt this applies also to the olfactory sense and to touch. In the same way that a specific colour therapy can be used to treat an ailment by Virtual Scanning Colour Therapy, Ayurvedha, Kinesiology, etc; sound can also be used therapeutically [166]. Proponents of aromatherapy, massage and the other sensory-based therapies will undoubtedly be in agreement with these general principles.

Sound perception is affected by age and by stress factors such as extreme noise which affect the hearing function. It is also affected by health conditions which decrease or increase sound perception.  It remains questionable whether hearing loss is due to noise, or to natural aging effects, or the effect of other factors associated with the modern way of life in developed countries. To illustrate the point Rosen [170] discovered almost no signs of presbycusis (age-related hearing loss) among the Mabaan tribe of the Sudan, irrespective of their age. He attributed this to their peaceful lives and good health.

As light is responsible for an estimated 85% of sensory input it represents by far the most powerful of the senses. It can be precisely measured and applied whereas the other sensory-based therapies have inherent theoretical and practical limitations).

Using the software programme developed by Grakov, which involves the mathematical modelling of data derived from the cognitive test procedure, the outcome is an unprecedented level of our understanding of physiology, and that our physiology is regulated by systems which regulate the function of the various systems and organs.

Repeated short-term exposure to stress-effects become the norm and dominate the long-term regulation of the physiology which is responsible for homeostasis (see figure 2). There is therefore a synergy between the function of the autonomic nervous system and the levels of biochemicals which raise or depress immune system function.

# Figure 2:

## Data from the External environment

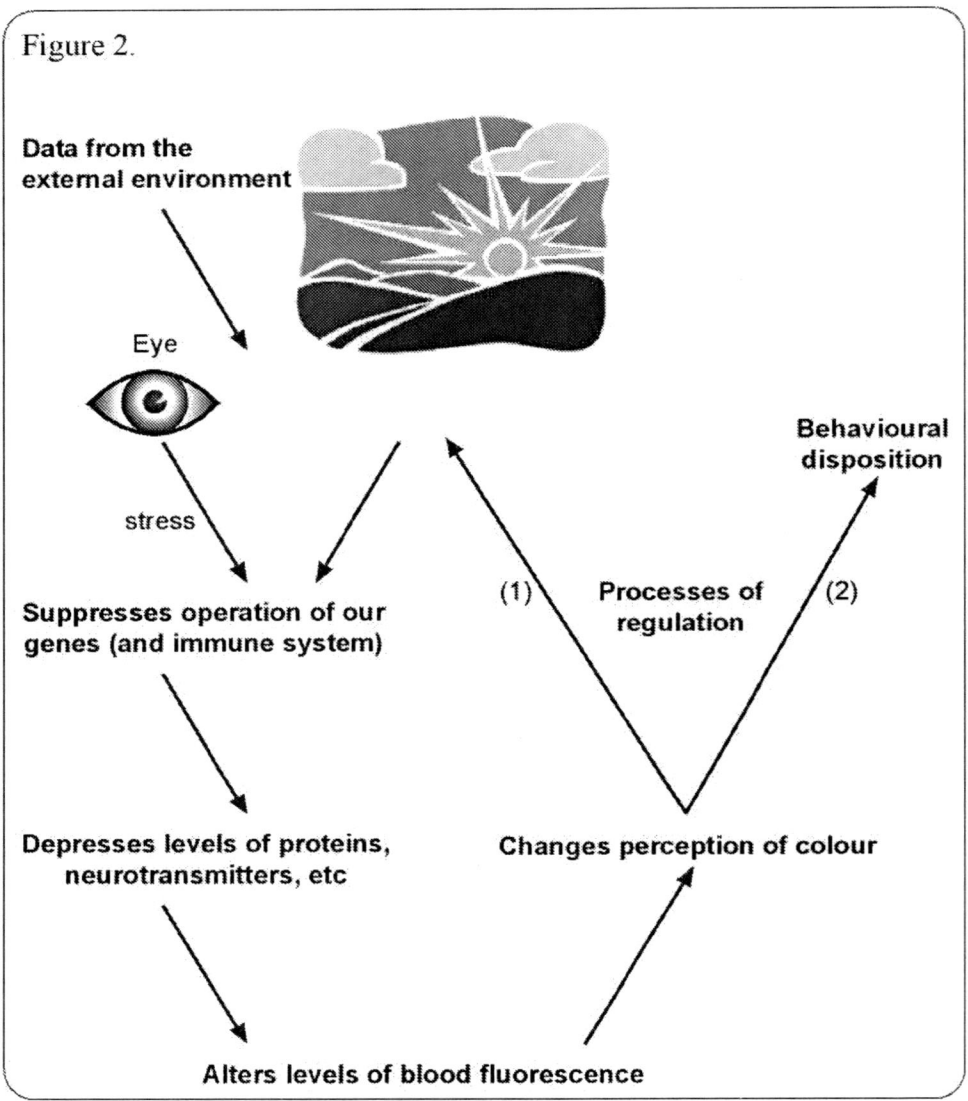

# Extracts of Articles by Russian Medical Researchers

*Translation of an article by Professor Yuri Vysochin, Director, Lesgaft Institute, Extracts of*

The experimental and theoretical investigations of Russian researchers 3 have proven 'that programmes of functional adjustment provide an adaptive mechanism for the human physiology'. N.N. Vasilevskiy emphasized that the adaptive mechanisms should be considered as 'controlling systems which are provided with rigid and flexible programmes as well as tracking systems which appear to elaborate initiating signals and withdraw from the memory an appropriate succession of controlling signals and programmes which are included in the regulation of the component'.

Further reports of experimental data by researchers (P. D. Gorizontov, 147; V. I. Medvedev, 149-152; I. A. Sapov 155, V. S. Novikov, 153-154; N.N. Vasilevskiy) illustrate that it is a disruption of the regulating role of the central nervous system and hormonal system that can cause a reduction of protective mechanisms and the development of pathological conditions.

Research carried out by N.H. Bekhtereva elucidated the neuro-pathological processes and features associated with their function. It was concluded that there appears to be the formation of new intracellular structures which were fixed in a corresponding matrix of long-term memory which gives the new pathological process stability.

Based upon these ideas G. N. Kryzhanovskiy 161 developed a concept of a pathological functional system (PFS) as one of the most common mechanisms underlying numerous central nervous system pathology forms.

Unlike the physiological FSs described in detail by P. K. Anokhin, the pathological functional system (PFS) is an accumulation of nervous formations, which have allostatic significance. The PFS illustrates how a pathogenic factor can cause further development or initiation of the given or a new pathological process. PFS as well as physiological FSs cause inhibition of other related systems. This has significant pathogenic importance, for it is connected with disintegration of nervous system activity and suppression of the regulatory and reparative mechanisms which for example subsequently distort the oxygen and carbon dioxide ratio in the organism.

# Homeostatic and Behavioural Limits Change with Age

*It is inevitable that our health starts to decline with age. Consider how our ability to deal with change adapts throughout our lives.*

From birth our lives are devoted to dealing with change. In our youth when perception is our dominant neural function we deal with change on a regular basis. Almost every experience is new. In fact we actively seek change in our rapidly maturing lives – through travel, exhilarating experiences, sporting challenges, etc.

As we age our neural function changes and progresses to reflect our altered priorities and physical capabilities. Imagination becomes more important as we seek to 'mate' and 'memory and associative thinking' as we seek to raise our family however with advancing years our ability to deal with change declines. Our body becomes less adaptable and less flexible, our behaviour becomes more predictable, and we make the decisions which pose less risk and require less biochemical change (see figure 3).

Figure 3. The effects of age on behavioural limits

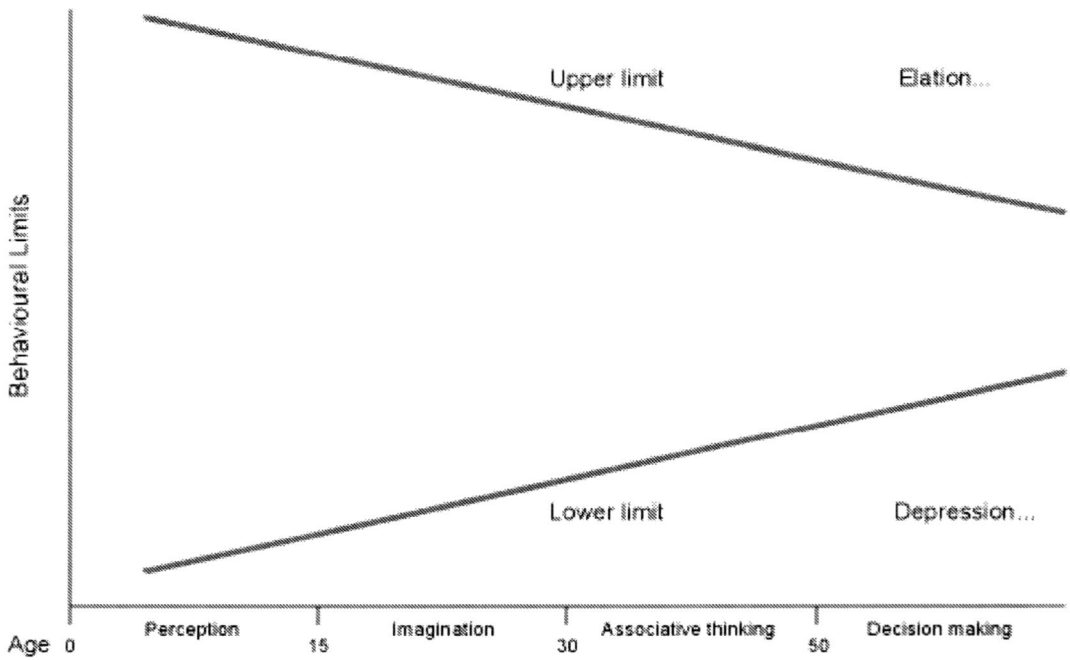

# The Justification for Physiological Systems

*A complex system can only work if there is a hierarchical mechanism which regulates its function.*

Grakov has identified that there are 14 PHYSIOLOGICAL SYSTEMS in the body whereas modern medicine accepts only that the body has various SYSTEMS of operation 163 i.e. their effect and structure is poorly understood. The fact that such issues are poorly understood is recognised in research programmes of the European Union (document FP7, Health-2007-2.2.2-2)

The structure of these systems have been precisely determined and involve a network of interconnected organs which are regulated by the autonomic nervous system. The brain and blood system are involved in most systems whilst others are part of only several systems.

Grakov has established in precise terms that the function of our physiological systems, organs, and the levels of our cellular and molecular biochemistry are regulated by light and colour.

**Figure 4.**

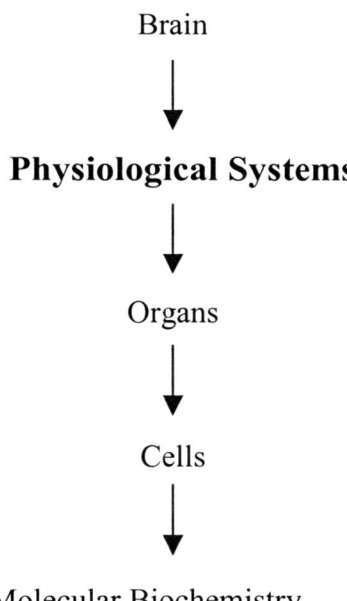

Brain

↓

**Physiological Systems**

↓

Organs

↓

Cells

↓

Molecular Biochemistry

By contrast to the conventional approach which ignores the significance of the body's physiological systems and focuses upon identifying and measuring the progression of pathologies, Virtual Scanning measures the effect of stress on the stability of the body's physiological systems and organs, and how this affects the levels of biochemicals at the cellular level. It determines the processes which are responsible for the development of pathology and measures their development from the pre-symptomatic level.

Medical conditions arise from the effect of stress-related, or psychosomatic, factors on the stability of the body's physiological systems. These systems are regulated by the brain's delta waves (frequency). By identifying the precise colour deficiencies and most affected functional systems it is possible to stimulate the compensatory response for the medical condition of concern. This results in the enhanced levels of chemicals in the immune system and the progressive elimination of the symptoms of illness.

The logic of the hierarchical nature of the human physiology as illustrated in figure 4 is inescapable. A complex system can only work if there is a hierarchical mechanism which regulates its function.

# The Holistic Nature of the Human Physiology

*Any holistic or biofeedback system involves the exchange of signals which regulate the system's function.*

It is indisputable that the body functions holistically in which the body's systems, organs and the brain are effectively in regular communication – how else could we function if this were not so? This holistic or biofeedback system involves the exchange of signals from the brain to the organ and vice versa.

Some researchers speculate upon the regulatory functions of hormones 15 as a means of regulating body weight.

Virtual Scanning provides us with evidence for the hierarchical and holistic nature of the human physiology which can be proven by selecting patients with a number of unique factors e.g.

- where there is no significant pathology and the dominance of the processes of compensation e.g. in a healthy child

- where there is a lack of compensation and the prevalence of pathology e.g. in an older person with failing health

- where a patient has had an organ removed

- where a patient has had an organ transplant i.e. they are using an organ which has the DNA of another person

- where the person's compensatory response has failed e.g. where someone has had a severe stroke and is partially paralysed

- considering examples which illustrate the development and recession of a medical condition and the ability to predict the occurrence of a medical condition

# How Stress Affects our Health.

*Consider how stress affects our mental health and our physical health. Our mind and body function in an inter-related and inter-dependent manner.*

The credibility of any theory is its ability to explain all of the observed phenomena yet in modern healthcare theories are used which have distinct limitations and which are unable to explain all of the phenomena and symptoms which are associated with illness.

In this battle for intellectual supremacy in which Psychology vies with Neurology and Computational Neuroscience, medical researchers working in the disciplines of pathophysiology, psychoneuroimmunoendocrinology, and psychoneuroimmunology, have come to recognise the inter-relatedness of behaviour with health and wellbeing.

Instead of expanding into ever more diverse areas of specialism, biomedical research is in fact converging.

**The following examples illustrate how stress affects our health:**

- Psychoneuroimmunoendocrinology: takes the holistic view of the mind/body/spirit as a synergistic interchange. This new field of research claims to provide evidence which suggests we are far more than a human machine.

- [17] Depression worsens the outlook of coronary heart disease patients: In a study of heart patients, those who were depressed suffered twice the level of poor health and three times worse quality of life than those with a more positive attitude.

- [18] Depression increases mortality rate after heart attack: In a study of those who survive an acute heart attack, depressed patients were three times more likely to die within the first year than those who had a balanced attitude, although all patients had the same level of care.

- [19] Sense of hopelessness causes atherosclerosis: A study of men with a 'high' sense of hopelessness found that their arteries thickened by nearly 20 per cent compared with those who had a positive attitude.

- [20] Anger can lead to coronary heart disease: People who are frequently very angry are twice as likely to suffer heart disease than those with infrequent anger outbursts.

- [21] Anger could trigger coronary heart disease: Anger can cause myocardial ischemia, and could be an independent risk factor for coronary artery disease. In a study of men who had expressed or concealed anger or irritability their chances of developing heart disease increased by four times.

- 22 Grief can cause a heart attack: A group of men and women were interviewed a week after suffering a heart attack, and researchers discovered that many had recently suffered the death of a close family member or friend. Researchers estimate that the risk of a heart attack increased 14 times during the first 24 hours, reduced to eight times the risk during the following 24 hours, six times in the third 24 hours, and then to 2-4 times for the ensuing month.

- 23 Social isolation and heart disease: People in social groups of less than three people were over twice as likely to suffer a fatal heart attack than those in larger groups.

- 24 Relaxation reduces your risks: Relaxation and breathing techniques reduce the risks of coronary heart disease. Researchers tested the theory on a group of people of 35 and 64 years with high levels of cholesterol who were smoking more than 10 cigarettes a day. Half were advised how to stop smoking and reduce animal fats in their diets, and participated in eight one-hour lessons on breathing, relaxation and meditation, whereas the rest of the group were only given information about smoking and diet. Those in the meditation group had lowered blood pressure, and fewer cases of angina, coronary heart disease, and fatal heart attack.

- 25 Heart disease is the main cause of death in western society although its cause is not understood. While obesity, high cholesterol and smoking are implicated, by contrast up to 50% of heart attack patients don't have these symptoms.

  The influence of stress and depression: c30 years ago a landmark study determined that a 'type A' personality i.e. those who are anxious about timekeeping, high-achievers and hostile, is 50% more likely to develop a heart condition than a 'type B personality' i.e who is easy-going and passive.

  Researchers from Northwestern University, Chicago tested the theory with a group of young adults of 18 - 30 years. They specifically assessed whether impatience, competitiveness, hostility, depression and anxiety in the group was related to their chances of developing hypertension, or high blood pressure. Hostility was the only behavioural trait that could dramatically influence hypertension.

- 26 Researchers from Institute of HeartMath reported on 'the Influence of Cardiac Afferent Input on Heart-Brain Synchronization and Cognitive Performance'.

- 27 Psychosocial factors such as chronic stress, depression, cynicism and distrust, are related to increased levels of inflammation markers (interleukin-VI, C-reactive protein and fibrinogen) which are linked to increased risk of cardiovascular disease.

- Stress affects the immune system 28 and hence interferes with wound healing, recovery from surgery, etc

# Consider How Nutritional Deficits can Cause or are Related to Behavioural Problems

*Nutritional deficits are related to a medical conditions but are often not the cause of the condition.*

- [29-31] Zinc and Mg deficiencies are well known to cause immune system problems coupled with fidgeting, anxiety, loss of coordination, learning difficulties et al

- [32,33] Lead can be responsible for aggression and poor concentration. Copper and Aluminium can be responsible for hyperactivity. Is this a surprise to electrochemists who would recognise that the presence of excess levels of one mineral/metal could lead to depletion of the level of another mineral/metal! (Tartrazine, now banned due to its association with hyperactivity in children, is believed to bind Zinc!).

- [34-37] The use of Omega-3 fatty acids are associated with improved concentration and reduced levels of aggression however, it is generally accepted that the results do not appear to be long-lasting i.e. that upon termination of a course of supplementation there is a reversal of the condition - the improvements are not sustained.

- The use of probiotics to treat deficiencies in gut flora [38]

- Depression is often linked to Vitamin B12 deficiency [39]

Nutritional supplementation addresses the nutritional deficit(s) which result from illness but they address only the SYMPTOMS of illness and do not address the fundamental CAUSE which has been responsible for its development.

# Why did the symptom occur?

## *What was it that led to the development of the symptoms?*

The medical system is largely based on the reductionist approach, based upon the study of pathophysiology, which has dominated the medical agenda for past decades. There are researchers who recognise that the reductionist approach has fundamental limitations and that the body functions in complex manner which cannot be addressed by the simplistic reductionist approach. As a result this has led to the growth of various multi-disciplinary approaches which involve the study of psychology with other medical disciplines e.g. psychology with neurology and/or with immunology, endocrinology, oncology, mathematics, etc. Many now recognise that the brain regulates our physiology and that the brain and body operates as a hugely complex multifunctional biofeedback system.

Perhaps this is already recognised to some extent within the pharmaceutical industry through their research into the role of the genes and of their interest in pharmaco-genetics yet the limitations of this approach appear glaringly evident. Consider the comments of acknowledged world-leading researchers such as Dr J.Craig Venter [117].

**"In everyday language the talk is about a gene for this and a gene for that. We are now finding that that is rarely so. The number of genes that work in that way can almost be counted on your fingers, because we are just not hard-wired in that way."**

**"You cannot define the function of genes without defining the influence of the environment. The notion that one gene equals one disease, or that one gene produces one key protein, is flying out of the window."**

Of the estimated 35,000 genes in the human genome, it is estimated that circa half to three-quarters of these go into the brain's makeup yet it is difficult to develop drugs which pass the blood-brain barrier. It appears unlikely therefore that many drugs will be able to treat illnesses which are related to the brain's biochemistry.

In recognition of this, some drug companies are now developing drugs which stimulate the body's immune system [40] thereby focusing upon the mechanisms which induce wellness instead of the conventional mechanisms which reduce the progress of pathology. This ignores (1) the effect of drugs upon the body's physiological stability and hence of their influence upon the levels of proteins and other immunochemicals (2) that drugs alter the brain waves perhaps to the extent that the changes are contrary to the patient's health.

The work of Psychologists, Neurologists and Neurobiologists exists at the frontier between psychology and health [41]. The issue becomes that of which brain waves to use i.e. those which are involved in the regulation and function of our behaviour or those which are involved in the management and regulation of our health.

The relationship of psychology to health is certainly not in dispute.

## How does our Behavioural Disposition Change as we Grow Older?

### *Further discussion of how behaviour changes with age*

There is not a 'Theory of Developmental Psychology' which meets all viewpoints. There are however many theories, each with a different emphasis, which describe the age-related changes which occur in our lives e.g.

- Baltes' life-span approach [42] hypothesized that development is not completed at adolescence but is continuous and extends across the entire life, and that each age period (childhood, adolescence, maturity, and old age) has its own developmental tasks.

- Gould [43] hypothesized that the age range 17-22 yrs is important to forge identity, 22-28 yrs attain goals, 28-34 yrs question life, 35-43 yrs create stability

- Levinson [44] hypothesized that the age range 17-22 years is important for the transition to independence; 22-28 years, to establish adult roles; 28-33 years, to reflect and make new choices; 33-40 years to consolidate career & family goals

- Piaget [45] hypothesized that there are specific age-related changes in a child's development which occurred at ages 2 years, 7 years and 11 years which affected their ability to process data and make logical decisions

- Jung's [46] observations and conclusions (listed below) appear more objective and developed than Freud's more esoteric conclusions. He considered a number of issues which appear more typical of the brain wave states.

  1. the **'ego'** is explained as the wakened or behavioural state – indicative of the beta state

  2. the **'personal unconscious'** as that which is not presently conscious although it could be – indicative of the alpha state

  3. the **'collective unconscious'** – indicative of the theta state

  4. 'the **shadow'**: the difference between good and evil and that they are a part of an archetype which derives from our prehistoric origins, when we were pre-occupied with survival and reproduction, and when we weren't self-conscious.

  5. the **'principle of entropy'** in which all existence is finite.

- Jung suggests that we have four functions which enable us to deal with the world: sensing, thinking, intuition and feeling.

Researchers have reflected upon the changes which appear to affect our ability to make decisions during our lives e.g. (1) how during the transition from adolescence into adulthood the person apparently forms a dream, mentor relationships, occupation, marriage and family, which leads to identity & intimacy; or (2) how during the transition from adolescence to maturity the person readjusts the young-old balance, the destruction-creation balance, the masculine-feminine balance, the attachment-separateness balance, which leads to clarified values.

Grakov's work has essential similarities to the work of researchers such as Jung and Baltes. He identified that the body has four significant physiological stages which occur in childhood (until 15 years), adolescence (from 15-30 years), adulthood (from 30-50 years) and maturity (over 50 years); and that each of these stages corresponds with distinct changes to our physiology and hence affects the way which we receive and process data. There is a remarkable line of logic and reason to these observations.

Evidence for these conclusions:

- in childhood our lives are dominated by the need to learn how to conduct our lives in order to survive;

- in adolescence we learn how to attract a mate;

- during the period of adulthood we learn how to cope with the huge number of competing influences when raising a family;

- during the period of maturity we use our experiences of life to make decisions and perhaps to compensate for our declining physical capabilities.

Furthermore Grakov has identified the significance of the brain waves and how they are involved in the processes which regulate our health, growth, function, behaviour i.e. the ways in which we process data and act.

The different brain waves [139] play a key role coordinating the complex functions of our mental and physiological processes.

Most psychology is essentially subjective and based upon simplistic models which associate identified behavioural traits with past experiences. Grakov has developed a mathematical model which compensates for the effect of age and hence defines the psychological, psychoemotional, and health profiles of the person. This sophisticated model considers how a person's neurological development – influenced by their medical condition - reflects their ability to perceive, imagine, memorise, process data, make decisions and act.

# Is it Right to Trust Purely Biomedical Conclusions?

*Consider the wider psychosomatic influences which affect our health.*

Could we determine how a computer works if we knew the detail of the components and circuitry? The answer is, of course, a resounding NO. We have to understand the software in order to make it work. The same is true of the human physiology. The software is the regulatory mechanism which we recognise as the homeostatic and allostatic mechanisms which regulate the physiological systems which control our health.

In any other major industry the complexity of the problem would have led to the introduction of mathematical modelling in order to make sense of the apparent chaos and disorder. There are many cases where this has been used to process the huge amounts of data e.g. which has been generated by advanced diagnostic technologies, into an intelligible format. Mathematical modelling is also being used in research to predict cell function [50]. These examples illustrate its steady progress into biomedical research.

Biochemistry is based upon the fundamental assumption or misassumption that we can determine the extent of an ailment by measuring one biochemical component yet there is a number of medical conditions which clearly do not correspond to this simplistic assumption. For example there are up to 16 different tests for diabetes, if not more, yet none appears to be a truly reliable indicator of this medical condition. For each of us the levels of the biomarker may differ. In some cases the levels may be comparable and within the considered biomedical limits but in others the levels may be significantly different. Perhaps at a level which could cause concern but which would not (yet) be affecting the person's health.

There are a wide range of medical conditions which have a number of contributory causes therefore the diagnosis and treatment of the condition must take into account the complex nature of the condition and the complex nature of the human physiology - yet if you cannot understand the cause of an ailment how can you do something about it?

The medical community appears not to have agreement on some of the basic issues e.g.

(1) in Germany medications to improve blood circulation (aspirin and ginkgo biloba) are two of the three largest selling medications; yet in the UK, and presumably the same applies in the US and other territories, high blood pressure is considered to be the greatest evil.

(2) 'statins' are used to lower blood cholesterol in order to reduce stroke yet there is no conclusive evidence that the lowering of blood ldl-cholesterol reduces the incidence of stroke. Furthermore low levels of ldl cholesterol are now associated with increasing prevalence of Parkinsonism [51]

111

# A Summary of Current Research

*The study of cognition is being taken seriously and research projects are underway at universities and world-leading health institutes.*

Since before the turn of the last century the most eminent computational neuroscientists have focussed upon elucidating the computational architecture of the brain. The ability to use the most modern techniques of neuroscience, computing and mathematics has for many years been envisaged by computational neuroscientists [54,55]. Much of this work appears focussed upon the development of systems, devices, technologies and machines which act more and more like humans rather than on systems which have a role in medical diagnosis or which have a therapeutic application.

When considering that this approach could have a human application in medical diagnosis and therapy [56,57] it has been considered that the brain could function in the manner of a data processing matrix and/or which use computational principles and algorithms to process the information of the autonomic nervous system [162].

To note how current research is progressing consider the following:

- Major software companies [52, 176] recognise the significance of cognition and are pouring millions of dollars into Psychology research

  *'Continuously recruiting world-class researchers from a diversity of backgrounds - psychologists and sociologists to anthropologists and mathematicians - to find answers to computer science's grand challenges'.*

- There are projects underway in most psychology departments of the leading universities [47, 48] which focus upon the relationship of cognition to mental and physical health e.g.

  *'....developing, testing and applying new approaches and algorithms for modeling from numeric, symbolic and pictorial data. ........ collaborates with psychologists, physicians, biologists, physicists and chemists. A notable aspect of much of this research is its application to problems in image analysis, medical diagnosis, ecological modeling, alternative medicine, ........'*

- Computational Neuroscience [49] projects are attempting to elucidate the neural structures and to understand more about the brain's synchronisation, processing speed, timing, robustness, modular construction, learning in context, information representation, information transmission, etc

- the US government has decreed that the 21st century should be known as the 'Century of Brain' and that research should have an emphasis upon brain function. Creation of the virtual physiological human is a part of this research.

112

- Research programmes under the European Union FP7-Health & ICT programmes include research into the significance of the body's physiological systems (Health-2007.2.2.2-2) and virtual physiological human (ICT-2007.5.3)

- A company [179] has been established to adopt astrological techniques to determine the emission of coloured biophotons from protein-substrate reactions. This uses fluorescence detector technology, based on a cryogenic super-conducting tunnel junction (STJ or Josephson Junction) device. This is able to detect the arrival of a biophoton and its colour. Used to capture light from distant galaxies, this is being modified for use as an instrument to replace conventional biochemical assays.

An illustration of the scope of current research, and hence of the recognition of the significance of brain function and cognition, can be understood by reading typical curriculum vitae of leading researchers e.g.

*'investigating the development and application of realistic models for the analysis and understanding of brain function, and, combining mathematical and computational tools with neurophysiological, neuroanatomical, or neurochemical techniques in order to decipher the mechanisms which underlie specific neuronal and behavioral systems'.*

This program also supports research projects focusing on understanding the computations made by nerve cells and groups of nerve cells in orchestrating behaviour.

Researchers are now considering how the neuronal processes are linked to cognitive capabilities. Consequently the most eminent of researchers are now aware of the need to consider the systems which regulate function at the cellular and molecular levels and of the need to consider how the brain's processing is synchronized [177, 178]. Further research is now considering the computational modeling of physiological systems [58,59] and of algorithmic models for physiological systems [78]. Nevertheless in their attempts to relate cognition to medical diagnosis researchers [56,57] are inhibited by the lack of a structured theoretical concept [163] that enables them to develop their understanding of information processing and brain function.

Further insights into the principles come from researchers studying the use of mathematical matrices to model how we perceive and memorise colour, and of the effect of age and weight upon colour perception [60]. According to Olafur Eliasson [61], an artist who caught the public's imagination with his 2003 exhibition at the Tate, 'The Weather Project', which specialised in working with colour *'people experience colour differently. Colour involves memory, perception and recognition. It is influenced by our emotions, sex and experience, even politics and ethics. Colours are like markers in our emotional histories. Certain hues can act as Proustian triggers, detonating lost moments from the past'.*

Grakov's work, already at a fully commercialized level, indicates that such concepts are very real and that they were established in 1985. Moreover it illustrates how far in advance is Grakov's research by comparison with current research.

113

# Virtual Scanning

**Virtual Scanning** demonstrates how complex mathematics and mathematical modelling can be used to determine a person's psycho-emotional profile, psychological profile and their health profile

Virtual Scanning sets the standard for this new generation of technologies. It demonstrates the need for a **paradigm shift** in medical thinking and emphasises the need to progress away from the diagnosis and treatment of symptoms to the diagnosis and stimulation of the processes which are responsible for the maintenance of our health and stability. It demonstrates the need to stimulate the natural processes which regulate our health i.e. of compensation and repair, rather than suppressing the processes of pathology.

Whereas research into the virtual physiological human is based upon the biochemical model for each organ Dr Grakov has understood how the brain regulates system, organ and cell function.

The therapy uses a form of audiovisual stimulation [150], [151], (or flashing light therapy) to treat the precise psychological or physiological condition. It focuses solely upon the deltawave frequency of 1-4 hz – the frequencies which regulate the body's physiological systems - and is remote from frequencies (6-8hz) which are associated with photo-sensitive migraine or epilepsy.

# The need to understand the implications of change in our Society

*Any new technology will be embraced by those
who want change and challenged by those who do not. Evolutionary change
allows us to consider the issues and to adapt whilst revolutionary change
creates uncertainty because of its potentially disruptive effects.*

Consider how new theories have been introduced in the past e.g. it was considered that the world was flat or how people scoffed at the Wright brothers experimentation with flight. Einstein's theory of relativity has stood the test of time for almost one hundred years although this theory may need to be modified to explain phenomena which does not conform to Einstein's model. If Einstein's theories are not sacrosanct why should any other theories be beyond reproach - especially those that are unsatisfactory and which have unsatisfactory levels of success?

'Claude Bernard' considered by many to be the father of pathophysiology, explains what makes a good or bad scientific theory:  *"Theories are only verified hypotheses, verified by more or less numerous facts. Those verified by the most facts are the best, but even then they are never final, never to be absolutely believed."* It takes just one inconsistent or contradictory observation to discredit a theory.

This is the progressive approach which has enabled civilization to develop, to develop and debate new theories, and to introduce the new technologies which have been of benefit to mankind. To explain as much as possible and then to allow the evolution of the theory taking into account new technologies, new theories, and factors which cannot be explained by the prevailing viewpoint.

Despite this medical theories which have inherent limitations are allowed to prosper e.g. the theory which links cholesterol to obesity and heart disease which is dismissed in the reference article 53. The author expertly dispels the link between low levels of cholesterol and heart disease and illustrates that cholesterol is in fact heart protective. Moreover she illustrates how low levels of cholesterol - cholesterol is the body's raw material for production of the neurotransmitter acetylcholine which is required for memory function - are clearly related to cognitive-decline in the aged e.g. in Parkinsonism.

The challenge therefore is to overcome the entrenched scepticism of the medical community and of those who, through their advancing years and experiences, have become less open-minded and hence are increasingly resistant to change.  They have the responsibility to marry their experience with the changes affecting western society arising from the revolution which has been created by the computer and internet 62.

Perhaps Virtual Scanning is too revolutionary. It is certainly required by politicians who seek to reduce the cost of providing healthcare and it is certainly required by those who seek to address the limitations of conventional healthcare.

# The Limitations of Biomedicine

*If all of the claims for biomedicine were true we would have eradicated illness from the surface of our planet yet the burden of illness increases every year.*

The prevailing biomedical viewpoint considers that inhibition of the pathological processes associated with an illness or ailment can eradicate the medical problem. This predominantly reductionist approach has fundamental limitations for a number of reasons including:

- it does not deal with the factors which were responsible for the development of the condition.
- the occurrence of Drug side-effects

- the re-occurrence of symptoms

- that 90% of drugs are ineffective in 50% of the population [75]

- it ignores the differing biological characteristics of demographic groups including age and the differing genetic characteristics [73]
- the clinical trials, upon which effectiveness is determined, are subjective

The implications are, using medical industry statistics, that e.g.

- 30% of medical conditions are of an undiagnosable nature [63]

- a GP's misdiagnosis can range from 20-80% (depending upon the medical journal selected and the remit of the review article) [64]
- various accepted and long-established diagnostic procedures have inherent limitations and that these limitations overlooked in the process of diagnosis.
- an estimated 21% of drug prescriptions are for use where the drug is not authorized [65]
- there are significant number of 'incidents' in the health services which damage the future quality of life of the patient [66]
- the cost of dealing with misdiagnosis and adverse effects of therapies is a significant factor in the cost of running our medical services

The seriousness of the adverse effects summarized above can be illustrated by reference to UK government figures published in July 2006 [66] which highlight that there are 974,000 recorded accidents by GPs and hospitals and 250,000 serious adverse drug reactions each year.

Prof David Webb, Professor of Therapeutics and Pharmacology at the University of Edinburgh [67] commented: "*It's an alarming situation that is worrying medical students, who have privately expressed their concerns about their lack of prescribing knowledge*". He is also reported to have commented: "*Patients are becoming ill and some are dying as a result of poor prescribing. There is no doubt about that. A substantial proportion of that is undoubtedly avoidable,*"

Biomedicine adopts a simplistic approach to diagnosis and treatment. It fails to consider that our physiology is a highly complex system and that the simplistic association of one biochemical with another is insufficient to elucidate the mechanisms which are responsible for illness. It assumes that the extent of an illness can be measured by determining the level of a biomarker. This is a fundamental mis-assumption. It is not the level of the biomarker which is important – it is the rate of reaction which is significant.

(reaction conditions)

Biomarker + substrate ⟶ products + light (colour/intensity)

The conventional approach ignores that the levels of the biomarker are not precise but instead vary across a range thereby demonstrating that maintenance of the body's stability is a relative function and that the body is a dynamic system. It also ignores that often the levels of the biomarker can be outside the normative range and yet the person may be healthy. The use of biomarkers enables us only to have a crude assessment of the degree of progression of an illness and/or the extent of the symptoms. There is therefore considerable scope for inaccuracy in such measurements. The rate of reaction (and hence the processes of health and illness) are relatively stable and can be monitored by measuring the light-emitted by protein/biomarker-substrate reactions. The colour being unique for each reaction and the intensity being proportional to its concentration.

To further complicate matters the mechanisms of c40-70% of drugs [68-71] are based upon our limited understanding of the function of G-protein coupled receptors (GPCRs) which are intimately involved with our sensory processing [25] and which are considered to be fundamental receptors in the processes of sensory perception. This illustrates that biochemicals involved in our sensory processing may also be simultaneously involved in organ function.

This approach ignores the possibility that complex systems could apply to the regulation of our physiology, that a hierarchical system could apply and that this could regulate our physiology. In addition this viewpoint ignores the effect of factors such as age and weight which have a fundamental effect upon our health.

The process of diagnosing the symptoms of illness and prescribing a drug to alleviate the symptoms fails to identify which reason actually caused the development of the symptom. If we do not understand the fundamental cause of a problem treating the symptom with a drug will not address the fundamental issue i.e. that the cause for the condition remains untouched. In such cases the symptoms could reoccur - which is often the case.

Our biochemistry and our sensory perception, health and behaviour, wellbeing and mental outlook, are inextricably inter-related and inter-dependent (fig 5)

## Figure 5

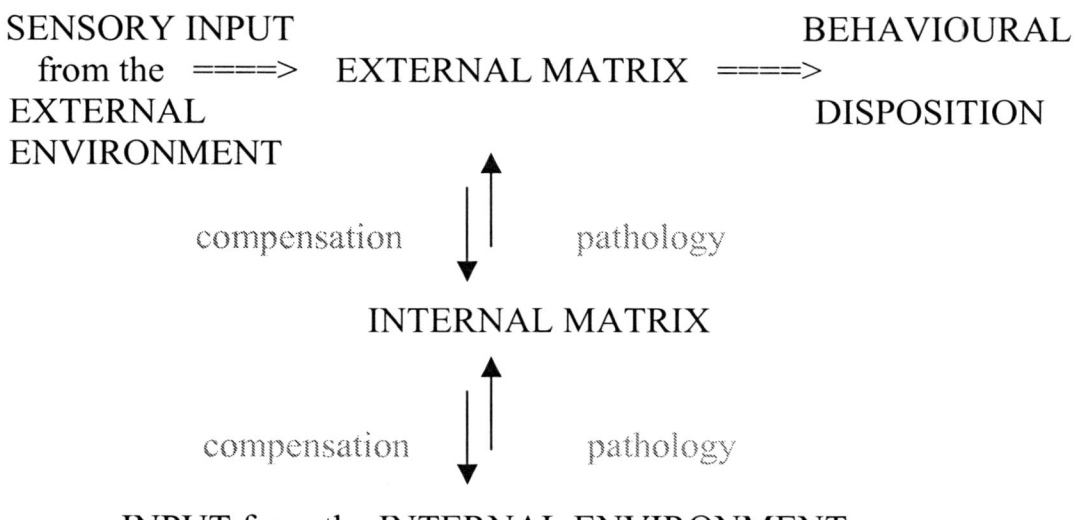

SENSORY INPUT from the EXTERNAL ENVIRONMENT ====> EXTERNAL MATRIX ====> BEHAVIOURAL DISPOSITION

compensation / pathology

INTERNAL MATRIX

compensation / pathology

INPUT from the INTERNAL ENVIRONMENT

There are a number of psycho-medical disciplines such as neurobiology, psychoneuroimmunology, psychoneuroimmunoendocrinology, computational neuroscience, neuro-oncology, etc; which recognise the inter-relatedness of the differing disciplines. There can be significant benefits to be gained by considering the relationship of our biochemistry with our psychology, cognition, visual perception, and brain waves.

Psychologists recognise the on-going progress of neuroscience [72] yet the significance of a number of key issues appears not to have been fully considered e.g.

- that our sensory perception and behaviour are completely unique to each individual and that we function in a 'relative' manner [73]. By contrast the reductionist approach considers that we function in an 'absolute' manner.

- although MRI scans record the regions of the cerebrum which are associated with specific events, memories, actions, etc; by contrast people with damage or partial removal of these regions of the brain can retain these memories.

- the discovery of mirror neurons casts doubts on claims that individual regions of the brain are solely responsible for memory, actions, etc; but instead is indicative of a more complex mechanism of sensory processing and memory involving more than one region of the brain and perhaps also of the body.

Our sensory perception will be affected if the blood flow to our skin, our eyes, our ears, our nose, tongue and throat is affected and this will also be the case if the cell content of our blood varies, perhaps when our immune system is low, and if our blood pressure is affected. Memory and concentration are affected by stress as a result of impaired blood flow to the brain so the function of our neural processes is affected by our physiological systems.

Consider:

- Stress is experienced by the senses – of which vision is our dominant sense.

- It affects the autonomic nervous system which depresses the immune system and initiates a wide range of effects such as the restriction of blood vessels which affects the flow of blood to the spinal chord and the brain.

- This affects the flow of oxygen and blood glucose which affects our memory, concentration, ability to react, etc.

- This affects the function of our senses including our vision, hearing, smell, taste and touch which can be detected as deficiencies to our visual, vocal, taste and audiological spectra.

- Our interpretation of language is considered to be a relative function (as assessed in psychometric analyses). This is unique to each person and their personal experiences.

- Our sensory perception and cognition is affected by illness. This affects our ability to function, visual perception, hearing, taste, speech, receptiveness to touch, etc.

The use of drugs is clearly associated with changes to our sensory perception which is often noted only as a side-effect which is reported in clinical studies and patient notes. Viagra for example works by inhibiting the function of the enzyme PDE6. This has a significant effect upon our perception of colour (making our vision a blue-green until the effect of the drug declines) because it is involved in the process of transduction in the retina. In fact most drugs are known to affect our sensory perception and behaviour to some extent. Researchers Berezin & Martinek [74] illustrated how the activity of enzymes can be stimulated or suppressed by the action of light and colour.

As drug-protein interactions release light of different colours, depending upon the precise nature of the drug and protein, it becomes clear that the rate of reaction between protein and substrate has an effect upon our sensory perception and vice-versa.

Drugs are c50% effective [75] thereby illustrating the fundamental limitations of the biomedical theory of illness which considers that stress exacerbates illness whereas stress in its various guises is actually the fundamental cause of illness [76]. This would appear to leave c50% of patients to the psychologist, to study the ailments which are considered to have a psychosomatic basis, or to the complementary therapist.

# Complementary Health

*We have seen how our sensory perception is related to our biochemistry. Is this able to cast light upon the mechanisms associated with the various complementary health approaches?*

Irrespective of the proliferation of studies and reports which attempt to denigrate the role of the complementary health therapist there is indisputably a substantial body of data which recognises the **positive beneficial effect of the sensory-based approaches** which involve light, sound, smell, touch and positive thought.

**LIGHT** is one of the most undervalued therapeutic agents and is recognised to have a positive therapeutic effect in the treatment of over 100 medical ailments [77]

**SPEECH,** including our vocal capabilities, are known to be affected by our health.

**HEARING,** including not just our ability to hear a particular frequency but our ability to discern the spoken word is known to be affected by our health

**TOUCH,** and in particular massage certainly has the ability to relax, and of course the touch of a loving partner can do wonders for your feelings of wellbeing

**SMELL,** through the power of aromatherapy, perfumes, oils and spices are certainly able to inflame feelings related to passion, appetite, relaxation, vigour, etc.

**POSITIVE THOUGHT, through meditation, yoga, cranial osteopathy and the positive effects of the PLACEBO effect** clearly support the contention that the body has a healing mechanism which is not directly dependent upon our biochemistry.

Sceptics in the medical community focus upon the apparently unscientific basis of complementary health techniques and of the apparent unreliability of the technologies which are used by practitioners of variable knowledge and experience.

The challenge is therefore to prove the scientific principles upon which complementary health and the sensory functions are based and hence to improve the specificity and reliability of these techniques.

## How can we Explain the Relationship between Cognition and Health?

*We have illustrated how our cognition is related to our health in the most subjective terms. Now consider the factors which are involved.*

The brain waves are perhaps the most undervalued components in our physiology because biomedical researchers have not yet discerned their function, yet the most eminent of medical researchers now recognise the limitations of the molecular and cellular basis of biomedicine and of the need to consider approaches which take into account e.g.

- the physiological SYSTEMS of the body [78,84];

- the need to relate cellular and molecular processes to the cognitive processes [24]; (3) the need to consider the 'software' of the brain and of the brain's function in terms of flow of data rather than the biological 'wetware' [55];

- the need to consider the function of the brain waves [139]

- the need to relate the physiology of our organs to the function of our brain;

- the need to understand what makes our physiology work [54, 79]

- the need to understand how our brain affects the function of the body and vice versa.

The only logical explanation which fits the facts is that it is 'the levels' of biochemicals and proteins in our physiology which affect our health and cognition, sensory perception, behaviour, emotions and wellbeing.

We know that our brain waves are involved with our health because the beta and alpha waves function when we are awake whereas the delta and theta waves function 24 hours per day therefore the delta and theta waves perform a function which is related to our health and physical preparedness whereas the beta and alpha waves are involved in our physical function, thought and behaviour. (Fig 6)

**Figure 6**

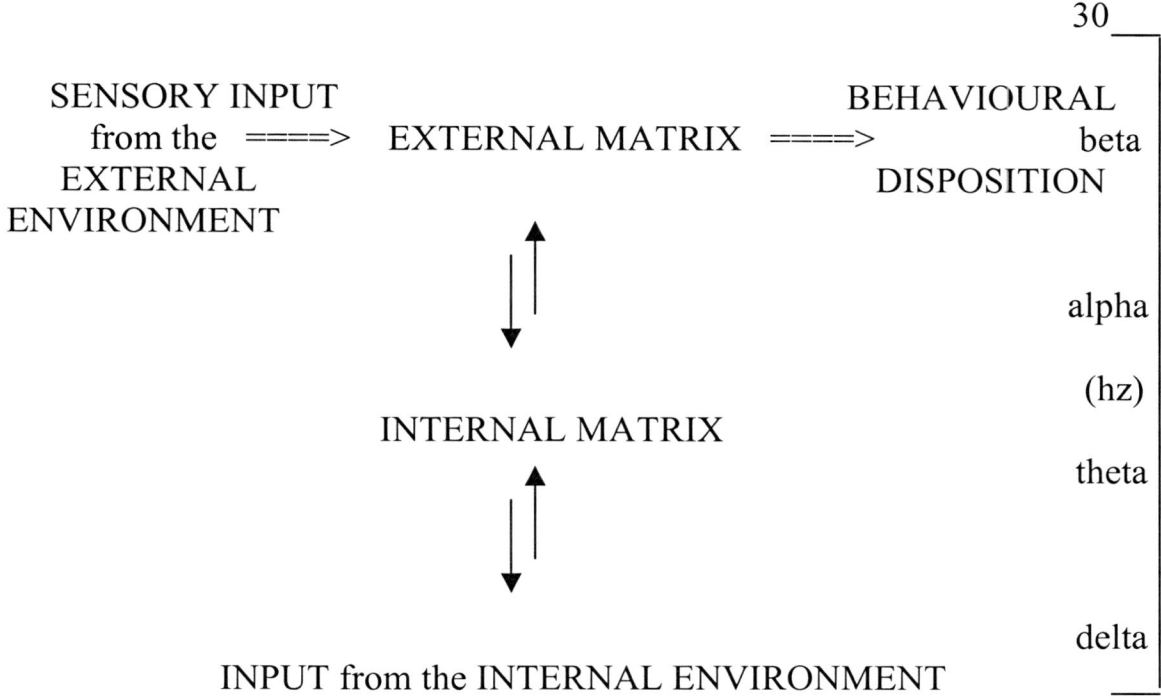

It is logical to consider that the human physiology functions through a hierarchical structure and that there are regulatory systems which monitor and regulate the function of the brain, the physiological systems and the organs.

That people being treated for one ailment report that another, apparently unrelated ailment, has healed  - such effects are known as **photomodulation** - illustrates that the body functions in a complex manner which affects physiological systems and that these systems operate in an inter-related manner.

For example

- a lady treated for leg ulceration reported that the eczema which had affected her arms, elbows and legs, had improved.

- an 11 yo girlbeing treated for dyslexia reported that her eczema which had effected her for many years had cleared.

The challenge is to provide evidence for these physiological systems.

Moreover there is little doubt that all aspects of our physiology are connected through the Autonomic Nervous System to the brain which regulates our health i.e. that the human physiology is a complex biofeedback system.

Consider how blood transfusions and organ transplants bring changes to our mental character [80-83], personality and health. The only plausible explanation is that our behaviour, emotions, personality i.e. our psychology; is the result of the complex interaction and feedback between our bodily organs, and brain. This includes the cumulative effect of stresses encountered during our lives and their effect on brain and organs.

# If Physiological Systems Exist What Do They Control?

*Instead of considering how our biochemistry has changed consider how the physiological systems which regulate our health have been affected by stress thereby affecting our biochemical stability.*

The physiological systems control the obvious e.g. digestion – to regulate the passage of our food and its interaction with the components of our digestive system. The same would apply to our excretive system, breathing, blood glucose, sleeping pattern, blood pressure, temperature – in fact all of the obvious factors which we recognise are involved with our function (see table 1 & 2). For each of these systems we can recognise the existence of deviations from normal operation i.e. at the hyper level or the hypo level – when it functions above or below the normal levels. The same applies to each organ where we can recognise e.g. too high or too low levels of thyroid function, of blood cell content , of minerals in the blood, of organ function, etc (see table 3).

The existence of the body's physiological systems is not in doubt and is recognised in every medical textbook [84]. What is in doubt is the precise nature of the body's physiological systems.

Each of the body's physiological systems is regulated by the brain's delta waves which in turn regulate the function of our organ and of the levels of biochemicals which are produced by each organ. The destabilising effect can clearly be demonstrated by noting how a pharmacologically active drug substance can be used to raise or lower the brain waves. The problem for our physiology is when long-term exposure - to effects which change our biochemistry - have a long-term effect upon our body's stability i.e. that the process changes from homeostasis (management of stability) to allostasis (management of instability) and of the subsequent effect upon the long-term memory which is involved in the process of regulating our health and hence of our behaviour.

If systems were to regulate our functional systems and the related organs we would not witness the occurence of side-effects - and this is the case with the sensory-based therapies. If our health improves naturally, perhaps as a result of having a holiday, we get well without side-effects.

By stimulating the brain using precisely selected delta waves it is possible to ensures co-ordinated or synchronised function of each of the organs in each system. This is analogous to the way that the engine timing in a vehicle regulates the efficiency of the combustion.

Such conclusions do not contravene any biochemical research but instead explains how our physiology changes under the effect of stress and how these changes are subsequently manifest as changes to our biochemistry i.e. as pathology, and hence as the symptoms of illness.

124

Each system comprises a structure in which the brain is connected via the autonomic nervous system to each of the listed organs…….. see figure 7.

- optimal cell content of blood

- optimal volume of circulating blood

- optimal pH level

- optimal Level of Osmotic Pressure in the Body

- optimal quantity of glucose in blood

- optimal level of blood pressure

- optimal breathing levels

- optimal digestion levels

- optimal body temperature

- optimal extraction level

- optimal sexual functions

- optimal position of body in the environment

- optimal sleeping pattern

- optimal locomotion, communication, etc.

# Examples of the structure of the physiological systems

## 1.    That which sustains optimal cell content of blood

Organs and Functional Systems monitored:
Brain                          Pituitary gland            Thyroid Gland
Adrenal Glands                 Blood and Peripheral blood vessels
Spleen                         Skeletal & Muscular system

## 2.    That which provides optimal volume of circulating blood

Organs and Functional Systems monitored:
Brain                          Pituitary gland            Thyroid Gland
Adrenal Glands                 Heart
Blood and Peripheral Blood Vessels                        Kidneys

## 3.    That which sustains optimal pH level

Organs and Functional Systems monitored:
Brain                          Pituitary gland            Thyroid Gland
Adrenal Glands                 Liver                      Pancreas
Blood and Peripheral Blood Vessels                        Lungs and Bronchi
Skin                           Stomach                    Duodenum
Small Intestine                Large Intestine            Kidneys

## 4.    That which Determines the Optimal Level of Osmotic Pressure in the Body

Organs and Functional Systems monitored:
Brain                          Pituitary gland            Thyroid Gland
Adrenal Glands                 Blood and Peripheral Blood Vessels
Spleen                         Lungs and Bronchi          Skin
Oesophagus                     Stomach                    Duodenum
Small Intestine                Large Intestine            Kidneys

## 5.    That which sustains optimal quantity of glucose in blood

Organs and Functional Systems monitored:
Brain                          Pituitary gland            Thyroid Gland
Adrenal Glands                 Liver                      Pancreas
Blood and peripheral blood vessels  Small Intestine       Kidneys

## 6.    That which sustains optimal level of blood pressure

Organs and Functional Systems monitored:
Brain                          Pituitary gland            Thyroid Gland
Adrenal Glands                 Liver                      Heart
Blood and Peripheral Blood Vessels                        Spleen

## 7.    That which sustains optimal breathing levels

Organs and Functional Systems monitored:
Brain                          Pituitary Gland            Thyroid Gland
Adrenal Glands                 Nose                       Lungs and Bronchi
Heart                          Blood and Peripheral Blood Vessels
Skin                           Small Intestine            Kidneys

## 8.    That which sustains optimal digestion levels

Organs and Functional Systems monitored:

| | | |
|---|---|---|
| Brain | Pituitary Gland | Thyroid Gland |
| Adrenal Glands | Liver | Gall Bladder |
| Pancreas | Blood and Peripheral Blood Vessels | |
| Oesophagus | Stomach | Duodenum |
| Small Intestine | Large Intestine | |

## 9.    That which sustains optimal body temperature

Organs and Functional Systems monitored:

| | | |
|---|---|---|
| Brain | Pituitary Gland | Thyroid Gland |
| Adrenal Glands | Blood and Peripheral Blood Vessels | |
| Lungs and Bronchi | Skin | Kidneys |

## 10.    That which sustains optimal extraction level

Organs and Functional Systems monitored:

| | | |
|---|---|---|
| Brain | Pituitary Gland | Thyroid Gland |
| Adrenal Glands | Blood and Peripheral Blood Vessels | |
| Peripheral Nervous System | Kidneys | Urinary Bladder |
| Skin | Lungs and Bronchi | Small Intestine |

## 11.    That which sustains optimal sexual functions

Organs and Functional Systems monitored:

| | | |
|---|---|---|
| Brain | Pituitary Gland | Thyroid Gland |
| Adrenal Glands | Blood and Peripheral Blood Vessels | |
| Ovaries | Testicles | Womb and Appendages |
| Prostate Gland | Penis | Mammary Glands |

## 12.    That which sustains optimal position of body in the environment

Organs and Functional Systems monitored:

| | | |
|---|---|---|
| Brain | Spinal Cord | Peripheral Nervous System |
| Pituitary Gland | Thyroid Gland | Adrenal Glands |
| Blood and Peripheral Blood Vessels | | Skeletal and Muscular System |

## 13.    That which sustains optimal sleeping pattern

Organs and Functional Systems monitored:

| | | |
|---|---|---|
| Brain | Pituitary Gland | Spinal Chord |
| Peripheral Nervous System | Ear and Nose | |

## 14.    That which sustains optimal locomotion, communication, etc.

By comparison the conventional approach considers that the body is regulated by a series of physiological systems comprising:

- **Endocrine system**: comprising pituitary, thyroid, adrenal and ovaries/testes.

- **Cardiovascular system**: comprising heart, blood vessels and blood

- **Respiratory system**: comprising nose, mouth, pharynx, trachea, diaphragm, abdominal muscles and lungs

- **Digestive system**: comprising oral cavity, oesophagus, gall bladder, liver, stomach, duodenum, pancreas, small intestine, large intestine,

- **Renal system**: comprising kidneys, ureters, urinary bladder and urethra

- **Reproductive system**: comprising ovaries, testicles, uterus, penis, prostate

- **Immune system**: which can be affected by disease – caused by genetic defects, hormonal imbalances, nutritional deficiencies,

- **Central Nervous System:**

- **Sensory System:**

This illustrates how the conventional explanation is far too simplistic. For example

- brain function affects the regulation of all physiological systems.

- most physiological systems are dependent upon the quality, quantity and pressure of blood.

- the digestive system is dependent upon the cell content, quantity and pressure of blood, blood type

- the function of our biochemistry is dependent upon the fine regulation of temperature and pH

Unsurprisingly the physiological structures proposed by Grakov and used in the development of Virtual Scanning appear to have far greater sophistication and underlying logic than the approach favoured by conventional medical research.

**Figure 7:**

## Typical illustration of a functional system comprising the inter-relationship of the digestive system

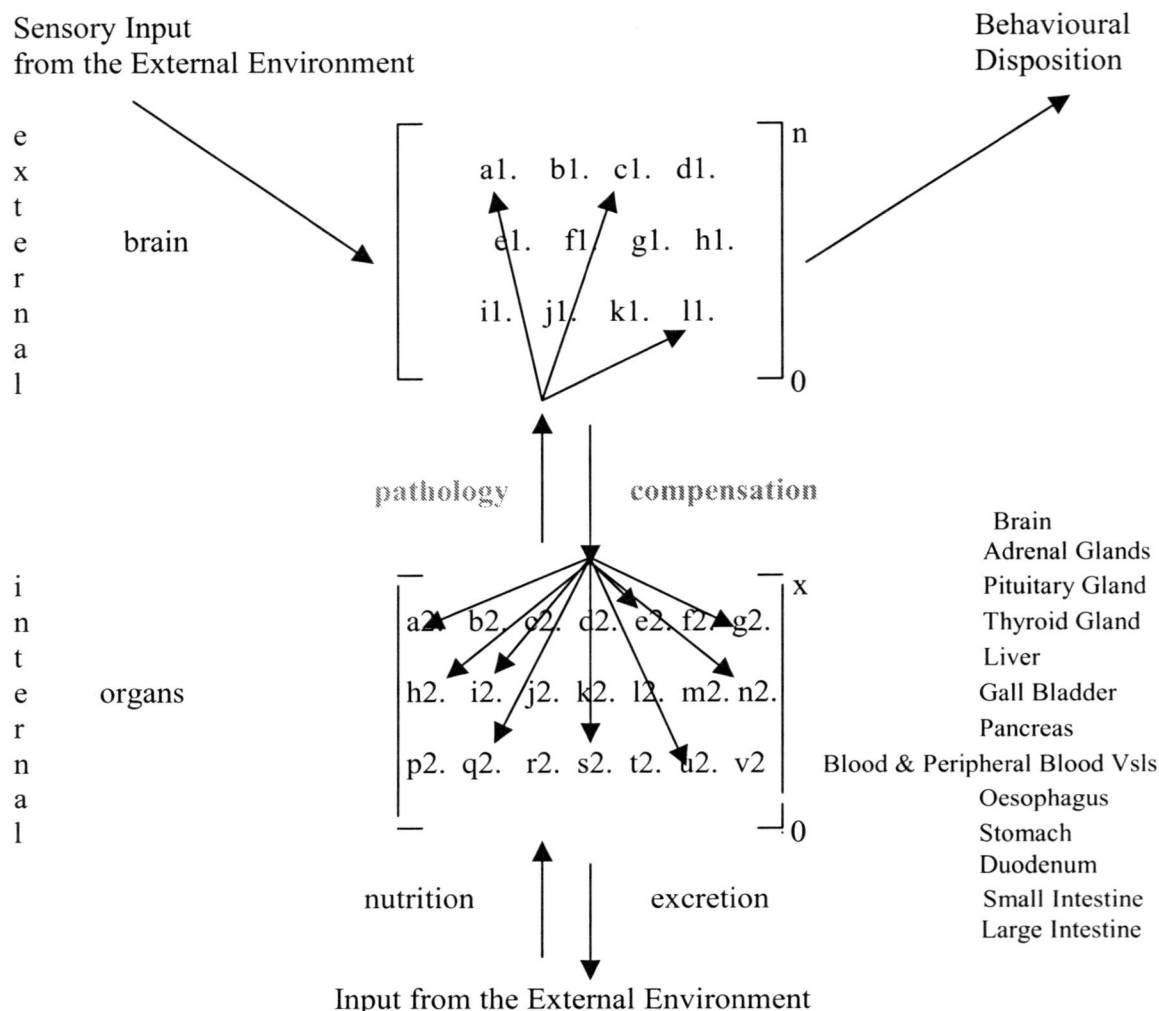

Long-term disturbances to our regulatory function result in stable pathology which is associated with the destabilized functional system. Problems with the biochemistry of one organ affect the brain waves and hence function of other related physiological systems and organs. This explains the phenomena known as photomodulation e.g. whereby a person with a heart problem could have a leg ulcer which refuses to heal.

Using this approach we can explain the function of almost all therapies including meditation, hypnosis, yoga, and ayurveda; behavioural therapies including sport; the sensory-based therapies including music and sound therapy, aromatherapy; of systems which work on the body's meridians e.g. acupuncture; and of herbal remedies, nutrition, and many drugs/medications (see fig 8)

**Figure 8**

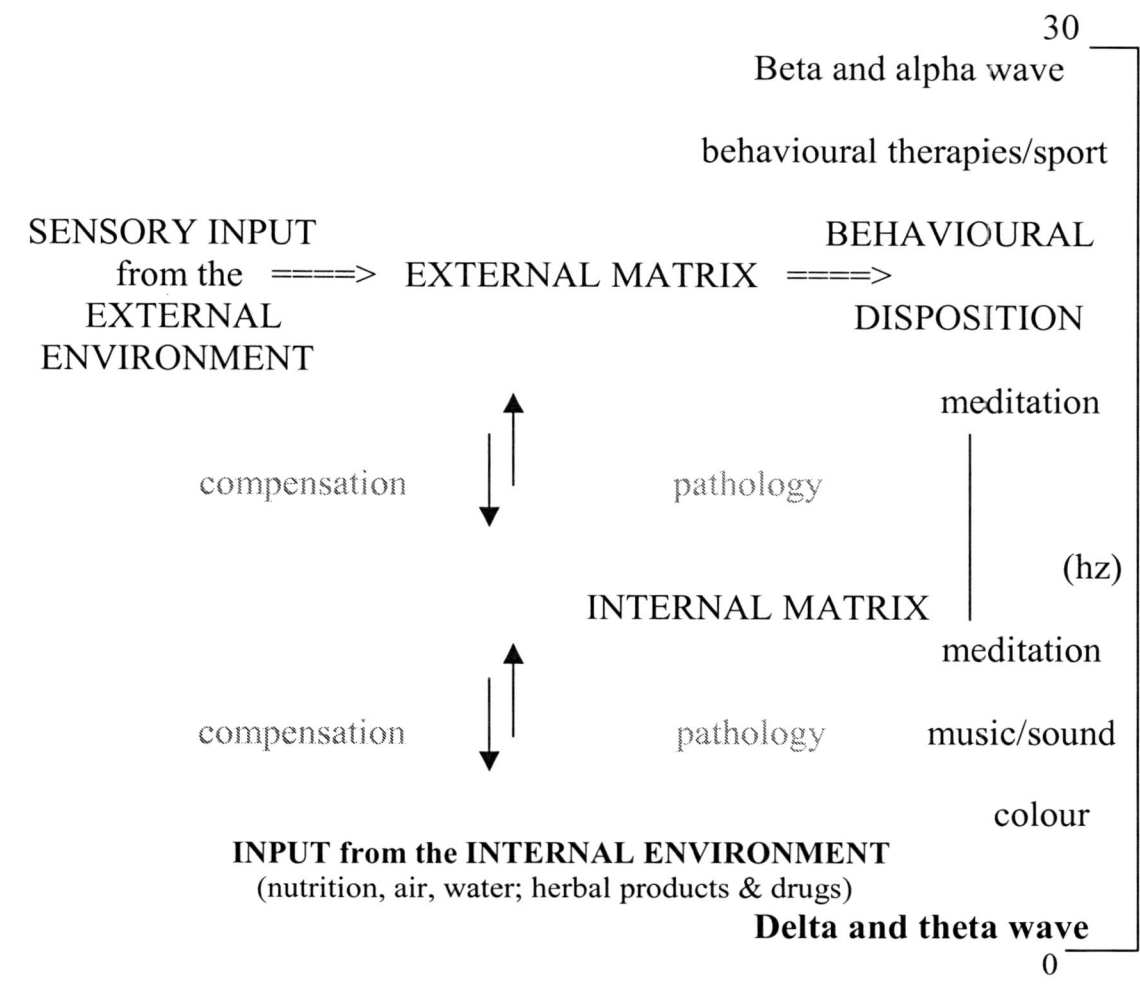

Our behaviour is regulated by the beta wave which scans at typically 15-30 hz i.e. receiving data 15-30 times per second. This rate of scanning is appropriate essential for behavioural function, movement, action, response, etc.

This data is disseminated through the other brain waves to affect thought, long-term behavioural patterns, learning and, at the most extreme levels, our health.

If our health were to be regulated at this frequency and the beta wave it would be difficult to maintain stability. Accordingly our health is regulated by the delta wave, at typically 1-4 hz, which appears more appropriate for maintaining the stability of a complex system.

Grakov's approach has enabled him to create the biomathematical model of our physiology (figure 9) and to identify deviations for the norm (figures 10 &11) which can be related, through the algorithms of the programme, to the precise medical deviations which we recognise as the symptoms or pathologies of a 'medical condition'.

**Figure 9: Man as a Digital System**

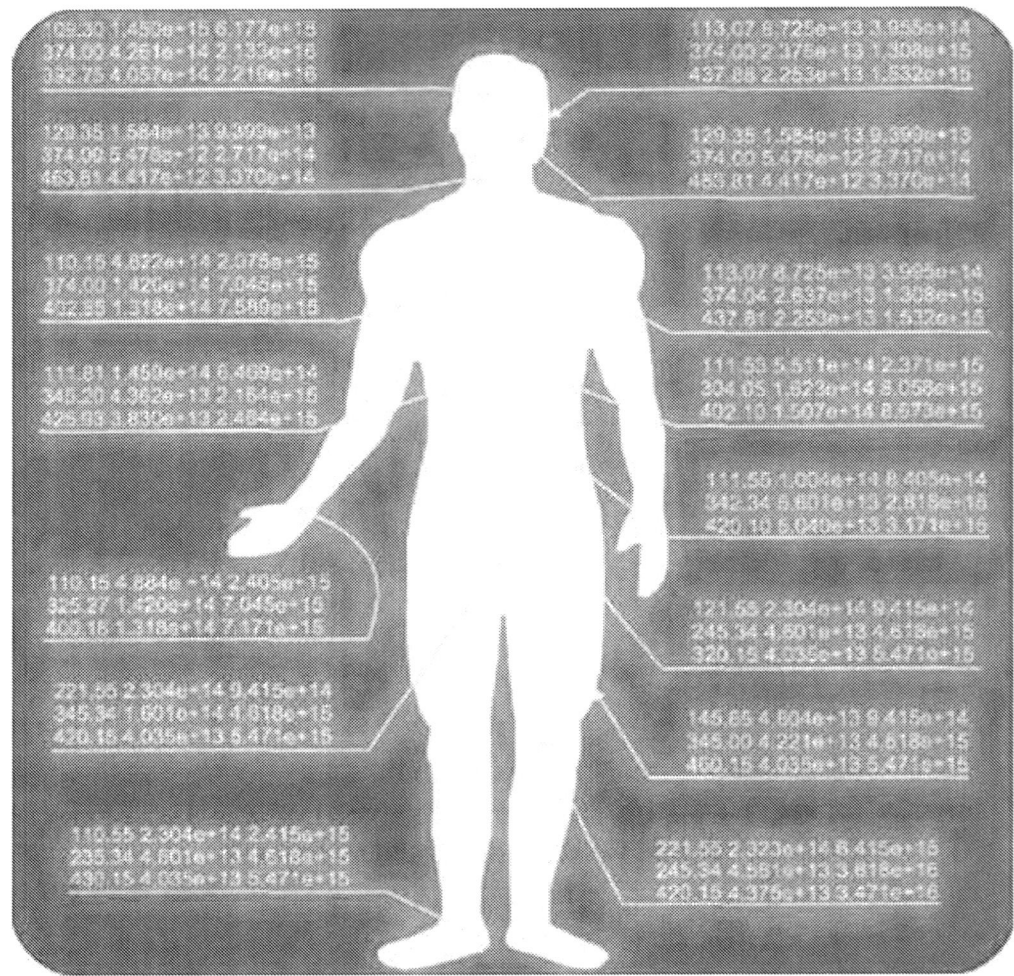

**Figure 10: Man as a Digital System – Deviations from the Norm**

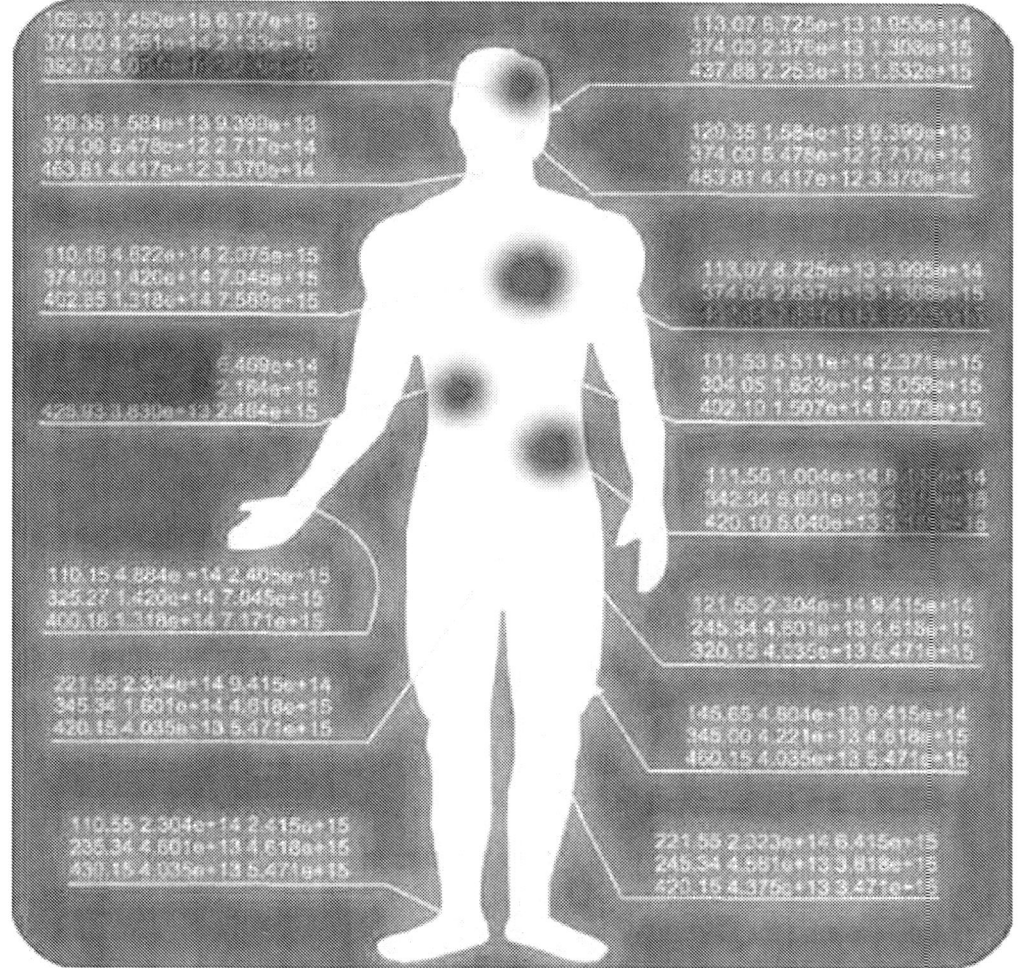

132

# Figure 11:  Man as a Digital System – Deviations from the norm

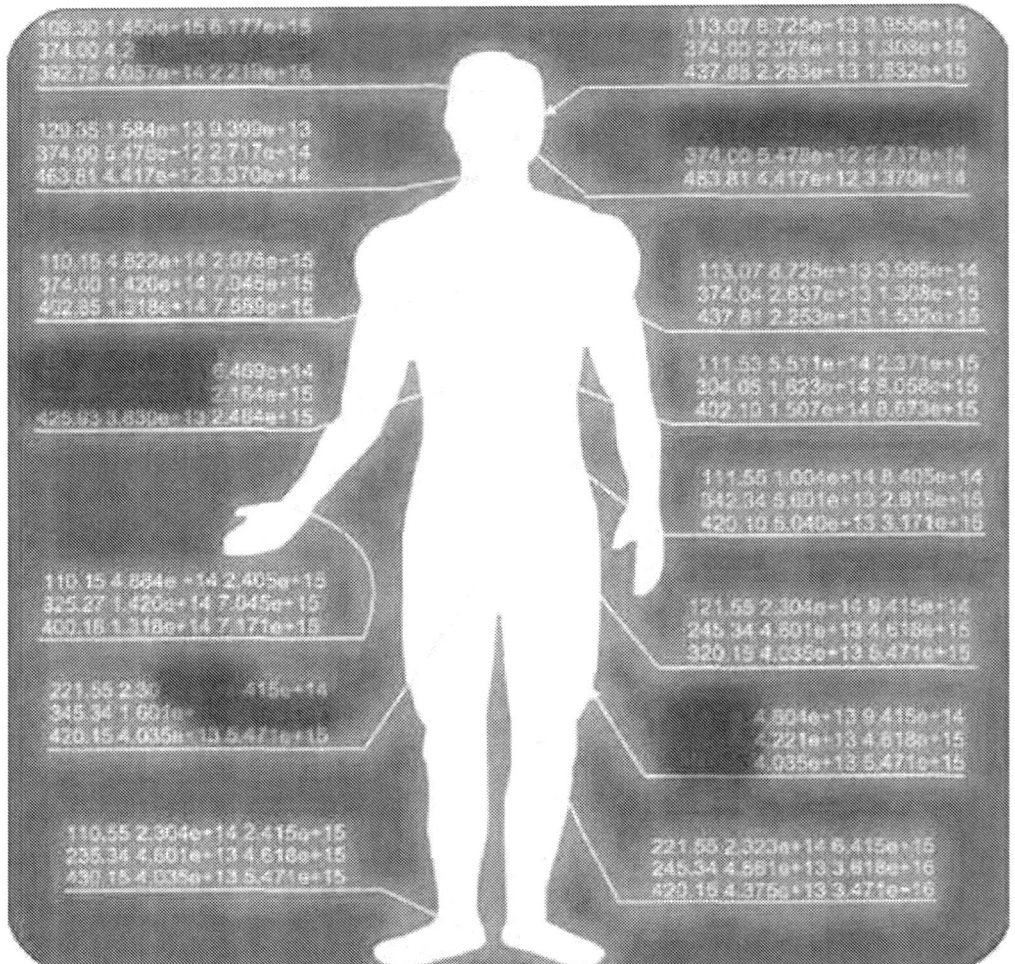

An intriguing and untypical example of how an understanding of the body's physiological systems can be used to improve health has arisen [138].

Sleeping sickness, **trypanosomiasis**, affects both humans and livestock and is endemic in sub-Saharan Africa where it is estimated that there are more than 70,000 sufferers. The disease which is is transmitted by the tsetse fly, is caused by the parasite *Trypanosoma brucei* (*T. brucei*) and results in neurological damage and death.

Researchers have identified that by exposing the parasite to physiological stress e.g. **low pH**, can trigger the pathway. Triggering the pathway, which the researchers have named SL-RNA silencing (SLS), halts the production of mRNA molecules and leads to the parasite's death.

# Does This Explain the Function of Other Complementary Health Therapies?

*Are complementary therapies the result of as yet unexplained phenomena? Does they involve the passage of signals from the brain to the organs and vice-versa? Can this be related to observations and precedents?*

Sensory stimulation is associated with processes and systems, which regulate our health and behaviour i.e. which send signals from the brain to our organs. Stress enhances the production of the stressor chemicals, such as the adreno-corticosteroids, which depress the function of the body's physiological systems, organs, immune system, and the cells.

It affects the ability of the digestive system to absorb nutrients.

If the exposure to stress is relatively minor, or short-term, stability will be re-established and normal function will return. However if exposure is long-term the production of stressor chemicals will continue. This will influence the stability of the pathological functional system which, through the autonomic nervous system, inhibits normal function. This alters the stability of the brain waves, and consequently affect mental attitudes, physical capabilities and health.

Selection of the appropriate brain frequencies (mainly in the delta or theta ranges) enables the use of hypnotherapy, meditation and other techniques, to induce behavioural changes with beneficial effects to health.

By selecting the appropriate colour and frequency or, in the case of sound and music: the note and frequency; it is possible to enhance the health of the patient and hence to positively influence their behaviour. As light comprises an estimated 85-90% of our sensory input it becomes 'glaringly obvious' that light and colour represent the best way to influence our health.

This indicates that sound and music have a beneficial effect upon health and wellbeing [46]. and explains why we can be energized when listening     to types of music which appeal to us. As our exposure to music is relatively short-term, and comprises only c5-10% of our sensory input, it has limited ability to provide a significant long-term benefit to health.

All aspects of our sensory input can be harnessed to influence our function. Ayurveda and other traditional medicines include selections of colour, taste and nutrients therefore it is entirely reasonable to expect that this can have a beneficial effect. The appropriate selection of influences which affect our sensory perception and the brain waves can, directly and indirectly have a positive effect upon our health.

There is a close correspondence between the chakras and the centres of the body [7,41] which have enriched concentrations of neuropeptides which regulate processing between brain and the immune system.

Similarly failures in the form of anosmias illustrates how the olfactory sense is affected by health-related factors [86,87].

Acupuncture [88] is believed to act by suppressing the processes of pathology and hence alleviating the symptoms of illness. There are several hypotheses to consider

(1) that its actions on processes of pathology and alleviation of symptoms result from its action on the endocannabinoid receptors in the brain [47a] involved in regulating pain, anxiety, hunger, etc.

(2) that by its action it relieves the 'psychosomatic influences' associated with the pain response and hence enables the system to achieve stability/homeostasis, therefore enhanced function of the body's physiological systems is a side-effect of the acupuncture process (see figure 12). The pain response depresses brain function and hence the function of the body's natural compensatory processes therefore its removal enables the body's stability to be restored.

(3) it directly stimulates the body's natural compensatory processes.

Options (1) and (2) are consistent with current thinking which considers that Acupuncture effectively inhibits the pain receptors i.e. it inhibits the natural pain-receiving function of the brain but fails to recognise the signalling function of the organs.

This fails to address the possibility that acupuncture's effect upon the body's physiological systems may disrupt the passage of signals from the organ to the brain (and vice versa) and hence could have a positive and negative outcome.

This would explain why acupuncture is mostly associated with its ability to treat pain, addictions, nausea and vomiting [91]. Other conditions which are believed to respond to Acupuncture include experimental pain, neck pain, headache/migraine, osteoarthritis, inflammatory rheumatic disease, stroke, addictions, asthma.

The effects of acupuncture, particularly on pain, are at least partially explicable within a conventional physiological model [90] i.e. that acupuncture is known to stimulate A delta fibres entering the dorsal horn of the spinal cord. It is considered that this mediates inhibition of pain impulses carried in the C fibres and subsequently enhances the inhibition of C fibre pain impulses at other levels of the spinal cord. This explains why acupuncture needles in one part of the body can affect pain sensation in another region.

The Skenar/InterX system is also believed to stimulate A Delta and C fibres.

Acupuncture is also known to stimulate release of endogenous opioids, the endorphins and endocannabinoids, and other neurotransmitters such as serotonin. This is likely to be another mechanism for acupuncture's effects, such as in acute pain and in substance misuse.

**Figure 12 :** **Typical illustration the effect of acupuncture upon the physiological systems**

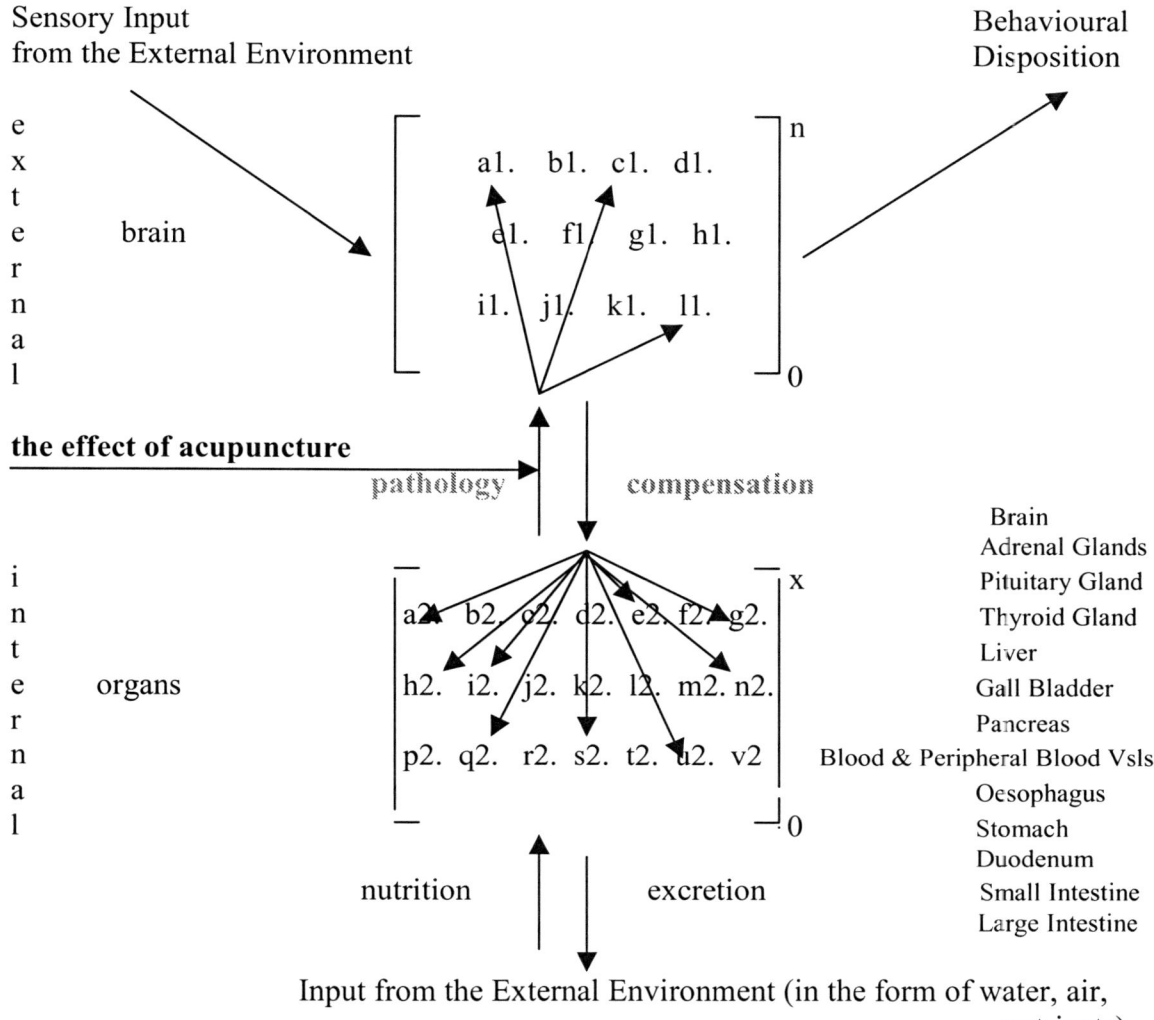

Sensory Input
from the External Environment

Behavioural
Disposition

the effect of acupuncture

Brain
Adrenal Glands
Pituitary Gland
Thyroid Gland
Liver
Gall Bladder
Pancreas
Blood & Peripheral Blood Vsls
Oesophagus
Stomach
Duodenum
Small Intestine
Large Intestine

Input from the External Environment (in the form of water, air, nutrients)

Virtual Scanning appears to show that Acupuncture cannot be directly enhancing the immune system but that such effects are only a side-effect of Acupuncture. Moreover such effects could be either beneficial or deleterious.

If beneficial it poses interesting implications for the independence of brain function. Whereas Acupuncture considers the human body to be controlled by a life energy 'Qi' , which flows around the body via the 12 meridians, Virtual Scanning is based upon the existence of 14 physiological systems and of the processes which regulate their function.

Behavioural therapies [96] have the ability to alter long-term patterns of response. Hence they can reduce the basic stimulus which may be causing behavioural and health problems.

The above observations are consistent with the concepts outlined throughout this book i.e. that the body is a complex biofeedback system comprising the body's biochemistry, the autonomic nervous system and a reciprocal system which is involved with the feed of signals from the organs to the brain.

Such a viewpoint is not new. Whilst researching the mechanisms of self-repair Dr Robert Becker [93] found what appeared to be a primitive 'DC current' system which probably preceded the 'evolved' AC system recognised by modern medicine. He claimed to have found that the meridians had similar electrical characteristics to transmission lines [94] and postulated that acupuncture points are 'amplification points' for this DC 'nervous system', which facilitates transmission over the distances from brain to periphery. Dr Becker was expert in the field of biological electricity and regeneration, and has twice been nominated for a Nobel Prize.

This property would also hold for the points in a system of nerve fibres which feed electrical impulses from the organs to the brain e.g. A delta and C fibres. This would be analogous to the function of the physiological system, which feeds signals from the brain to the organs through the autonomic nervous system. The amplification points would presumably be where the signals from the organs came together in the biofeedback system. It does not however explain how the brain could distinguish between the various neural impulses which originated from different parts of the body.

The idea that the meridian system is a component of a biochemical feedback system which has electrical characteristics is consistent with the development of magnetic acupuncture [95] which could only be effective if there were the presence of an electrical field.

There is little evidence to support the contention that acupuncture directly affects the body's physiological systems but, perhaps, instead works at the cellular and molecular level. As the simultaneous use of acupuncture and virtual scanning appears in some cases to be contra-indicative this indicates the presence of two different modes of action i.e. that Virtual Scanning works upon the compensatory mechanisms which maintain our health and that acupuncture acts upon the mechanisms associated with pathology.

Acupuncturists defend their technology with the same vehemence that physiologists defend biomedicine – as if the acupuncture meridians were intended merely for the purpose of inserting acupuncture needles (yet overlook the fact that acupuncturists are human and humans make mistakes. The act of inserting needles is dependent upon the knowledge, expertise and abilities of the acupuncturist). Like biochemistry it manipulates a natural phenomenon which exists to convey data regarding damage, disruption from our organs to the brain e.g. disruption of blood flow; skin damage; pain in joints, muscles, nerves, etc. The brain uses this information to adjust the body's physiological systems. If the flow of this information is disturbed e.g. by acupuncture or related effects, it is logical to assume that this will have an effect which could be both positive and negative.

## Placebo effect & Positive thinking [97].

*Consider how psychosomatic influences affect groups of people.*

Consider the same basic schematic, outlined in figures 1 – 4, in which we discuss the processing of sensory data by the brain.

**Figure 13**

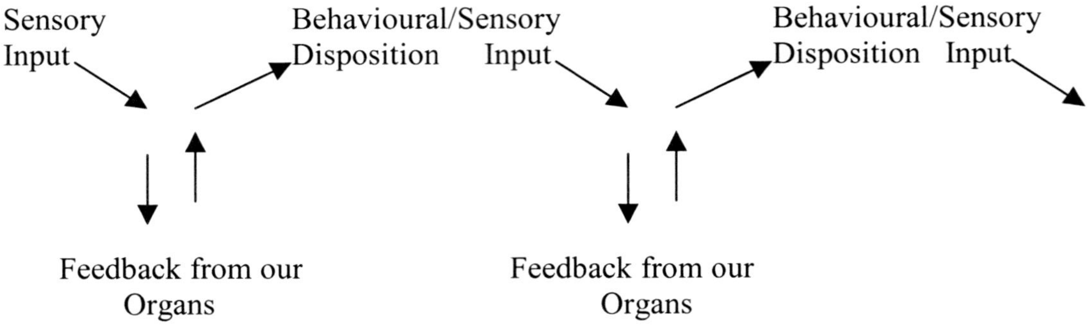

Sensory Input
Behavioural/Sensory Disposition Input
Behavioural/Sensory Disposition Input
Feedback from our Organs
Feedback from our Organs

Moreover as data is cumulative we can assess the interaction between people or effects.

**Figure 14**

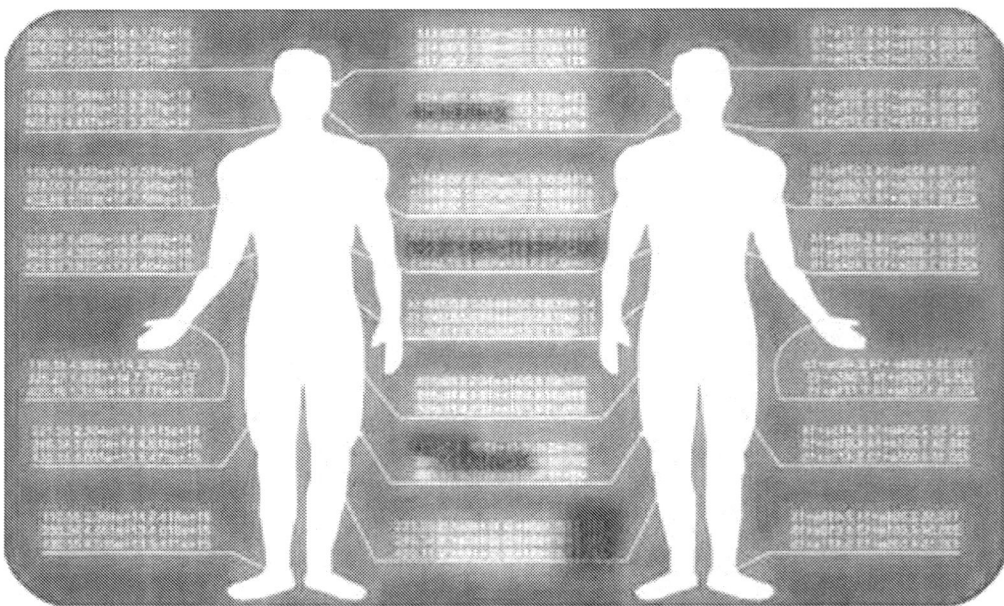

Research [98] suggests that severe and long-term stressors, such as that which results from caregiving, may leave carers vulnerable to a range of health-related problems. These effects persist well beyond the end of the stressful situation i.e. after the caring activities have ceased. The tendency to get good emotional support is associated with high NK cell activity in a study [99] of breast cancer patients.

By contrast a study of patients with Alheimers [100] disease showed a greater degree of depression and lower life satisfaction than the comparator group; and upon wound repair [101] , regulation of the sympathetic nervous system [102], on defects in NK cell function [103] and on reactions to flu vaccine [104]

These affects were also shown to apply to couples in marital conflict [105-107].

# What Proof Can be Offered for the Fundamental Concepts Outlined?

## *What is conjecture and what constitutes proof?*

Virtual Scanning offers the most compelling evidence for a hierarchical system as outlined. It uses many of the principles outlined in this article and employs mathematical modeling and algorithms to relate the information from a cognitive test procedure to our psychological profile and hence to our health.

In figure 15 below the health report (selected organs) of a lady with migraine illustrates how we are able to identify the issues which contribute to her migraine such as Impairment of Spinal Circulation, Vertebral Artery Syndrome, and Spinal Osteochondrosis.

The balance of compensatory signals, in blue, and pathology signals, in red, illustrate the holistic or biofeedback nature of our physiology.

**Figure 15:**      Organ Reports for a Lady of 59 years with Migraine.

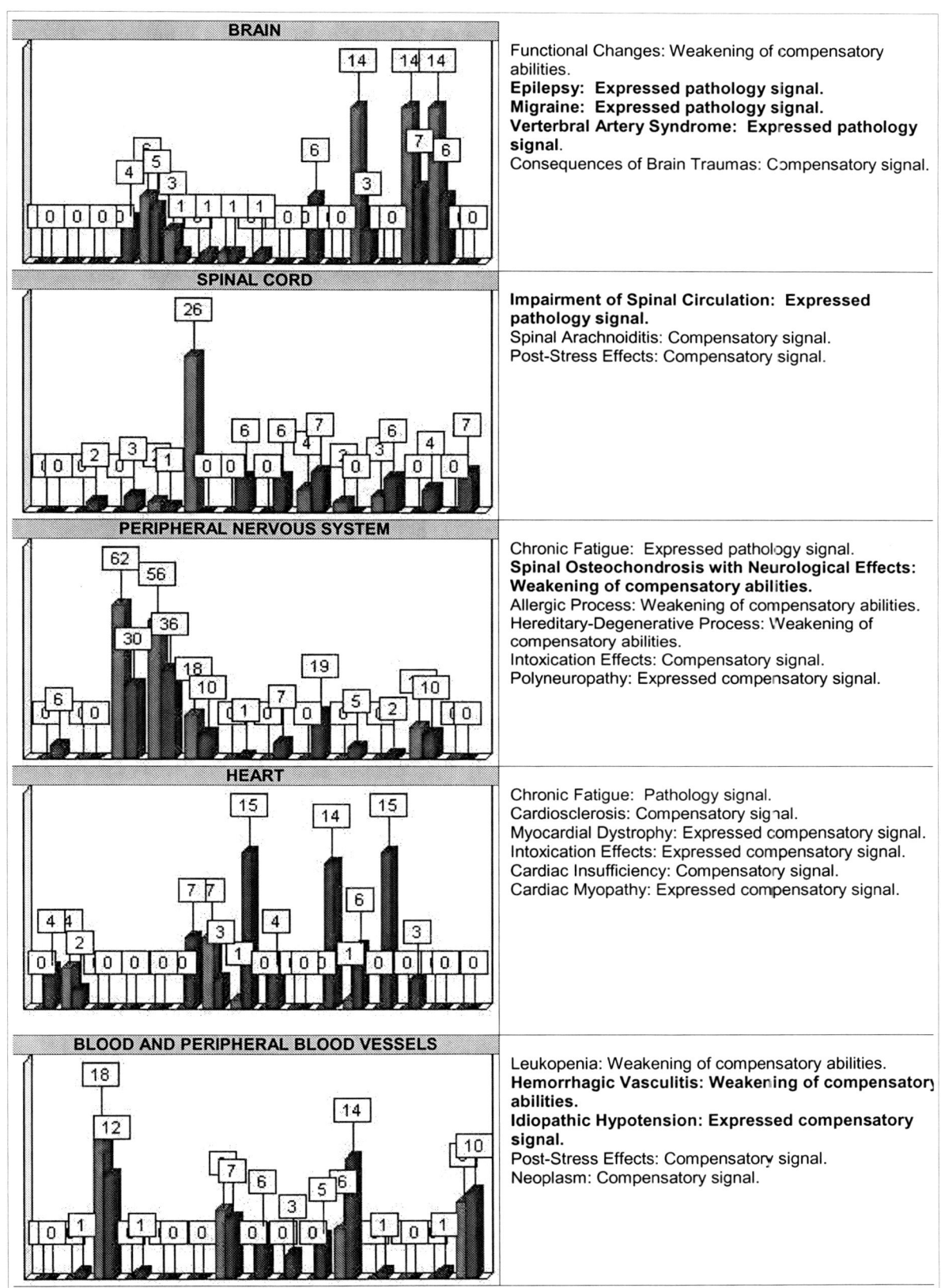

**BRAIN**

Functional Changes: Weakening of compensatory abilities.
**Epilepsy: Expressed pathology signal.**
**Migraine: Expressed pathology signal.**
**Verterbral Artery Syndrome: Expressed pathology signal.**
Consequences of Brain Traumas: Compensatory signal.

**SPINAL CORD**

**Impairment of Spinal Circulation: Expressed pathology signal.**
Spinal Arachnoiditis: Compensatory signal.
Post-Stress Effects: Compensatory signal.

**PERIPHERAL NERVOUS SYSTEM**

Chronic Fatigue: Expressed pathology signal.
**Spinal Osteochondrosis with Neurological Effects: Weakening of compensatory abilities.**
Allergic Process: Weakening of compensatory abilities.
Hereditary-Degenerative Process: Weakening of compensatory abilities.
Intoxication Effects: Compensatory signal.
Polyneuropathy: Expressed compensatory signal.

**HEART**

Chronic Fatigue: Pathology signal.
Cardiosclerosis: Compensatory signal.
Myocardial Dystrophy: Expressed compensatory signal.
Intoxication Effects: Expressed compensatory signal.
Cardiac Insufficiency: Compensatory signal.
Cardiac Myopathy: Expressed compensatory signal.

**BLOOD AND PERIPHERAL BLOOD VESSELS**

Leukopenia: Weakening of compensatory abilities.
**Hemorrhagic Vasculitis: Weakening of compensatory abilities.**
**Idiopathic Hypotension: Expressed compensatory signal.**
Post-Stress Effects: Compensatory signal.
Neoplasm: Compensatory signal.

By contrast we note in figure 16 the complete absence of the compensatory signals which regulate our physiology i.e. that in the patient who had experienced a stroke resulting in severe paralysis that there is evidence to suggest that the brain's controlling mechanism had completely failed and was no longer able to feed the necessary levels of stimulus which could regulate the function of all organs. Consequently we note the steady development of pathologies throughout the body.

**Figure 16:** Total Failure of Compensatory Signals in a male patient of c60 years following stroke

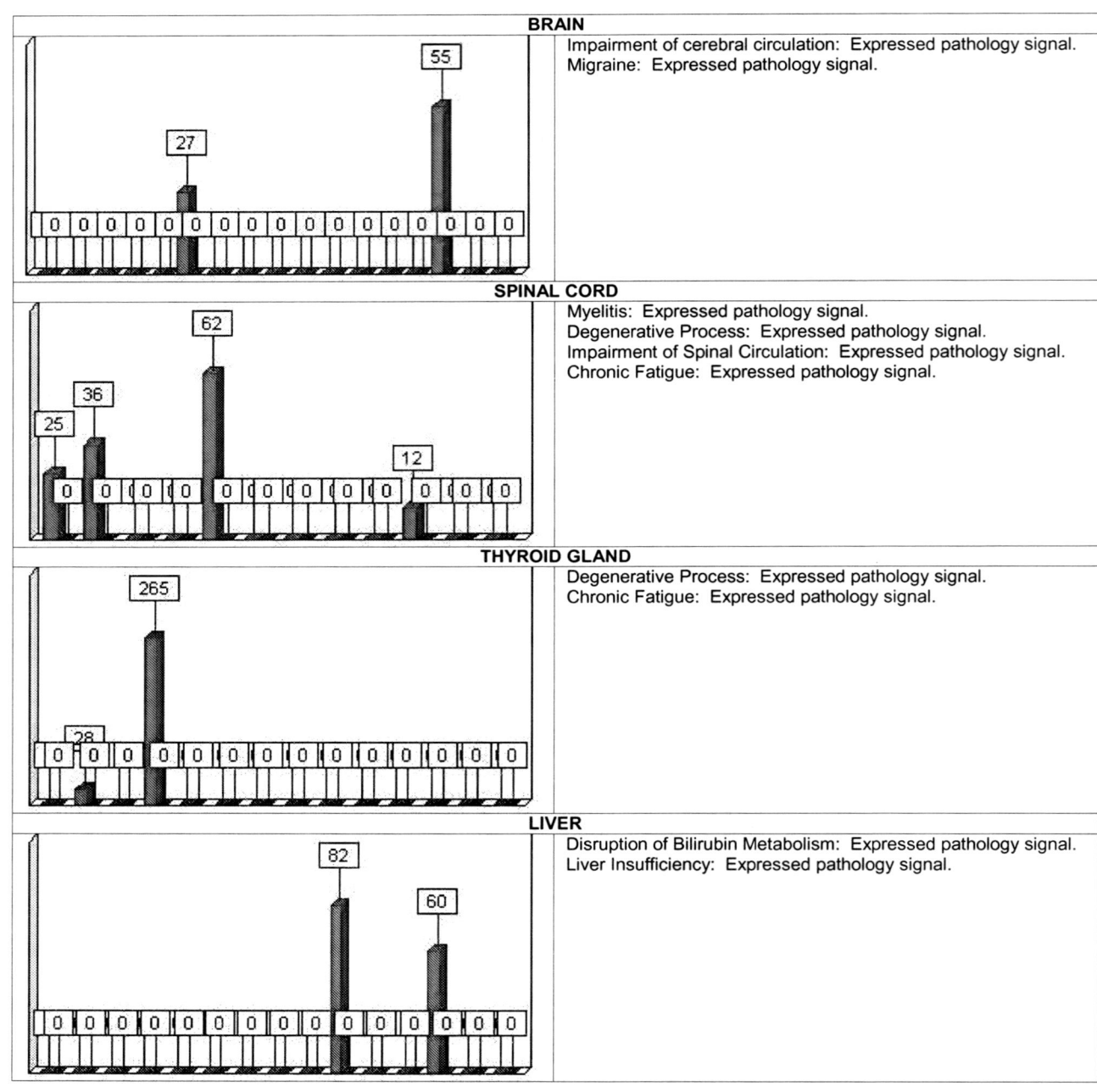

143

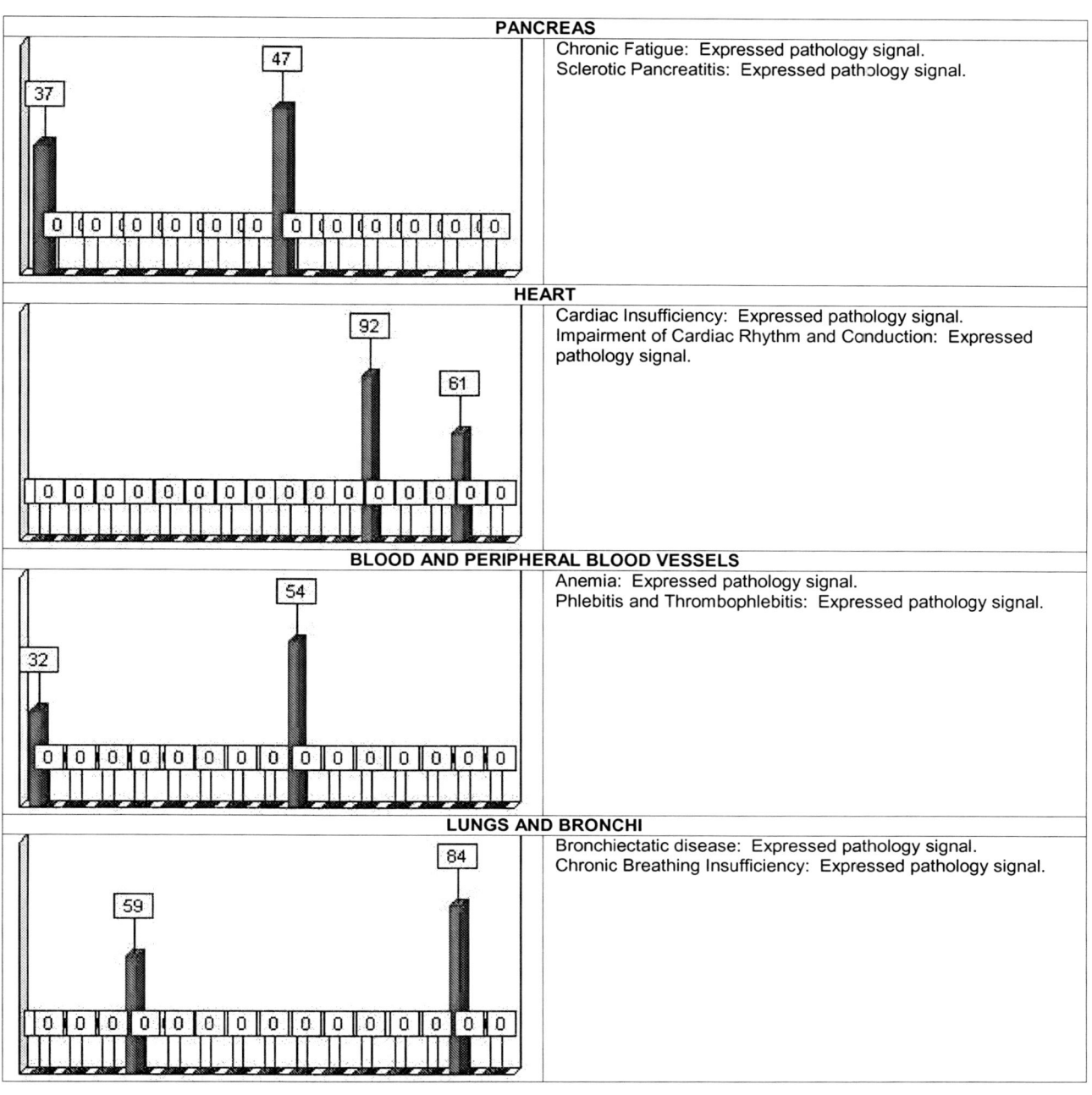

| PANCREAS | |
|---|---|
| | Chronic Fatigue: Expressed pathology signal.<br>Sclerotic Pancreatitis: Expressed pathology signal. |
| **HEART** | |
| | Cardiac Insufficiency: Expressed pathology signal.<br>Impairment of Cardiac Rhythm and Conduction: Expressed<br>pathology signal. |
| **BLOOD AND PERIPHERAL BLOOD VESSELS** | |
| | Anemia: Expressed pathology signal.<br>Phlebitis and Thrombophlebitis: Expressed pathology signal. |
| **LUNGS AND BRONCHI** | |
| | Bronchiectatic disease: Expressed pathology signal.<br>Chronic Breathing Insufficiency: Expressed pathology signal. |

And finally in figure 17 we note the almost complete absence of any signals in the mammary gland of a patient who had undergone a mastectomy which supports the contention that there is a steady flow of signals from the brain to the organ and vice versa which forms the basis of a hierarchical or biofeedback system which regulates our physiology. The absence of signals would of course be expected if there was no longer an organ present to be part of this biofeedback system.

144

# Figure 17:

Lack of signals from and to the breast in a patient who had undergone mastectomy

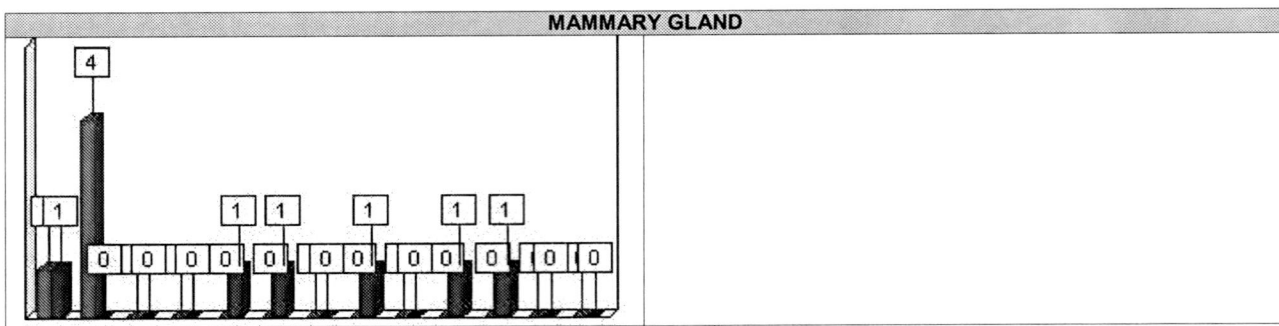

# The Influence of Light and Colour upon our Health

*We undoubtedly feel better during the summer when there is less prevalence of illness. Why should this be so? Let us consider the facts.*

In northern climes, winter often brings the blues. A simple and proven remedy is the use of powerful light.

1. According to researchers Seasonal Affective Disorder can be cured by sitting in front of bright light (10,000 lux) for c30 mins in the morning and evening [108,109].

2. This activates the pineal gland which regulates the production of melatonin and serotonin. These are associated with sleeping and waking. Darkness stimulates the production of melatonin which is necessary during sleep and is conducive to healing and longevity. If levels of melatonin are not reduced by the morning light, lethargy and depression can arise. The opposite effect may reduce the sexually inhibitive effect of melatonin and lead to earlier puberty in adolescents.

3. In a comparative study for the treatment of Seasonal Affective Disorder light therapy was demonstrated to be more effective than Prozac [110].

4. Until the 60`s babies born prematurely suffered a life-threatening condition of jaundice, which may have necessitated a blood transfusion. Now, due to research by R.J.Cremer [111] all that is required is exposure to light. This results from the chemical breakdown of bilirubin by full spectrum or uv light

5. Dyslexia sufferers are now enabled to read comfortably with tinted glasses or overlays; black and white is often too harsh for them to see clearly. Coloured lenses [112] are known to improve reading and help to prevent migraines in a small number of patients.

6. Some flashing-light therapies, of an empirical nature, are also used to treat dyslexia although expensive and with variable outcomes.

7. Colour is also used in the assessment and treatment of Dyslexia and Autism although it is not considered to be a cure. (SNOOZELIN [134,135])

8. Blue light has been used to treat Arthritis [140] and red light to stop migraines [141].

9. UV B is useful for Vitamin D production in the skin but it is not good to get too much exposure.

10. Curtis & Hurtak [113] suggest that in addition to the circulatory systems of blood, lymphatic system and Nervous System that there is the emergence of a further concept based around the body's receptiveness to light and its ability to energise. This has been termed the electromagnetic body which 'may be a vehicle of consciousness projection'

11. Others such as S.V.Krakov [115] examined colour perception and its relationship to the autonomic nervous system. He established that the colour red stimulated the sympathetic nervous system and the colour blue stimulated the parasympathetic nervous system.

12. Gariaev [116, 143-145] and coworkers refer to the body as an energy biocomputer rather than a molecular machine. They question some of the basic assumptions associated with genetic and molecular biology i.e. that only 2% of our DNA is significant and that the remaining 98% is considered to have little biological significance. They consider that such assumptions, to which biomedicine is prone, are a significant omission in biomedical research.

   Their research has allegedly demonstrated that light plays a significant role regulating the function of DNA and that

   o   this been experimentally demonstrated to enhance the rate of metabolic reactions.

   o   the implication is of a electromagnetically-based language which communicates between DNA and the cells.

   They conclude the existence of a quantum-based approach in which light regulates the function of DNA and hence of cellular processes. If so these findings change our understanding of the workings of DNA and undermine the present biotechnological dogma which allows for its chemical manipulation.

13. The proponents of these new concepts can cite the work of Nobel Laureate Dr Niels Ryberg Finzen [118].

14. In 1941 Dr Frank Apperly [119], discovered that sunlight appeared to have a protective effect against many cancers, including breast, lung, prostate and colon. By studying cancer statistics for North America, he noted that people who live nearer to the equator have a lower incidence of cancer. Many studies have confirmed these observations. Unsurprisingly sunlight stimulates production of vitamin D by the skin and is the greatest source of Vitamin D. He discovered that it was not sunlight that caused skin cancers, it was the high temperatures which were associated with excess exposure which did the damage. High exposure to sunlight in cooler climates with mean temperatures below 5.5 degrees C (42 degrees F) was not associated with increased incidence of skin cancer.

15. Two further studies confirm the vital role that the vitamin D plays in preventing breast cancer. In the first, carried out by Imperial College London [120], women who had higher intake of vitamin D - from sunlight, cod liver oil or milk - between the ages of 10 and 29 had a 40 per cent reduced risk of developing breast cancer later in life.

16. Artificial light induces the production of stressor chemicals [121].

17. Researchers have reported on the use of light to treat cancerous tumours [122]. In the treatment of over 3,000 patients – patients who had been previously treated by surgery, chemotherapy, etc; a 70-80% success rate has been claimed. Further research has reported on the use of light to treat AIDS and leukaemia. [123]

18. In the second study [124], women with high levels of vitamin D in their blood had a 50% lower risk of developing breast cancer, however the greatest protective effect occurred when levels were 52 nanograms per millilitre of vitamin D, which equates to a daily intake of 1,000 IU, a level which is difficult to obtain by purely dietary means. The best food sources of vitamin D include eggs, liver, and fish.

19. Astronauts lose on average 1-2% of bone mass each month during space flights.

20. Finally, a doctors' ability to diagnose is affected by their health which affects their colour vision [125].

Other biological effects which can be achieved as a result of light stimulation [126] include:

- Increased ATP production

- A significant increase in protein synthesis within the cells of the body [127]

- Increased multiplication of collagen fibres

- Increased production and/or activity of enzymes, and improved function of the lymphatic systems which are involved in cell regeneration

- Development of Blood Vessels

The immunological effects of light from laser and non-laser sources [128] were shown to increase in serum IgM levels of over 26% within 10 days.

As always these concepts reduce to the biological level and to the level of persons trying to understand the actual processes rather than their significance.

The biochemical approach of anatomical dissection, and the analyses of biochemical reactions in the body, has been based on increasing the level of understanding of the complex human structure yet the reverse appears to have happened. At each step more and more information, often contradicting previous findings, becomes known yet the understanding of the processes within the body appears to become less and less. Increased knowledge appears to be leading to greater understanding of the body's biochemistry but by less understanding, and greater obfuscation of the complex processes which regulate our function. It appears more logical therefore to consider the function of structured processes, the passage of data to the brain, and the ability to regulate the body i.e. as a steady state.

Medical researchers and philosophers now contemplate theories to explain the apparent flow of energy in the body yet are they guilty of making the same mistakes as many others previously of confusing symptoms with effect and not seeking the CAUSE for the symptoms.

Is it possible that despite the mass of information which is published in the scientific press each year that much of this research is a waste of time because it is selectively absorbed or discarded according to the priorities of the day. Researchers such as Popp F.A, [129-132] was able to identify that light and biophotons were involved in the regulation of the various biological processes. Perhaps he, like Grakov, was too far ahead of his time!

## Accreditations:

1    Russian Academy of Natural Science, Silver Medal of the Academy

2    Ministry of National Health of the Russian Federation, Approval Certificate

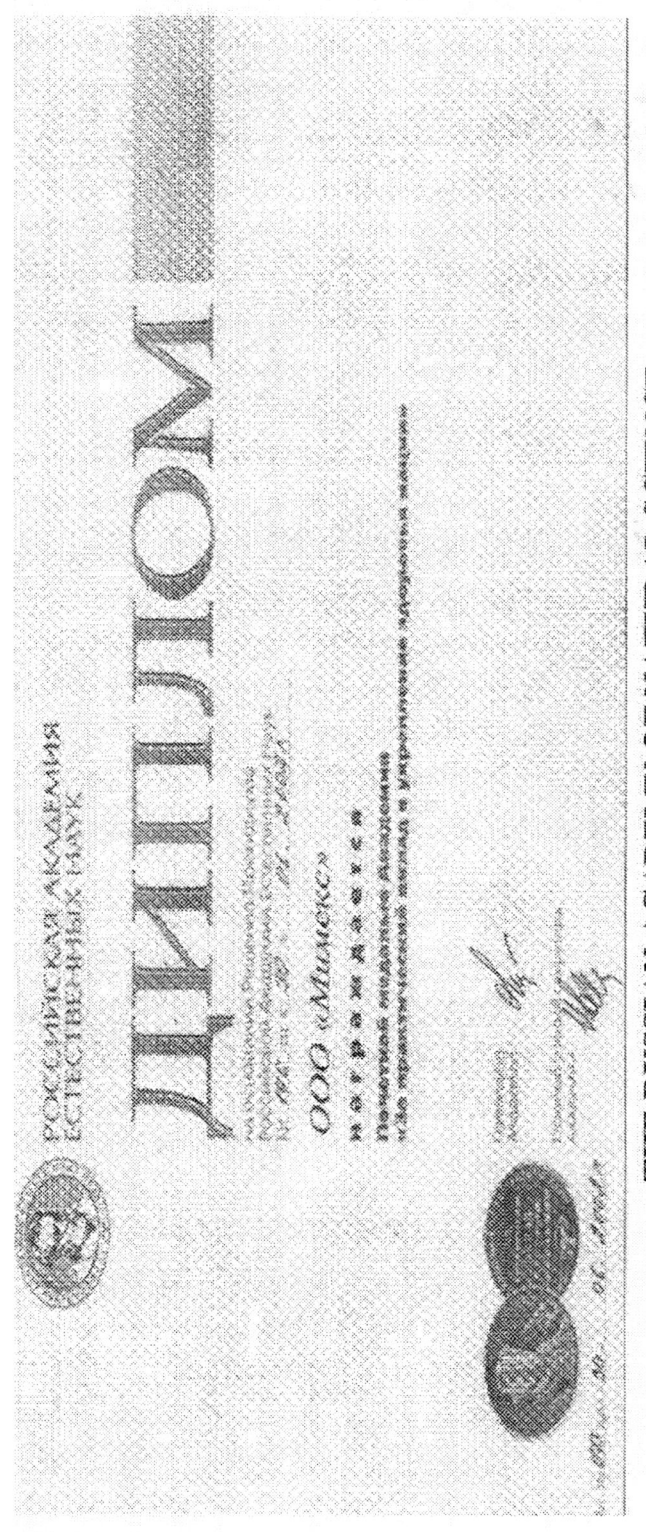

**THE RUSSIAN ACADEMY OF NATURAL SCIENCE**

**DIPLOMA**

THE PRESIDIUM OF THE RUSSIAN ACADEMY OF SCIENCE AWARDED

**SCIENTIFIC ORGANISATION 'MIMEX'**

**WITH THE SILVER MEDAL OF THE ACADEMY**

'FOR DEVELOPMENT IN MEDICINE, SCIENCE AND NATIONAL HEALTH'

PRESIDENT OF THE ACADEMY                         SIGNATURE

SCIENTIFIC SECRETARY OF THE ACADEMY        SIGNATURE

REGISTER No 202        27  June   2001

150

By the order of NHS of
The Russian Federation

# MINISTRY OF HATIONAL HEALTH OF THE RUSSIAN FEDERATION
No 036                    19-01-00

THIS IS TO CERTIFY THAT SOFTWARE 'STRANNIK' OF MIMEX COMPANY- INFORMATION AND CONSULTING PROGRAMME

IS FULLY APPROVED AND CAN BE USED IN THE NATIONAL HEALTH SERVISE OF THE RUSSIAN FEDERATION.

**Grounds for approval:**
Protocol of Technological Tests   No13-01/00/2-т

Protocol of Expertise       No 17-01/00/2-3
Valid till                  19-January-2005
State Secretary
Deputy Minister             Dedkov E D -
signature

# References:

1.  '*Why we get sick*': Nesse R.M, Williams C.W: pub Vintage

2.  Anokhin, PK. *Internal Inhibition as a Problem of Physiology (in Russian).* Moscow: Medgiz, 1958; **Anokhin, PK.** General principles of formation of adaptive-defense adjustments. *Proc Acad Med Sci USSR* 17: 16-28, 1962; **Anokhin, PK.** *Biology and Neurophysiology of the Conditioned Reflex.* Moscow: Medicina, 1968.

3.  K. V. Sudakov, 156-159; P. D. Gorizontov, 146-148; N.N. Vasilevskiy,; G. N. Kryzhanovskiy 161; V. I. Medvedev, 149-152; I. A. Sapov 155, V. S. Novikov, 153-154

4.  *Neuroscience,* 27th October 2005, Williams.D, Hofer.H, **www.medicalnewstoday.com/medicalnews.php?newsid=32597**

5.  *Journal of the Optical Society of America,* June 1942, Krakov.S.V, Colour Vision and Autonomic Nervous System

6.  Gerard.R.M, Differential Effects of Coloured Lights on Psychophysiological functions, Ph.D. dissertation, 1958

7.  comments attributed to Dr Candace Pert

8.  comments attributed to David Krech, psychologist

9.  Goldin.P, Colormetrics: www.colormetrics.com

10. Paulus    http://orlab.optom.unsw.edu.au/ICVSFolder/programme99

11. http://www.umm.edu/men/viagra.htm

12. http://www.chronicneurotoxins.com/info/vision_rationale.cfm

13. *Age and Ageing* 2003, 32, 26-32

14. *British Psychological Society, Scottish branch annual conference* 24th November 2006, Shipley B., reported in the Daily Mail 25th November 2006.

15. Penn State project sponsored by the NIMH; H.J.Leidy, J.K. Gardner, B.R. Frye, M.L. Snook, M.K. Schuchert, E.L. Richard

16. http://www.nhsdirect.nhs.uk/articles/article.aspx?articleId=541&PrintPage=1

17. *Journal of the American Medical Association,* 2003; 290: 215-21, Ruo B, Rumsfeld JS, Hlatky MA, Liu H, Browner WS, Whooley MA

18. *Psychosomatic Medicine,* 1999; 61: 26-37

19. *Atherosclerosis, Thrombotic and Vascular Biology,* 1997; 17: 1490-95

20. *Circulation,* 2000; 101: 2034-9

21.    *Archives of Internal Medicine*, 2002; 162: 901-6)

22.    *Family Practitioner News*, 1996; 26: 8

23.    *Psychosomatic Medicine*, 2001; 63: 267-72

24.    *British Medical Journal*, 1985; 290: 1103-6

25.    *Journal of the American Medical Association*, 2003; 290: 2138-48

26.    **International Journal of Psychophysiology** *2002; 45(1-2):72-73. McCraty,R, presented at the 11th World Congress of Psychophysiology, July-Aug. 2002,*

27.    *Archives of Internal Medicine* 2007, 167 (2):174-181, Psychosocial Factors and Inflammation in the Multi-Ethnic Study of Atherosclerosis, Ranjit.N.

28.    Kiecolt-Glaser, Page, Marucha, MacCallum & Glaser 1998

29.    Linus Pauling Institute, http://lpi.oregonstate.edu/infocenter/minerals/zinc/

30.    *Journal of Nutrition 1981*;111:1876-1883, Rayssiguier Y, Gueux E, Weiser D. Effect of magnesium deficiency on lipid metabolism in rats fed a high carbohydrate diet.

31.    *Am J Med 1994* Jan;96(1):63-76, Magnesium and its therapeutic uses: a review, **McLean RM.**

32.    *Physiol Behav* 1991 Oct;50(4):757-64, Lead effects on food competition and predatory aggression in Binghamton HET mice: Hahn.M.E, Burright.R.G, Donovick.P.J.

33.    **http://www.nsc.org/issues/lead/healtheffects.htm**

34.    *J. Med Hypoth*, 1981, 7, 673-99  link between adhd, asthma, eczema and other allergic symptoms /consistent with a deficiency of Essential fatty acids;

35.    *Prostaglan Leukotr Essent Fatty Acids*, 2000, 63, 1-9  difficulty in processing fats;

36.    *J Pediatr*; 1994, 125, s39-47 deficiency of omega-3-fatty acids;

37.    *Proc Natl Acad Sci USA*; 1986; 4021-5 deficiency of omega-3-fatty acids

38.    Dr Natasha Campbell-McBride: '*Gut and Psychology Syndrome: Natural Treatment for Autism, ADD/ADHD, Dyslexia, Dyspraxia, Depression, Schizophrenia*' pub Be Healthy books.

39.    *Journal of the American Family Physician*; Vol 67, no5, 1st March 2003

40.    *European Cancer Research meeting in Prague*, (reported Nov 2006), Chesney.J, University of Kentucky; *The Lancet*, November 2002, Korzenik.J, Dieckgraefe.B,

41. Dr Candace Pert: www.angelfire.com/hi/TheSeer/Pert.html

42. http://www.mpib-berlin.mpg.de/en/aktuelles/nachruf_pbb.htm

43. http://en.wikipedia.org/wiki/Stephen_Jay_Gould

44. http://www.mspp.edu/index.asp?action=29&what=100058

45. http://en.wikipedia.org/wiki/Carl_Jung

46. Lekander.M., Karolinska Institute

47. *Emergent Computational Neural Architectures based on Neuroscience*; Wermter.S., Austin.J., Willshaw.D

48. **http://www.tlc2.uh.edu/News/NIHGrantsmanshipSeminar2**

49. ***Journal of the Proceedings of the National Academy of Sciences***, January 29th January 2007, researchers from the University of California

50. ***Movement Disorders***, published on-line on December 18, 2006.

51. **http://research.microsoft.com/aboutmsr/overview/default.aspx**

52. *CAM* March 2007, Vol 6, no 8 p38-44, Cambell-McBride.N

53. *UKCRC Grand Challenges Workshop*, November 2002, 'The Architecture of Brain and Mind', Denham.M

54. *UKCRC Grand Challenges Workshop*, November 2002, 'A Theory of the Brain', Borisyuk.R

55. *Applied Artificial Intelligence*, 7: 317–337, 1993, I. Kononenko. Inductive and Bayesian learning in medical diagnosis.

56. I. Kononenko: Machine learning for medical diagnosis: History, state of the art and perspective, Invited paper, *Artificial Intelligence in Medicine* – ISSN 0933-3657, 23(1): 89–109, 2001.

57. 'Modeling Cognitive Development in the Human Brain'; Coward A.L; Australian National University, Department of Computer Science

58. *Physiological Genomics* 23:1-3 (2005) American Physiological Society; Computational modeling of physiological systems; Beard.D.A, Bassingthwaighte.J.B, Greene.A.S

59. www.iscc.org/jubilee2006/Presentations/Oicherman.pdf

60. **http://www.findarticles.com/p/articles/mi_qn4158/is_20060814/ai_n16649199**

61. *Physiological Genomics* 23:1-3 (2005)1094-8341/05, Computational modeling of physiological systems Beard.D.A, Bassingthwaighte J.B, and Greene A.S.

62.   *CAM*, March 2007, Vol 6 (8) p 38-44, 'Time to get scientific: let's scrap the diet-heart-cholesterol hypothesis', Cambell-McBride.N

63.   comments attributed to Dr David Green, Civitas

64.   *The Lancet, New England Journal of Medicine, The Mayo Clinic*

65.   **Journal of the American Medical Association**, 2005; 293: 1348-58

66.   **British Medical Journal** 2006, 333:59, Leigh

67.   comments attributed to Prof David Webb, Professor of Therapeutics and Pharmacology at the University of Edinburgh

68.   *Journal of Cell Science* 116: 4867–4869; Kroeze, W.K., Sheffler, D.J., and Roth, B.L. (2003). "**G protein-coupled receptors at a glance**".

69.   *Med. Chem.* 7 (9), 861-888, Muller.G (2000) Towards 3D Structures of G-protein-coupled receptors: a multidisciplinary approach.

70.   *J Mol Med, 1995.* **73**(2): p. 51-63; Gudermann, T., B. Nurnberg, and G. Schultz, Receptors and G proteins as primary components of transmembrane signal transduction. Part 1. G-protein-coupled receptors: structure and function.

71.   *Nat Biotechnol,* 1996. **14**(11): p. 1516-8, Drews, J., Genomic sciences and the medicine of tomorrow.

72.   comments attributed to V.Wedderburn, President, *British Psychological Society* in **The Psychologist** 2004.

73.   http://en.wikipedia.org/wiki/Pharmacogenetics

74.   *Photochemistry and Photobiology,* pp. 637-649, 29, 1979, Martinek, K. & Berezin, I. Artificial Light-Sensitive Enzymatic Systems as Chemical Amplifiers of Weak Light Signals

75.   report attributed to Roses.A., Duke University

76.   http://www.pfizer.com.au/Media/Stress.aspx

77.   J. Liberman: *Light—Medicine of the Future*, pub, Bear & Co., Vermont, 1991; http://www.egt.bme.hu/!EnglishEducatio/Basic%20Dayl.%20Arch.pdf

78.   www.cbiol.leeds.ac.uk/algorithmic.html

80.   www.nexusmagazine.com/articles/CellularMemories.html;

81.   *Am J Psychiatry* 1967; 124:1190-1195, Lunde DT. Psychiatric complications of heart transplants

82.   *J Heart Transplants* 1988; 7:223-226, Kuhn WF et al. Psychopathology in heart transplant candidates.

83. Sylvia C, Novak W. *A Change of Heart*. New York, NY: Little, Brown, 1997.

84. http://www.knowledgehorizons.manchester.ac.uk/researchthemes/index.asp?areaID=21

85. http://www.knowledgehorizons.manchester.ac.uk/researchthemes/index.asp?areaID=21

86. *Psychological Science* 15 (3), 143–148. Djordjevic.J, Zatorre.R.J, Petrides.M, Jones-Gotman.M (2004), The Mind's Nose. Effects of Odor and Visual Imagery on Odor Detection

87. Lawless, H.T. (1997) Olfactory psychophysics. Beauchamp, G.K. and Bartoshuk, L. (eds), Tasting and Smelling. Academic Press, San Diego, CA, pp. 125–174

87. *British Medical Journal* 2001;323: 467-468 The safety of acupuncture

88. *Scientific American*, December 2004, 'The Brain's own marijuana', Nicoll.R.A., Alger.B.E.

90. *British Medical Journal* 1999;319:973-976, 'ABC of Complementary Medicine', Vickers.A, Zollman. C.

91. E. Ernst and A. White (1999), *'Acupuncture - A Scientific Appraisal'*, pub Oxford, Butterworth- Heinemann, pp107-127

92. **http://www.energyfields.org/science/becker.html**

93. Cross Currents, by Robert O. Becker MD.

94. Dr. Robert Becker, author of The Body Electric and Cross Currents

95. www.magneticacupuncture.com

96. http://www.cognitivetherapy.com/basics.html

97. comments attributed to Milgrom. L

98. Esterling, Kiecolt-Glaser, Bodnar & Glaser, 1994; *Physical Illness and Depression in Older Adults*, pub Springer ISBN 978-0-306-46269-6

99. Levy, S. M., Herberman, R. B., Lippman, M., & d'Angelo, T. (1987). Correlation of stress. factors with sustained depression of natural killer cell activity

98. *Proc Natl. Acad Sci USA*, 93:3043-3047, 1996, Esterling, Kiecolt-Glaser & Glaser, 1996; CHRONIC STRESS ALTERS THE IMMUNE RESPONSE TO INFLUENZA VIRUS VACCINE IN OLDER ADULTS, Kiecolt-Glaser JK, Glaser R, Gravenstein S, Malarkey WB, Sheridan J

99. *Canadian Psychology* August 1995, 'Stress, Aging, and Resilience: Can Accrued Wear and Tear Be Slowed?', Hawkley.L.C, Berntson G.G, Engeland.C.G, Marucha.P.T, et al

102. Mills.P.J, et al 1997

103. *Psychosomatic Medicine* 64:477-486 (2002), 'Health Consequences of Alzheimer's Caregiving Transitions: Effects of Placement and Bereavement', Grant.I, Adler.K.A, Patterson.T.L, Dimsdale.J.E, Ziegler.M.G and Irwin.M.R

104. *Proc Natl Acad Sci* U S A. 1996 April 2; 93(7): 3043–3047, 'Chronic stress alters the immune response to influenza virus vaccine in older adults', Kiecolt-Glaser.J.K, Glaser.R, Gravenstein.S, Malarkey.W.B, and Sheridan J.

105. Miller.G.E, Dopp, Myers, Stevens, & Fahey, 1999;

106. Kiecolt-Glaser et al 1997

107. *Psychom Med* 56:41-51, 1994, 'Hostile Behaviour during Marital Conflict alters Pituitary and Adrenal Hormones', Malarkey WB, Kiecolt-Glaser JK, Pearl D, Glaser R;

108. *American Journal of Psychiatry*, pp. 509-511, 148(4), 1991; Oren, D. et al, Treatment of Seasonal Affective Disorder with Green Light and Red Light

109. *Journal of Affective Disorders*, pp. 209-216, 20, 1990, Brainard, G. et al, Effects of Different Wavelengths in Seasonal Affective Disorder,

110. *American Journal of Psychiatry*, 2006; 163: 805-12

111. *The Lancet*, pp. 1094-1097, 1, 1958, Cremer, R. et al, Influence of Light on the Hyperbilirubinemia in Infants,

112. Wilkins.A; Patel R, Wilkins AJ and Evans BJW. Randomized controlled trial of the use of precision tinted lenses in migraine, including an investigation of the optometric correlates of migraines. *Child Vision Research Society*, 1999

113. *Journal of Alt & Complementary Medicine* Vol 10 No1, Curtis & Hurtak

114. *Journal of Clinical Pathology*, 2006, 17 October

115. *Journal of the Optical Society of America*, June 1942, S.V.Krakov 'Colour Vision and the Autonomic Nervous System':

116. Gariaev.P, 1994 143-145

117. Dr J.Craig Venter, quoted in The Times, Monday February 12, 2001 'Why you can't judge a man by his genes' **http://www.thetimes.co.uk/article/0,,2-82213,00.html**; *Time's Scientist of the year (2000).* recognized as one of the two most important scientists in the worldwide effort to map the human genome. 'The Genome Warrior', The New Yorker Magazine, June 12, 2000.

118. Nobel Laureate Finsen, N. The Red Light Treatment of Smallpox, *British Medical Journal*, pp. 1412-1414, 7, 1895

119. Dr. F.Apperly, University of Melbourne

120. http://www.guardian.co.uk/medicine/story/0,,1924059,00.html

121. *Ophthalmologica* 180, (4), 1980, 188-197; "The Effect of Natural and Artificial Light via the Eye on the Hormonal and Metabolic Balance of Animal and Man", Hollowich.F. et al.

122. *Seminars in Surgical Oncology* 5 (1989), pp6-16; "Photoradiation Therapy-New Approaches", Dougherty.T.J.

123. Engelman.R, "Light Kills AIDS Virus in Blood", *Scripps Howard News Service*, January 13th 1988.

124. University of California, women with high levels of vitamin D in their blood had a 50% lower risk of developing. *Nutra-Ingredients*, USA, 17 October 2006

125. *British Journal of General Practitioners*. 1999 June; 49(443): 469–475. Colour vision deficiency in the medical profession, Spalding.J.A, International Colour Vision Society

126. extracts from an article by Warren.S.W.; *Positive Health* December 2004

127. Baxter.G.D; *Therapeutic Lasers – Theory and Practice*. ISBN 0-443-04393-0 1997

128. *Photochem. Photobiol. Sci.*, 2004, 3, 102 - 108; The regulatory effect of polychromatic (visible and infrared) light on human humoral immunity; Zhevago.N.A, Samoilova.K.A and Obolenskaya K.D

129. The quantum naturopath: activating quantum healing with new flexoelectric technology. *Townsend Letter for Doctors and Patients*, March, 2003, Yannick.P

130. Popp FA et al: Advances in Biophoton Research. 1992, *World Scientific*, Singapore.

131. Popp, FA & Chang JJ Mechanism of interaction between electromagnetic fields and living systems. *Science in China* (Series C), 2000; 43:507-18.

132. *Biophotons - The Light in Our Cells*, Marco Bischof *pub* Zweitausendeins, Frankfurt, 1995. ISBN 3-86150-095-7

133. Dr Max Luscher: http://www.colourtest.ue-foundation.org/

134. Snoezelin: http://en.wikipedia.org/wiki/snoevelin; Chung J.C.C, Lai C.K.Y, Snoezelen for dementia. *The Cochrane Database of Systematic Reviews* 2002, 4. Art no: CD003152;

135. Lancioni G.E, Cuvo A.J, O'Reilly M.F, Snooezelen: an overview of research with people with developmental disabilities and dementia. *Disab.Rehabil*.2003; 2002; 24:175-84

136. *Journal of Neuroscience*, 27th October 2005; Williams D. University of Rochester, Allyn Professor of Medical Optics, Centre for Visual Science

137. en.wikipedia.org/wiki/Rhodopsin

138. ***European Molecular Biology Organization, Journal of,*** Michaeli.S et al Life Sciences Department of Bar-Ilan University in Israel

139. ***Science,*** 15th September 2006, Knight.R, Rauch E.

140. ***International Journal of Biosocial Researchy*** 3, (2) 1982 pp 49-54, McDonald. S.F, 'Effect of Visible Light Waves on Aerthritis Pain: A Controlled Study'

141. ***Brain/Mind Bulletin*** 15, (4), January 1990, p 1.

142. ***J Appl Physiol*** 92: 1378-1382, 2002; Vol. 92, Issue 4, 1378-1382, April 2002 Early contributions of Russian stress and exercise physiologists, **Viru.A.**

143. http://www.fractal.org/Life-Science-Technology/Peter-Gariaev.htm

144. http://www.emergentmind.org/gariaev06.htm

145. http://homepages.ihug.co.nz/~sai/quanbiol.htm. Gariaev.P.P, Birshtein.B.I, Iarochenko.A.M, Marcer.P.J, Tertishny.G.G, Leonova.K.A, Kaempf.U, "The DNA-wave Biocomputer"

146. Gorizontov P.D. Role of hormones in general adaptation syndrome and diseases of adaptation (in Russian). ***Klin Med (Mosk)*** 34: 20-29, 1956.

147. Gorizontov P.D (Editor). *Homeostasis.* Moscow: ***Medicina,*** 1976.

148. Gorizontov, PD. Disputable questions of adaptation diseases and the stress problems (in Russian). ***Klin Med (Mosk)*** 55: 3-11, 1977

149. Urazaev A.M, Kulakov Iu.A, Medvedev M.A; Physiological characteristics of adaptation processes which precede the restructuring of functional systems. ***Dokl Akad Nauk SSSR.*** 1987; 295(6):1509-12.

150. Zagulova.D.V, Podkopaeva T.I, Vasil'ev.V.N, Medvedev M.A, Effect of audiovisual stimulation on heart rhythm variability.***Bull Exp Biol Med.*** 2001 Mar;131(3):273-5.

151. Masterova E.I, Vasil'ev V.N, Nevidimova T.I, Medvedev M.A. Immunologic response of healthy individuals to audiovisual stimulation. ***Biull Eksp Biol Med.*** 1999 Aug;127(8):204-6.

152. Nesterenko AI, Vasil'ev VN, Medvedev MA, Robenkova TV., Physiological and psychological characteristics of dependency of the organism on the type of personality, ***Fiziol Cheloveka.*** 2003 Nov-Dec;29(6):79-85.

153. Novikov.VS, Sharmin IA, Bornovsky VN 1992 A trial of the Pharmacological Correction of Sleep Disorders of Sailors during a Voyage , **Military Medical Journal** 8, 47-49

154. Novikov VS. "Psycho-physiological Support of Combat Activities of Military Personnel". ***Mil Med J.*** 1996; No. 4, P 37-40.

155. Sapov IA, Kuleshov VI, Levshin IV, et al. The acid-base status of the human body during the breathing of air with an admixture of different concentrations of carbon dioxide. *Fiziol Cheloveka 1990 Jan-Feb; 16(1) :127-32*

156. Sudakov, VK. *General Theory of Functional Systems.* Moscow: *Medicina*, 1984.

157. *Neurosci Behav Physiol.* 1987 Nov-Dec;17(6):480-8. Oligopeptides in the formation of biological motivations. Sudakov.K.V. P. K. Anokhin Institute of Normal Physiology, Academy of Medical Sciences of the USSR, Moscow.

158. *Zh Evol Biokhim Fiziol* 1990 Jan-Feb;26(1):120-9. The genetic determination of functions: oligopeptides in the systemogenesis of behavioral acts Sudakov.K.V. Oligopeptides in the formation of biological motivations. *Neurosci Behav Physiol.* 1987 Nov-Dec;17(6):480-8.

159. *Fiziol Zh SSSR Im I.M.Sechenova* 1988 Jan;74(1):8-16. Gene determination of physiological functions: experimental approaches based on the functional systems theory. Sudakov KV.

160. Methodology of the theory of Functional Systems in the Design of Devices for Control of Human Physiological Systems, Yumatov Y. A. ; *Vestnik Akademii medicinskih nauk SSSR* (Vestn. Akad. med. nauk SSSR) 1997, n°12, pp. 40-45 pub. *Medicina*, Moskva, RUSSIE, FEDERATION DE (1946- 1992) (Revue)

161. http://www.the-aps.org/publications/tphys/legacy/1992/issue4/140.pdf

162. Analysis of complex physiological systems by information flow: a time scale-specific complexity assessment, Hoyer.D, Birgit F, Pompe.B, Schmidt.H, Werdan K, Müller-Werdan.U, Baranowski.R, Żebrowski.J.J, Meissner.W, Kletzin.U, Adler.D, Adler.S, Blickhan.R *Biomedizinische Technik/Biomedical Engineering*, 51, (2) Special Issue: Biosignal Processing, July 2006, pp41-48

163. Learning Qualitative Models from Physiological Signals (1994) D.T. Hau, Coiera.E.W, *AAAI Symposium on AI in Medicine - Interpreting Clinical Data*

164. Rev Chir Oncol Radiol O R L Oftalmol Stomatol Otorinolaringol. 1975 Oct-Dec;20(4):269-76. Audiogram changes in diabetes mellitus. Mosora.N, Prodan.N, Bota.D.

165. http://www.ieptherapy.com/page/17eod/Services/Auditory_Integration_Therapy.html

166. http://beingdyslexic.co.uk/forums/index.php?s=b7ef428accb45ba54cbede069a628829&showtopic=493&pid=4188&st=0&#entry4188

167. *European Archives of Oto-Rhino-Laryngology*, Volume 257, Number 3 / April, 2000, 124-127

168. *Circulation.* 2000;101:1812, Dilated Cardiomyopathy and Sensorineural Hearing Loss, Schönberger.J, et al

169. **http://www.drf.org/hearing_health/viewpoints/032304.htm**

170.  "Presbycusis Study of a Relatively Noise-Free Population in the Sudan," American Otological Society, *Transactions*, vol. 50, 1962, pp. 135-152. Rosen.S

171.  Medical Assessment and Treatment, *Evid. Based Complement. Altern. Med.*, Advance Access published on October 5, 2006;

172.  Virtual Scanning, *Journal of Alternative & Complementary Medicine*, Volume 13 no2, Ewing G., Ewing E., Hankey A.

173.  Joshi.K, Hankey.A, Patwardhan.B, Traditional Phytochemistry: Identification of Drug by 'Taste', **Evid. Based Complement. Altern. Med.**, Advance Access published on October 5, 2006;

174.  Hankey.A, Studies of Advanced Stages of Meditation in the Tibetan Buddhist and Vedic Traditions. I: A Comparison of General Changes *Evid. Based Complement. Altern. Med.*, Advance Access published on July 31, 2006;

175.  Hankey.A, CAM and Post-Traumatic Stress Disorder *Evid. Based Complement. Altern. Med.*, Advance Access published on July 6, 2006;

176.  "Cognition," Microsoft® Encarta® Online Encyclopedia 2007 http://uk.encarta.msn.com

177.  Kandel.E, Nobel Prize for Physiology 2000: *Scientific American Mind* May 2006

178.  Fields.D.R: 'Beyond the Neuron Doctrine': *Scientific American Mind* June/July 2006 p 21–27

179.  http://www.le.ac.uk/biology/phh4/bioastral/

# Chapter 4

# The Available Evidence

compiled and edited by

Graham Ewing

## 4.1 Government Approvals & Certifications

*Virtual Scanning is Approved in Russia, Ukraine, and other former Soviet republics.*

The "Virtual Scanner" system was evaluated by S.F.Vladimirskiy at the MONIKI Scientific Research Institute in Moscow. As a result, the Ministry of Health of the Russian Federation certificated the use (certificate no 036 dd 19.01.00) of the software by the public health service.

It obtained the official registration for computer programs; certificate no 980696 (dated the 7th of December, 1998); which was authorized by the Russian agency of patents and trade marks (Rospatent).

MIMEX, the originator company, was established on the 4th of December, 1989, though the staff formation and the start of technology development had commenced in 1986 at the University of Krasnoyarsk.

The Personal Biological modeling technology developed for this medical application has been used in laser therapy computing systems, and diagnostic systems "Virtual Scanner" versions 1 & 3 –7 [1].

In September 2006 Virtual Scanning became a CE-marked technology following 14 months consideration by the Medicines and Healthcare Regulatory Authority in the UK.

## 4.2 Performance of Virtual Scanning

1.      The first significant report on Virtual Scanning's diagnostic capabilities was in an article by Vysochin Y in 2002 (see appendix A), in which a team of medical researchers from the **Lesgaft Institute** 2 reported on the diagnosis of 370 patients.

The condition of 305 patients (23 medical categories including encephalopathies, arthropathies, hypertension, gastritis, cholecystitis and various digestive system disorders) were subsequently confirmed by conventional methods of medical diagnosis.

The remaining 65 were either false positives or were diagnosed at the earlier pre-symptomatic stage i.e. at a stage of development which was earlier than could be detected by conventional diagnostic test procedures.  The article concluded that Virtual Scanning is up to 21% more sensitive as a system of medical assessment than conventional laboratory methods (see table 1).

The same article reports on the therapeutic effectiveness of Virtual Scanning in a study of 1672 patients and of the positive recovery of 93.2% in patients with a wide and varied list of medical disorders (see table 2).

## TABLE 1: Evaluation of Virtual Scanning Diagnosis: 370 patients

| № | Diagnosis | № of Patients diagnosed by Virtual Scanning | № of Patients confirmed by conventional techniques | Effectiveness |
|---|---|---|---|---|
| 1 | Vegetative-vascular Distony | 14 | 10 | 71,4 % |
| 2 | Encephalopathy | 4 | 4 | 100,0 % |
| 3 | Cerebrovascular Disorders | 28 | 22 | 78,6 % |
| 4 | Acute Bronchitis | 12 | 10 | 83,3 % |
| 5 | Chronic Bronchitis | 11 | 9 | 81,8 % |
| 6 | Acute Rhinitis | 16 | 13 | 81,5 % |
| 7 | Tonsillitis | 13 | 11 | 84,6 % |
| 8 | Chronic Otitis | 3 | 3 | 100,0 % |
| 9 | Ankilosing Spondilitis | 6 | 5 | 83,3 % |
| 10 | Vertebral Osteoarthrosis | 34 | 30 | 88,2 % |
| 11 | Intercostal Neuralgia | 11 | 8 | 72,7 % |
| 12 | Polyneuropathies | 11 | 9 | 81,8 % |
| 13 | Ischaemic Heart Disease | 9 | 7 | 77,8 % |
| 14 | Hypertension | 33 | 27 | 81,8 % |
| 15 | Chronic Pyelonephritis | 6 | 5 | 83,3 % |
| 16 | Nephrolithiasis | 11 | 9 | 81,8 % |
| 17 | Chronic Gastritis | 29 | 24 | 82,8 % |
| 18 | Peptic Ulcer Diseases | 22 | 19 | 86,4 % |
| 19 | Chronic Pancreatitis | 16 | 12 | 75,0 % |
| 20 | Chronic Hepatitis | 5 | 4 | 80,0 % |
| 21 | Chronic Cholecystitis | 46 | 39 | 84,8 % |
| 22 | Cholelithiasis | 13 | 10 | 76,9 % |
| 23 | Diabetes Mellitus | 17 | 15 | 88,2 % |
| | Totals | 370 | 305 | 82,4 % |

## TABLE 2:   Evaluation of Virtual Scanning Therapy: 1672 patients

| № | Diagnosis | № of patients | № of therapy courses | Effectiveness |
|---|---|---|---|---|
| 1 | Chronic Fatigue Syndrome | 43 | 1 | 97,7% |
| 2 | Depressive and Anxiety Disorders | 54 | 1-2 | 96,3 |
| 3 | Organic Disorders/Diseases of CNS | 26 | 1-2 | 95,0% |
| 4 | Vegetative-vascular Distony | 96 | 1-2 | 85,0% |
| 5 | Cerebrovascular Disorders | 46 | 1+ massage | 97,8% |
| 6 | Spinal Circulation Disorders | 57 | 1+ massage | 100% |
| 7 | Cerebral Palsy | 12 | 1+ medications | 100% |
| 8 | Chronic Bronchitis | 37 | 1-2 | 100% |
| 9 | Bronchial Asthma | 12 | 2 | 91,7% |
| 10 | Chronic Tonsillitis | 7 | 1 | 100% |
| 11 | Chronic Otitis | 8 | 1 | 100% |
| 12 | Ischaemic Heart Disease | 63 | 1-2 | 90,5% |
| 13 | Chronic Cardiac Insufficiency | 11 | 1-2 | 81,8% |
| 14 | Cardiac Arrhythmias | 12 | 1-2 | 83,0% |
| 15 | Myocarditis | 30 | 1-3 | 93,3% |
| 16 | Hypertension | 120 | 1-2 | 87,5% |
| 17 | Chronic and Acute Gastritis | 105 | 1-2 | 98,1% |
| 18 | Chronic Duodenitis | 29 | 1 | 100% |
| 19 | Peptic Ulcer Diseases | 75 | 1-2 | 100% |
| 20 | Chronic Hepatitis | 53 | 1-2 | 92,5% |
| 21 | Chronic Cholecystitis | 58 | 1-2 | 98,3% |
| 22 | Dyskinesia Biliary Ducts | 52 | 2 | 100% |
| 23 | Cholelithiasis | 15 | 1-2 | 86,7% |
| 24 | Chronic Pancreatitis | 49 | 1 | 85,7% |
| 25 | Nephrolithiasis | 42 | 2 | 86,5% |
| 26 | Pyelonephritis | 26 | 2 | 84,6% |
| 27 | Hydronephrosis | 2 | 2 | 100% |
| 28 | Cystitis | 12 | 3 | 83,0% |
| 29 | Prostatitis | 70 | 2 | 94,3% |
| 30 | Disorders of Thyroid Gland | 73 | 1 | 93,2% |
| 31 | Hypofunction of Adrenal Cortex | 21 | 1-2 | 61,9% |
| 32 | Ovarian Cyst | 14 | 1 | 86,0% |
| 33 | Mastopathy | 18 | 2-3 + medications | 83,0% |
| 34 | Gynaecological Diseases | 40 | 1 | 100% |
| 35 | Diabetes Mellitus | 31 | 1-2 | 100% |
| 36 | Musculoskeletal Syst Disorders | 19 | 1 + medications | 100% |
| 37 | Vertebral Osteoarthrosis | 168 | 1-3 | 93,5% |
| 38 | Gout | 26 | 1 | 100% |
| 39 | Ankylosing Spondilitis | 40 | 1-2 | 95,0% |
| | Totals | 1672 | | 93,2% |

In the report, 'effective' is defined as a 'distinct and indisputable improvement in the condition'.

## The report's conclusions

1.  The clinical research, which have been carried out on a large number of patients (370 people – diagnosis; 1672 people – treatment), has proven

    - high accuracy of diagnosis (82.4% of findings confirmed by clinical diagnosis)

    - high efficiency of treatment (93.2% recoveries and significant improvements).

2.  Research involving electroencephalography (EEG) and polymyography (PMG) established that "Virtual Scanner" therapy results in

    - fast and considerable increase of adaptability and percentage of alpha rhythm

    - improved condition of the Central Nervous System due to increased **Development Rate and the force of Inhibiting processes (DRI)**, increased **Activity of Inhibiting Systems (AIS)**,

    - and that increased regulation of cerebral activity results in considerably increased stress rate, maximum force, relaxation rate and improved condition of the NeuroMuscular System.

3.  Significant and positive changes of Central Nervous System and NeuroMuscular System are accompanied by improved physical activity and condition of the Cardiovascular system.

    - After 20 "Virtual Scanner" system sessions the **Frequency of Cordial 4 Clonus in quiescence 5 (FCC$_q$)** and in period of **rehabilitation (FCCr)** decreased by 8.9% and 5% resp, while work capacity (**N$_p$**) and speed endurance increased by 13.2% and 12.8%resp.

    - **Heart Activity Efficiency Factor (HAEF), Pulse Recovery Rate (PRR)** and **General Efficiency (GE)** increased by 15.6%, 20% and 17.5% resp.

    - After 5, 10 and 20 "Virtual Scanner" sessions the **Possibility of Injury (IP)** and Musculoskeletal system diseases, and also the heart overstress decreased by 15%, 16.8% and 18.1% resp.

      *That enables us to conclude that "Virtual Scanner" therapy is an effective preventative measure for overstress, injury and musculoskeletal system disease and prevention of cordial overstress at hard physical and psycho-emotional load.*

4.  "Virtual Scanner" therapy improves the condition of the Central Nervous System. This is subsequently manifest as improved muscle relaxation, physical activity, heart function, coordination of system and organ activity (which limit physical

efficiency), and reduced susceptibility to injury, musculoskeletal system diseases and cordial overstress.

5. "Virtual Scanner" is a high-performance system and absolutely suitable for wide application not only in public health service (for treatment and prophylaxis of different pathological processes).

   It is effective *in any kinds of sport or professional human activity that requires correction for the influence of psychological stress; normalization of the regulatory system; inhibition of the Central Nervous System; increased muscle relaxation, economy and effectiveness of CardioVascular System activity, mental and physical activity, and survival under extreme conditions.*

6. Taking into account the minimum time spent for complex diagnostics is less than 10-15 minutes and that treatment sessions last typically 15-20 minutes, and also the main object of informational correction is normalisation of regulatory control of cerebral functions, it is anticipated that the *"Virtual Scanner" system will be applicable in all areas of human activity concerned with hard physical and psycho-emotional load; improved regulation of movement and coordination, physical activity, endurance; and improved stability stress-generating factors.*

   *This will be particularly relevant to those in* sport, choreography, ballet, rescuers, firemen, landing troops, emergency platoons, aviation, cosmonautics and others.

**2.    Various independent medical institutes in Russia have reported on their experiences with Virtual Scanning e.g.**

**(i)    Dr V.A. Ignatiev, Director and Urologist, Limited Company "Novator",** City of Siktivkar (Republic of Komy in Siberia):

Reports in a study of over 3,000 patients tested during the period 1999- 2004, confirmation of results by conventional diagnostic procedures in 98% of cases, and of positive response of 656 patients to Virtual Scanning therapy out of a total of 711 patients i.e. a 92.3% (see table 3).

## TABLE 3: Evaluation of Virtual Scanning Therapy: 711 patients

| No | DIAGNOSIS | No of Patients | Treatment Modules | No of Sessions | Positiv Results | Effectiv ness % |
|----|-----------|----------------|-------------------|----------------|-----------------|-----------------|
| 1 | Cerebrovascular Disorders | 49 | Brain | 49 | 47 | 95 |
| 2 | Chronic Fatigue Syndrome | 43 | Brain | 43 | 42 | 98 |
| 3 | Epilepsy | 4 | Brain&Spinal Cord | 4 + 2 | 4 | 100 |
| 4 | Migraine | 41 | Brain | 41 | 36 | 88 |
| 5 | Ankilosing Spondilitis | 28 | SC, PNS & SMS | 28+28+28 | 27 | 96 |
| 6 | Arthropathies – any joint diseases (expl.: arthritis.) | 22 | SMS | 22 | 14 | 64 |
| 7 | Musculoskeletal Disorders | 98 | SC, PNS & SMS | 102 | 96 | 98 |
| 8 | Myocarditis | 15 | Heart | 15 | 13 | 87 |
| 9 | Hypertension | 45 | Adrenal&Brain | 45 + 45 | 32 | 71 |
| 10 | Hypofunction of Thyroid | 22 | Thyroid Gland | 22 + 22 | 21 | 95 |
| 11 | Thyroiditis | 22 | Thyroid Gland | 22 + 22 | 20 | 91 |
| 12 | Chronic Bronchitis | 6 | Lungs&Bronchi | 6 | 6 | 100 |
| 13 | Chronic Sinusitis | 3 | Nose | 3 | 2 | 67 |
| 14 | Allergic Rhinitis | 8 | Nose | 8 | 5 | 63 |
| 15 | Chronic Otitis | 8 | Ear | 8 | 8 | 100 |
| 16 | Oesophagitis | 2 | Oesophagus | 2 | 2 | 100 |
| 17 | Chronic Gastritis | 63 | Stomach | 63 | 61 | 97 |
| 18 | Peptic Ulcer Diseases | 32 | Stomach&Duodenum | 12 + 32 | 32 | 100 |
| 19 | Chronic Pancreatitis | 11 | Pancreas | 11 | 11 | 100 |
| 20 | Chronic Cholecystitis | 13 | Gall Bladder | 13 | 13 | 100 |
| 21 | Postcholecystectomy Syndrome | 8 | Gall Bladder | 8 | 8 | 100 |
| 22 | Chronic Hepatitis | 6 | Liver | 6 | 6 | 100 |
| 23 | Dyskinesia Biliary Ducts | 16 | Gall Bladder | 16 | 16 | 100 |
| 24 | Chronic Gastroenteritis | 2 | Small Intestine | 2 | 2 | 100 |
| 25 | Chronic Colitis | 6 | Large Intestine | 6 | 5 | 83 |
| 26 | Chronic Pyelonephritis | 12 | Kidneys | 12 | 12 | 100 |
| 27 | Cystitis | 15 | Bladder | 15 | 13 | 87 |
| 28 | Nephrolithiasis | 13 | Kidney&Bladder | 13 +13 | 13 | 100 |
| 29 | Male infertility | 10 | BrainProstateBladd | 10+10+10 | 8 | 80 |
| 30 | Female infertility | 10 | BrainOvariesWomb | 10+10+10 | 8 | 80 |
| 31 | Chronic Prostatitis | 46 | Prostate & Bladder | 46 + 30 | 46 | 100 |
| 32 | Adenoma of Prostate | 12 | Prostate & Bladder | 36 + 36 | 10 | 83 * |
| 33 | Chronic Adnexitis | 6 | Ovaries & Womb | 6 + 6 | 6 | 100 |
| 34 | Menstrual CycleDisorder | 5 | Ovaries & Womb | 5 + 5 | 4 | 80 |
| 35 | Allergodermatitis | 9 | Skin & Liver | 9 + 9 | 7 | 78 |

* size of adenomas reduced from 2 cm and less)

**(ii)** **Dr Kolyanov V.G., Head of Neurology Department of Medical Rehabilitation Centre,** (Pyatigorsk City, Siberia):

reported on the diagnosis of >4,500 patients and of an 89% positive response to therapy in >1,600 patients treated using Virtual Scanning therapy

He commented:

(1) 'upon the ability of the system to reveal disorders from the early stages of illnesses, and to carry out informational therapy according to the individual condition of each patient. These were considered to be crucial in improving the effectiveness of preventative and rehabilitative medicine'.

(2) Effectiveness of informational therapy within patients undergoing this treatment as following:

- Significant improvement – 67,7%
- Improvement – 21,3%
- Insignificant improvement – 5%
- Without changes – 6%
- Worsening – 0%

(3) Especially interesting cases of "difficult" conditions such as migraine, depression, including endogenic, night wetting, phobias, etc. The treatment of vegetative syndromes of children is especially successful.

(4) Despite the fact that pathology, which is detected for the first time by VS, still needs to be confirmed by other conventional methods the system "VIRTUAL SCANNER" can be used as a tool for quick screening tests.

(5) Taking in consideration all foregoing, the system "VIRTUAL SCANNER" (especially it's latest versions) could be successfully used in complex methods of rehabilitation of patients.

**(iii) Dr Z.Sarsinbayeva and Dr S.Sarsinbayeva.**, Alma Ata, Kazakhstan:

reported on the diagnosis of 2077 patients (96.7% congruence with conventional means of diagnosis – table 4) and of a 95.1% positive response to therapy in 128 patients treated using Virtual Scanning therapy (see table 5).

## TABLE 4: Evaluation of Virtual Scanning Diagnosis

| No | DIAGNOSIS | № of Patients diagnosed by Virtual Scanning | № of Patients confirmed by conventional techniques | Effectiveness % |
|----|-----------|-----------|-----------|-----------|
| 01 | Encephalopathies | 22 | 20 | 90.9 |
| 02 | Cerebrovascular Disorders | 130 | 123 | 95.0 |
| 03 | Consequences of brain trauma | 8 | 8 | 100 |
| 04 | Arthropathies – any joint diseases (expl.: arthritis.) | 257 | 257 | 100 |
| 05 | Ischaemic Heart Diseases | 51 | 48 | 93.2 |
| 06 | Hypertension | 134 | 132 | 98.5 |
| 07 | Chronic Pyelonephritis | 117 | 115 | 98.3 |
| 08 | Nephrolithiasis | 72 | 65 | 72.7 |
| 09 | Chronic Gastroduodenitis | 215 | 213 | 99.0 |
| 10 | Peptic Ulcer Diseases | 28 | 24 | 85.7 |
| 11 | Chronic Pancreatitis | 29 | 25 | 86.2 |
| 12 | Chronic Cholecystitis | 337 | 337 | 100 |
| 13 | Cholelithiasis | 18 | 16 | 88.8 |
| 14 | Chronic Colitis | 115 | 110 | 95.6 |
| 15 | Diabetes Mellitus | 67 | 56 | 83.5 |
| 16 | Uterine Fibroids, Mastopathies | 13 | 11 | 90.3 |
| 17 | Anaemia | 260 | 250 | 96.0 |
| 18 | Thrombophlebitis, Varicose Veins | 78 | 76 | 97.6 |
| 19 | Allergodermatitis | 112 | 109 | 97.3 |
| 20 | Post operational scarring (adhesions) | 14 | 14 | 100 |

## TABLE 5: Evaluation of Virtual Scanning Therapy: 128 patients

| No | Diagnosis | No of Patients | Results of Treatment | | | | | |
| | | | Significant Improvement | | Improvement | | No changes | |
| | | | Abs. | % | Abs. | % | Abs. | % |
|---|---|---|---|---|---|---|---|---|
| 1 | Ischaemic Heart Disease | 12 | 7 | 58.3 | 4 | 33.3 | 1 | 8.4 |
| 2 | Hypertension | 19 | 10 | 52.6 | 4 | 21 | 5 | 26.4 |
| 3 | Cerebrovascular Disorders | 12 | 12 | 100 | - | - | - | - |
| 4 | Peptic Ulcer Diseases | 21 | 15 | 71.4 | 6 | 28.6 | - | - |
| 5 | Chronic Cholecystitis | 24 | 22 | 91.6 | 2 | 8.4 | - | - |
| 6 | Chronic Pancreatitis | 11 | 8 | 72.7 | 3 | 27.3 | - | - |
| 7 | Diabetes Mellitus | 2 | 1 | 50 | 1 | 50 | - | - |
| 8 | Musculoskeletal System Disorders | 27 | 20 | 74 | 6 | 22.2 | 1 | 3.8 |
| | | 128 | 95 | 71.35 | 26 | 23.85 | 1 | 4.8 |

# 3.    A Preliminary Analysis of the Effect of Virtual Scanning Therapy on Biochemical parameters of Patients

This is illustrated in the articles below. These illustrates that the changes in blood content i.e. improved phagocytosis activity, improved activity of granulocytes, improved lymphocyte population, increased killer cell population; and the improved functioning of the organism was subsequently confirmed by Vysochin in article.

Also, that EEG (electroencephalograph), PMG (polymyography) and other procedures were used to determine the claimed improvements that "Virtual Scanner" therapeutic sessions

- lead to the fast recovery and essential increase of adaptability;

- Frequency of Cordial Clonus in quiescence 3-5 decreases considerably;

- Efficiency and high-speed endurance increase;

- Heart Activity Efficiency Factor (HAEF) increases

- Pulse Recovery Rate (PRR) increases

- and General Efficiency (GE) of organs and systems increase.

Origin of the data: Moscow City Zelenograd Administrative District Public Health Service Office; Government Establishment Reg. No 000575; Out-patients' Clinic No 152:

The objective assessment was obtained by investigating blood content and correlative/comparative analysis of blood tests before and after the treatment. The research showed:

- The level of immunoglobulins (IgG, 19A, IgM -Mancini technique -single radial immunodiffusion) was within the normal reference range for all patients.

- Absolute quantity of lymphocytes was within the normal limits for all patients in the first investigation, and increased for 50% of patients in the second investigation.

- Phagocytosis activity of neutrophils with latex particles was within the normal limits and was not changed. Total phagocytosis activity averaged 1.42 for the group of patient in the first investigation and 1.53 in the second investigation, so far increased slightly.

- The amount of neutrophil-lysosomal-cationic proteins identifying non-enzymatic bactericidal activity of granulocytes (Shubitch M. G. method - cytochemical bioassay) was evaluated by the average-cytochemical coefficient (ACC). In the first investigation all patient had lower ACC values (group-average ACC=1.35), but in the second investigation -1.61 (was within the normal range of 1.5 to 1.7).

- Evaluation of lymphocyte population was carried out by indirect fluorescence staining immunoassay using mono clonal antibodies (Sorbent Ltd). Each patient had CD3 and CD4 subpopulation within the normal reference range in the first and second investigations but slightly elevated in the second investigation compared to the first investigation results.

- Natural killer cells' ( CD 16) subpopulation was slightly higher than normal in the second investigation.

The results indicate that Virtual Scanning light therapy has a positive effect on immune-system related measures in the blood stream [82].

**4. Virtual Scanning [6,7] appears able to diagnose medical conditions at a pre-symptomatic level i.e. BEFORE they manifest gross symptoms.**

- Conditions such as rhinitis, migraine, pneumonia, and prostate cancer have been diagnosed prior to onset of symptoms with subsequent confirmation by conventional diagnostic procedures at a later date.

- A duodenal ulcer diagnosed when a GP's repeat diagnosis failed to identify it was confirmed when the patient was hospitalized with the condition.

- Conditions can be monitored over time to note the progress of Virtual Scanning light therapy, or indeed any other therapy, and hence to track the regression of medical symptoms of concern.

- Many conditions for which forms of medical diagnosis are non-existent or inadequate can be diagnosed by Virtual Scanning e.g.

    Migraine
    Epilepsy
    Chronic Fatigue Syndrome
    Fibromyalgia
    Irritable Bowel Syndrome
    Dyslexia
    Asthma
    Chronic Obstructive Pulmonary Disorder
    Bronchiectatic Disease

- In several cases of these pathologies, it has proved possible to demonstrate that the patient has been predisposed to a medical condition throughout their adult life.

- There are few, if any, cases where Virtual Scanning version 7G has not been able to diagnose a medical condition, or has misdiagnosed a medical condition.

Indications of misdiagnosis using Virtual Scanning version 7G appear rare.

**5.** **In a number of cases, Virtual Scanning has been able to correctly diagnose medical conditions despite the failure of conventional diagnostic procedures and technologies to confirm the diagnosis.**

Example 1:     a lady who complained of duodenal problems. Her GP was unable to confirm the existence of any problems despite repeated examinations and dismissed the possibility that there could be a problem despite being advised that Virtual Scanning identified reasonable cause to doubt the diagnosis and of the possibility of a duodenal ulcer. The lady subsequently suffered from a perforated duodenal ulcer which required hospitalisation.

Example 2:     of a lady who, several years earlier, had a bone-marrow transplant and chemotherapy to treat leukaemia. Her blood samples indicated that she did not have a problem. Virtual Scanning identified changes, which seemed to indicate reoccurrence of her leukaemia including 'functional changes and neoplasm'. On the next blood sample leukaemia was diagnosed. The lady has subsequently undergone a further bone-marrow transplant and chemotherapy.

Example 3:     of a man of c85 years. Virtual Scanning identified type 2 diabetes. It took two further years before this was diagnosed by his GP.

## 6. On a number of occasions Virtual Scanning has diagnosed medical conditions *before* their symptoms subsequently manifested.

Example 1: a lady tested by Virtual Scanning and identified with **rhinitis** commented that she did not have rhinitis but phoned several days after the consultation to confirm that she had subsequently developed a cold/bacterial infection.

Example 2: a lady clearly suffering from breathing problems was identified to have **pneumonia**. The pneumonia manifested severely the week following the consultation and medical intervention was required.

Example 3: over a period of 1-2 years, regular tests on a man in his mid-fifties indicated steadily increasing preclinical levels of **migraine**. A **migraine** type event finally occurred in mid-2006.

Example 4: a man of c50 years was identified with advanced morphological changes in the **prostate gland**. These included indications of functional changes at a cellular level of the type that precede cancer, and neoplasm. Within a year prostate cancer was diagnosed.

Example 5: a lady of c50 years was identified with morphological change indicative of pancreatic cancer. These included indications of functional changes at a cellular level of the type that precede cancer, and neoplasm. Within two years pancreatic cancer was diagnosed.

## 7. Further discussion of the articles:

Virtual Scanning has been used to successfully treat patients with

(1)    Migraine, Chronic Fatigue Syndrome, Trigeminal Neuralgia, Headaches, Rheumatic aches and pains, Digestive system disorders, Dysarthria, Tinnitus, Slipped Disc, Depression, Eczema, Asthma and related breathing disorders such as emphysema;

(2)    Attention Deficit Disorder, Dyslexia;

(3)    Mood disorders, lack of motivation/lethargy, memory and concentration problems, lack of energy, etc.

(4)    Systems-related disorders e.g. Sleeping pattern disorders, Circulatory problems, Temperature regulation, Breathing disorders, etc.

but has had limited success treating ailments, which are due to

(1)    physical damage and are considered to be irreversible in nature

(2)    genetic characteristics

(3)    physiological deterioration, or which

(4)    are being treated by a cocktail of medications

It is necessary for patients to adhere to therapy as instructed. Best results seem to come from those with best adherence.

## 8. Examples of success measured as clearly evident, indisputably positive improvement in a patient's health:

- Significantly reduced frequency and/or magnitude of a migraine attack

- Recovery of the ability to speak

- Sleeping properly as compared to being completely unable to sleep at night

- Being able to breath without requiring an asthma inhaler

- Being freed from the discomfiture of irritable bowel syndrome

- Being freed from depression

- Being able to jog around their village whereas previously they had been chronically fatigued, listless and deprived of energy and motivation.
- Being able to read a book whereas by comparison they were previously unable to do so.
- Being freed from the tranquilising effect of epilepsy medication and hence being able to resume an active life.
- Being freed from the ringing-in-the-ears effect which is tinnitus

- Having significantly improved memory and concentration

- Being able to walk freely without pain or restriction whereas by comparison the patient was immobilized or had severely limited movement in the legs and/or back
- Having improved feelings of wellbeing

- Having reduced weight

- Dyslexia: able to read a book compared to previously being unable to do so.

- Epilepsy; cessation of medication, removal of its tranquilizing effects, and hence being able to resume an active life.
- Tinnitus: cessation of its ringing-in-the-ears effect

- Memory and concentration: significant improvements

- Disability: an immobilized patient with severely limited movement in legs and back became able to walk freely without pain or restriction

- Obesity: reduced weight

## 4.3    Virtual Scanning: Assessment and Treatment of Migraine

Migraine is responsible for an estimated cost to the UK economy of >£750M. The condition affects an estimated 1 in 8 persons. There are no medical technologies which are able to diagnose a person's predisposition to this most distressing medical condition. There are no drugs which can alleviate the symptoms and there are no therapeutic approaches which are able to alleviate the cause.

The only options are medications which reduce the severity and longevity of migraine attacks. The success of these medications is considered to be, at best, around 50%.

The fundamental basis for the migraine condition remains the subject of conjecture and leaves fundamental questions unanswered. Low-blood pressure is widely considered by researchers in Germany [85] to be as damaging to health as high blood pressure. In addition low-blood pressure is often common for patients with migraine and is considered to be a statistically significant precursor to stroke.

## The Medical Basis for Migraine

A number of theories [83] have been proposed to explain the origins of Migraine including.

- the Vascular Theory

- the Cortical Spreading Depression Theory [84]

- the Neurovascular Hypothesis/Neurogenic Dural Inflammation Theory

- the Serotonergic Abnormalities/Vascular Hypothesis

- the Integrated Hypothesis

or is

- the result of abnormal firing of brain neurons

- the result of a heart abnormality, a Patent Foramen Ovale (PFO)

## Theoretical Summary

In general the above theories are based upon the observed phenomena (electrical, biophysical and biochemical) which can be detected in patients with Migraine. They deal with the alleviation of symptoms rather than of identifying the factors which have caused its development. It is only by identifying the fundamental causes that can lead to the development of drugs or therapies which will prevent the occurrence of migraine-type events.

Of the above theories, only the Integrated Hypothesis includes practical consideration of the fundamental stress-related factors which could activate specific centres which subsequently initiate a migraine attack.

Whatever the origins or theories there is widespread acceptance that the depressed electrical activity in the brain activates the trigeminal nerves and nociceptors in the meningeal and cerebral blood vessels and that migraine attacks happen because of vasodilation in the cranial blood vessels.

Interestingly most, if not all, of the above theories are unable to explain the relationship of migraine with menstruation in some women [87].

**The Therapeutic Options**

In practical terms the medical profession has few, if any, drugs which are reliably able to address and relieve the symptoms of migraine [86]. Perhaps this is because the medical condition remains poorly understood and because the therapeutic approach is oriented towards the alleviation of symptoms rather than the prevention of further attacks.

This is illustrated by considering the case of a lady of 59 years who was taken to hospital in an ambulance due to the severity of a Basilar-type migraine attack. During the day in hospital she was administered orally seven types of medication and then released, in her words 'not feeling a great deal better'. No-one could tell her why her migraine attack had occurred, or why on this occasion it was so very severe, or what she should do to avoid further attacks. She was advised to sleep in a darkened room until the migraine had run its course.

Of course, the use of medications do relieve the symptoms to some extent otherwise they would not successfully complete clinical trials and become approved for use. Nevertheless it is widely accepted that migraine medication are only circa 50/52% effective (ref Allen Roses, GSK, 2003). Their effectiveness remains subject to debate. The modern 5-HT type medications (triptans) are known to relieve symptoms only to leave the patient vulnerable to further migraine events within periods of typically 12-72 hours.

Interestingly the older forms of medication e.g. ergotamine (which has unpleasant side-effects) and paracetamol are often most effective when used in combination with Caffeine (a stimulant which raises blood pressure) and/or Aspirin (which is known to thin the blood) which is consistent with the need for improved flow of blood to the brain.

Migraine triggers include chocolate, soft drinks, tea and coffee, all of which contain caffeine [103-105].

Migraine medications claim only to relieve the symptoms of migraine. There are no recorded claims that they can tackle the origins of the medical condition and eliminate the fundamental cause(s).

# Examples of Success using Virtual Scanning Colour Therapy

- A Latvian lady in her early 40's: had tried all forms of conventional therapy offered by her GP and hospital but had experienced little or no improvement in her migraines. She came to Virtual Scanning in a search for something to remove the fundamental cause of her migraines and prevent their reoccurrence.

  Within one month following commencement of therapy she reported her migraine attacks to have ceased; the second month she reported improved mental clarity and cessation of her tinnitus. Since commencing therapy she has not had any further migraine attacks.

- A lady of 59 years who had been experiencing **migraine** attacks throughout her life: the attacks had recently become increasingly severe, the latest event being the worst, resulting in her being admitted to hospital in a semi-conscious state. During her day in hospital she was given 7 different types of medication. Then, no better, she was released and told to go home and remain in a dark room. No one in the hospital could tell her what had caused her migraine attacks or what she might do to prevent their reoccurrence!

  A Virtual Scanning assessment indicated her attacks to have been due to a combination of a number of factors including (1) impaired spinal circulation (2) spinal osteochondrosis (3) vertebral artery syndrome (4) idiopathic hypotension (variable and/or low blood pressure) and a number of lesser indications: they appeared to have been caused by the lack of blood-supply to the brain.

  The lady undertook a course of Virtual Scanning therapy and has not experienced any further migraines. Her life has been completely transformed. She has much improved health, less stress, less anger, less irritation, more patience and more to give to her family and friends.

example 1: Migraine, woman 54 years, 64 kgs.

**BRAIN**

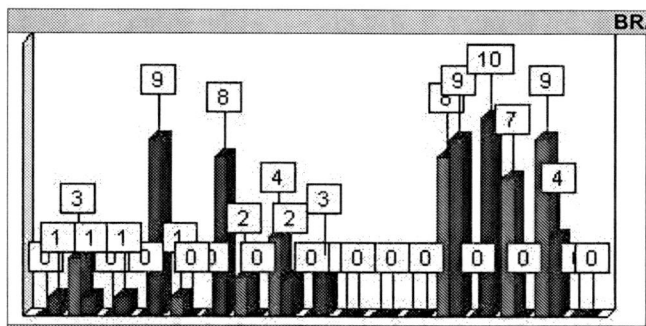

**Epilepsy: Compensatory signal.**
**Migraine: Pathology signal.**
**Verterbral Artery Syndrome: Expressed pathology signal.**
**Arachnoiditis: Expressed compensatory signal.**
**Impairment of cerebral circulation: Compensatory signal.**
Age-Related Changes: Expressed compensatory signal.

**SPINAL CORD**

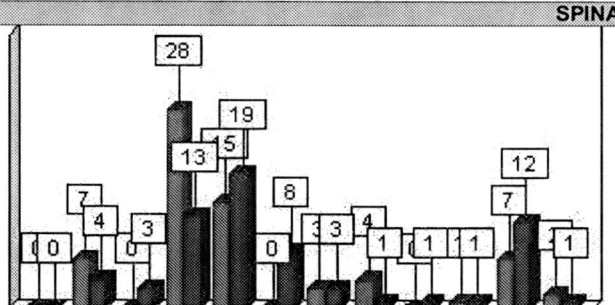

Degenerative Process: Weakening of compensatory abilities.
Allergic Process: Expressed pathology signal.
**Impairment of Spinal Circulation: Compensatory signal.**
Intoxication Effects: Compensatory signal.
Neoplasm: Compensatory signal.

**PERIPHERAL NERVOUS SYSTEM**

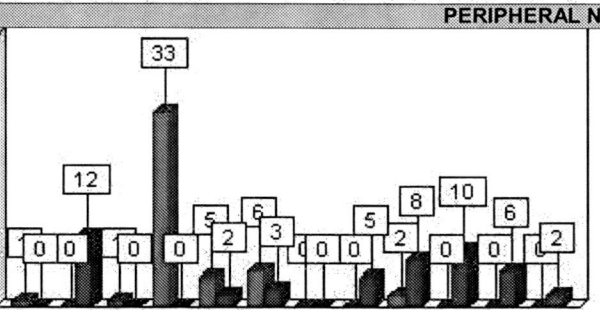

**Spinal Osteochondrosis with Neurological Effects:**
**Expressed pathology signal.**
Neuritis: Compensatory signal.
Age-Related Changes: Compensatory signal.
Radiculitis: Compensatory signal.

**EAR**

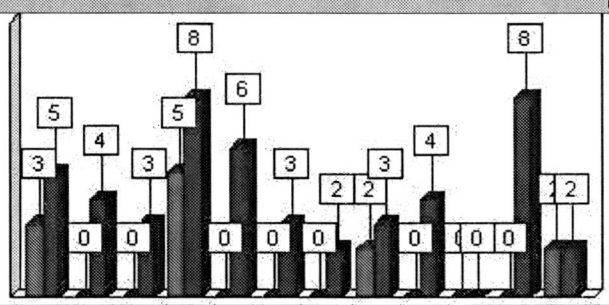

Degenerative Process: Compensatory signal.
Intoxication Effects: Compensatory signal.

**NOSE**

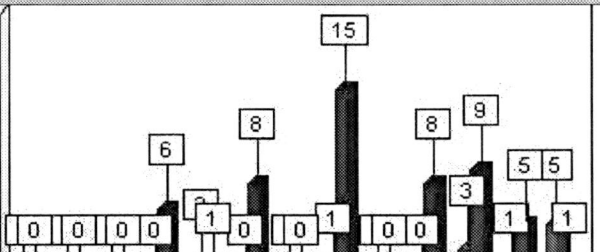

Intoxication Effects: Compensatory signal.
Age-Related Changes: Expressed compensatory signal.
Frontitis: Compensatory signal.
Degenerative Process: Compensatory signal.

**PITUITARY GLAND**

184

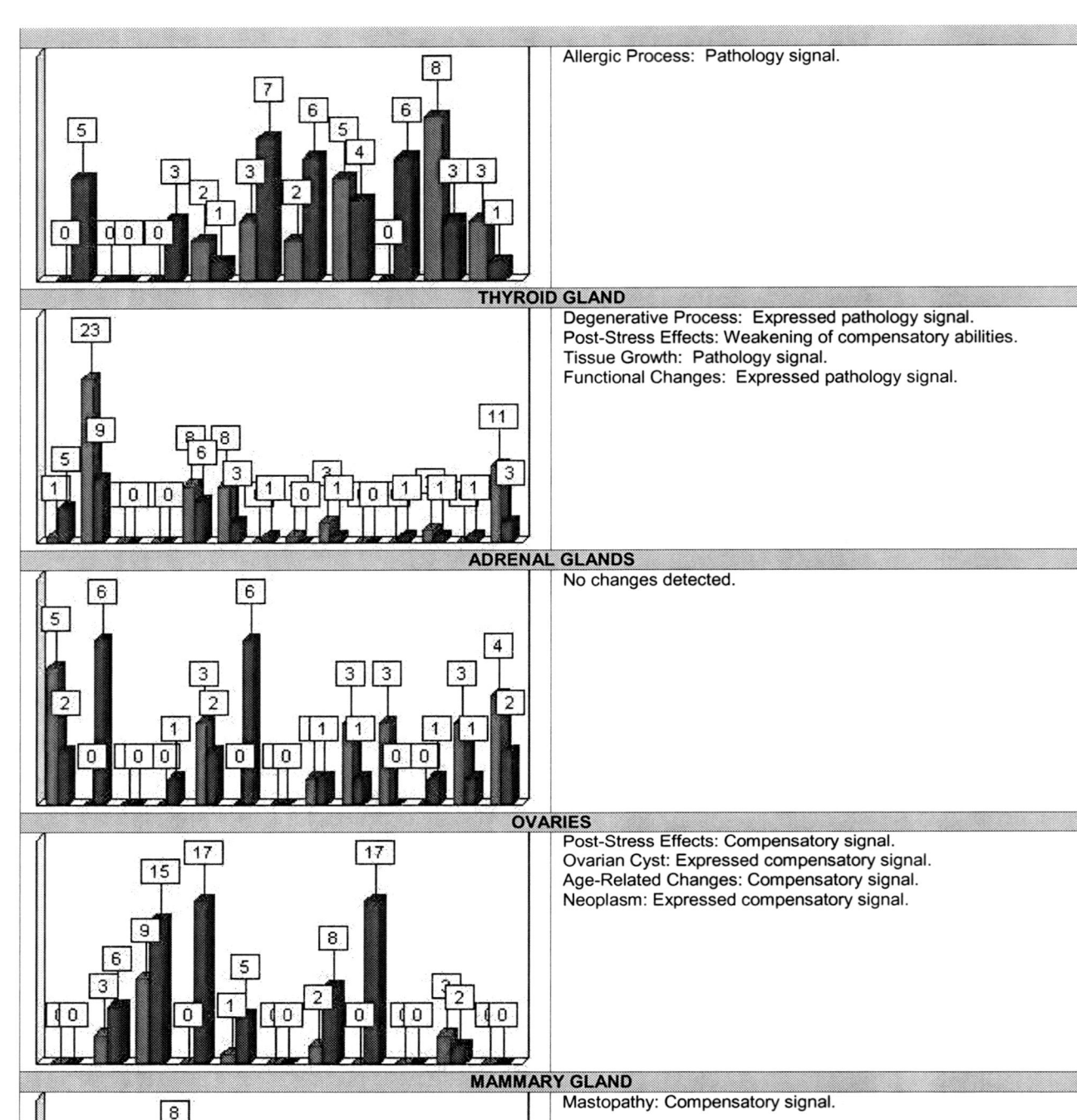

Allergic Process: Pathology signal.

**THYROID GLAND**

Degenerative Process: Expressed pathology signal.
Post-Stress Effects: Weakening of compensatory abilities.
Tissue Growth: Pathology signal.
Functional Changes: Expressed pathology signal.

**ADRENAL GLANDS**

No changes detected.

**OVARIES**

Post-Stress Effects: Compensatory signal.
Ovarian Cyst: Expressed compensatory signal.
Age-Related Changes: Compensatory signal.
Neoplasm: Expressed compensatory signal.

**MAMMARY GLAND**

Mastopathy: Compensatory signal.

185

## LIVER

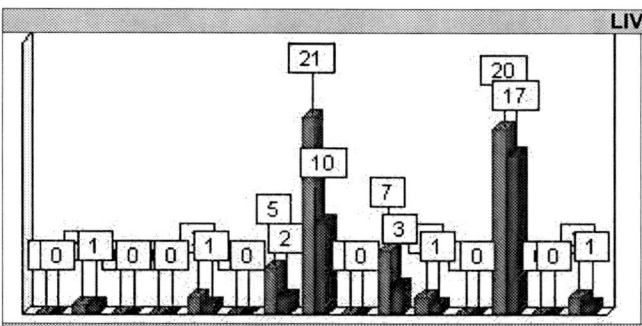

Degenerative Process: Expressed pathology signal.
Disruption of Bilirubin Metabolism: Pathology signal.
Liver Insufficiency: Weakening of compensatory abilities.

## GALL BLADDER

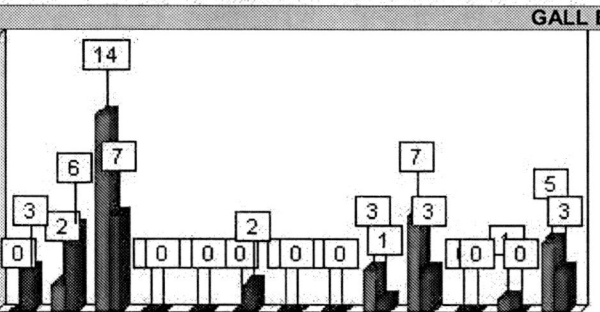

Post-Stress Effects: Expressed pathology signal.
Chronic Fatigue: Pathology signal.

## PANCREAS

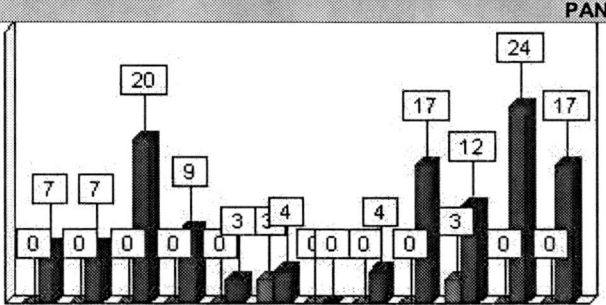

Tension of compensatory abilities.

## HEART

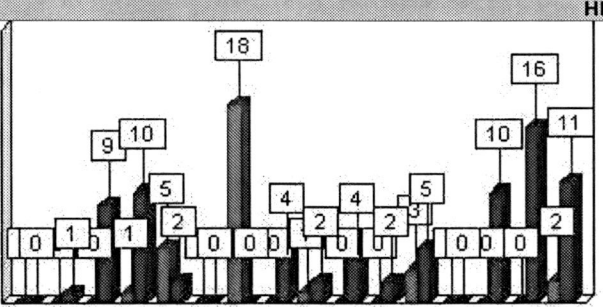

**Cardiac Infarction: Pathology signal.**
Chronic Fatigue: Expressed pathology signal.
Tension of compensatory abilities.

## BLOOD AND PERIPHERAL BLOOD VESSELS

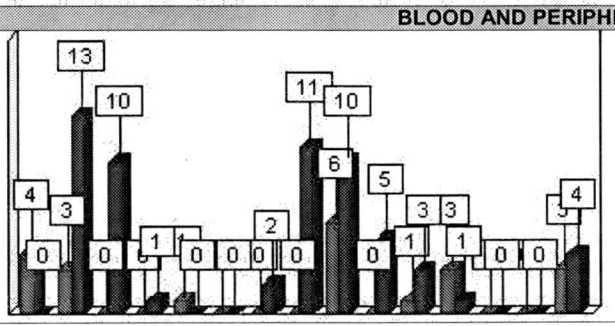

**Phlebitis and Thrombophlebitis: Compensatory signal.**
Age-Related Changes: Expressed compensatory signal.
**Leukopenia: Compensatory signal.**
Neoplasm: Expressed compensatory signal.

186

## SPLEEN

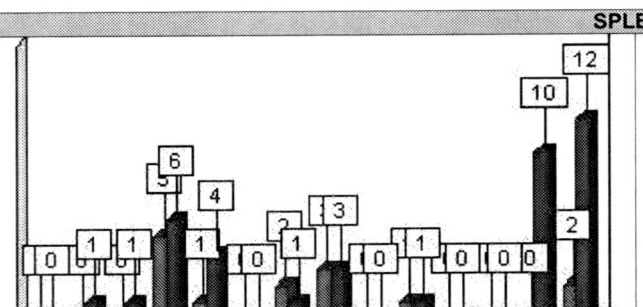

Functional Changes: Compensatory signal.
Neoplasm: Compensatory signal.
Tissue Growth: Expressed compensatory signal.

## LUNGS AND BRONCHI

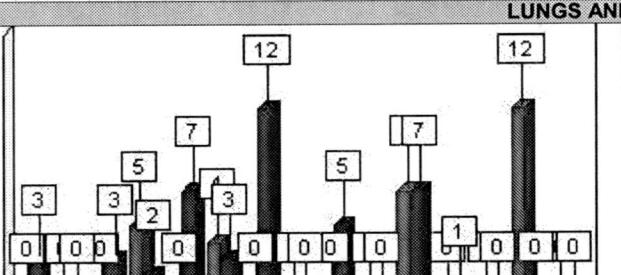

Chronic Fatigue: Compensated pathology condition.
Chronic Breathing Insufficiency: Expressed pathology signal.
Allergic Process: Compensatory signal.
Bronchial Asthma: Expressed compensatory signal.

## SKIN

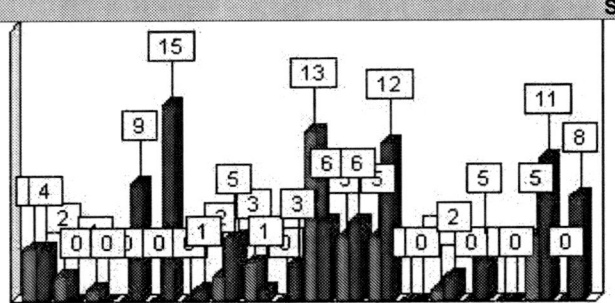

Chronic Fatigue: Expressed pathology signal.
Eczema: Compensatory signal.
Age-Related Changes: Expressed compensatory signal.
Herpes: Expressed compensatory signal.
Neoplasm: Expressed compensatory signal.
Psoriasis: Expressed compensatory signal.
Neurodermatitis: Compensatory signal.
Erythema: Compensatory signal.
Intoxication Effects: Compensatory signal.

## OESOPHAGUS

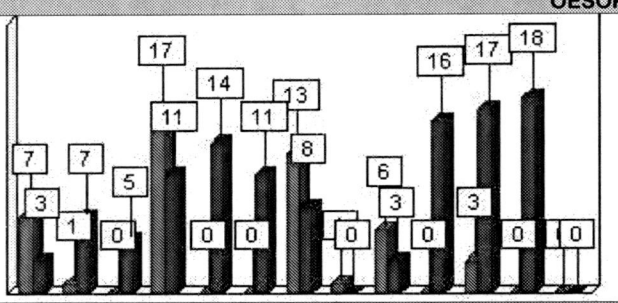

Functional Changes: Pathology signal.
Chronic Fatigue: Weakening of compensatory abilities.
Allergic Process: Weakening of compensatory abilities.
Tension of compensatory abilities.

## STOMACH

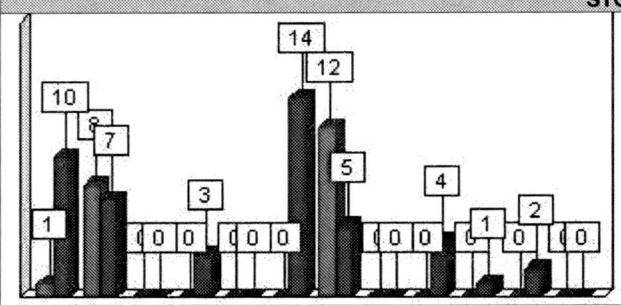

Allergic Process: Weakening of compensatory abilities.
Post-Stress Effects: Pathology signal.
Age-Related Changes: Compensatory signal.
Intoxication Effects: Expressed compensatory signal.

## DUODENUM

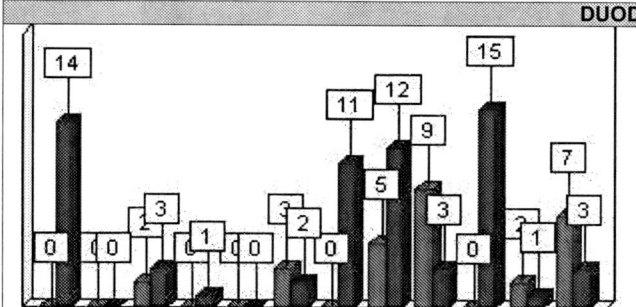

Post-Stress Effects: Pathology signal.
Chronic Fatigue: Pathology signal.
Neoplasm: Expressed compensatory signal.
Ulcerative Disease: Compensatory signal.
Allergic Process: Compensatory signal.
Dyskinesia: Expressed compensatory signal.

## SMALL INTESTINE

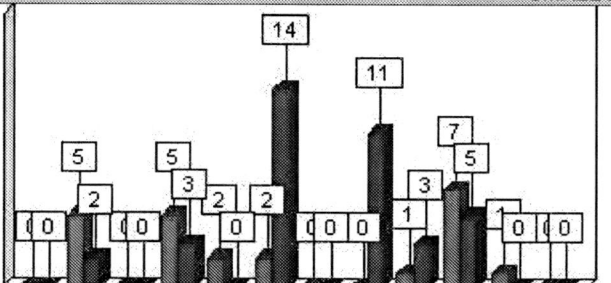

Diverticulae: Weakening of compensatory abilities.
Abnormalities of Development: Expressed compensatory signal.
Neoplasm: Compensatory signal.

## LARGE INTESTINE

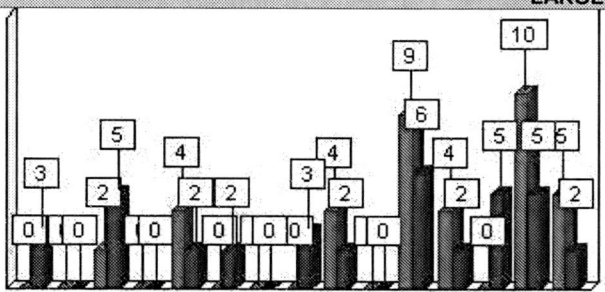

Functional Changes: Weakening of compensatory abilities.
Neoplasm: Pathology signal.

## KIDNEYS

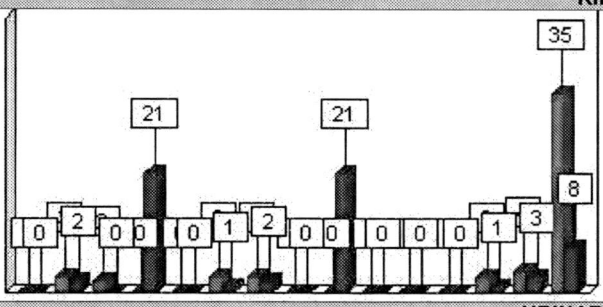

Functional Changes: Expressed pathology signal.
Pyelonephritis: Expressed compensatory signal.
Tissue Growth: Expressed compensatory signal.

## URINARY BLADDER

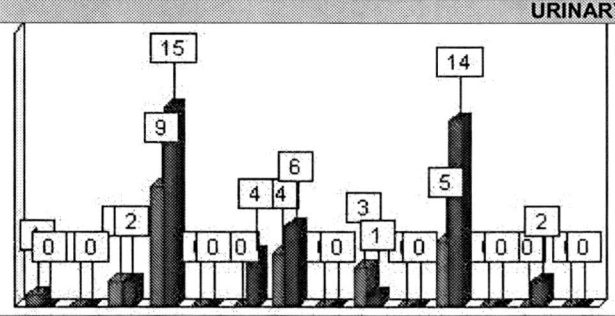

Post-Stress Effects: Compensatory signal.
Degenerative Process: Compensatory signal.
Allergic Process: Expressed compensatory signal.

188

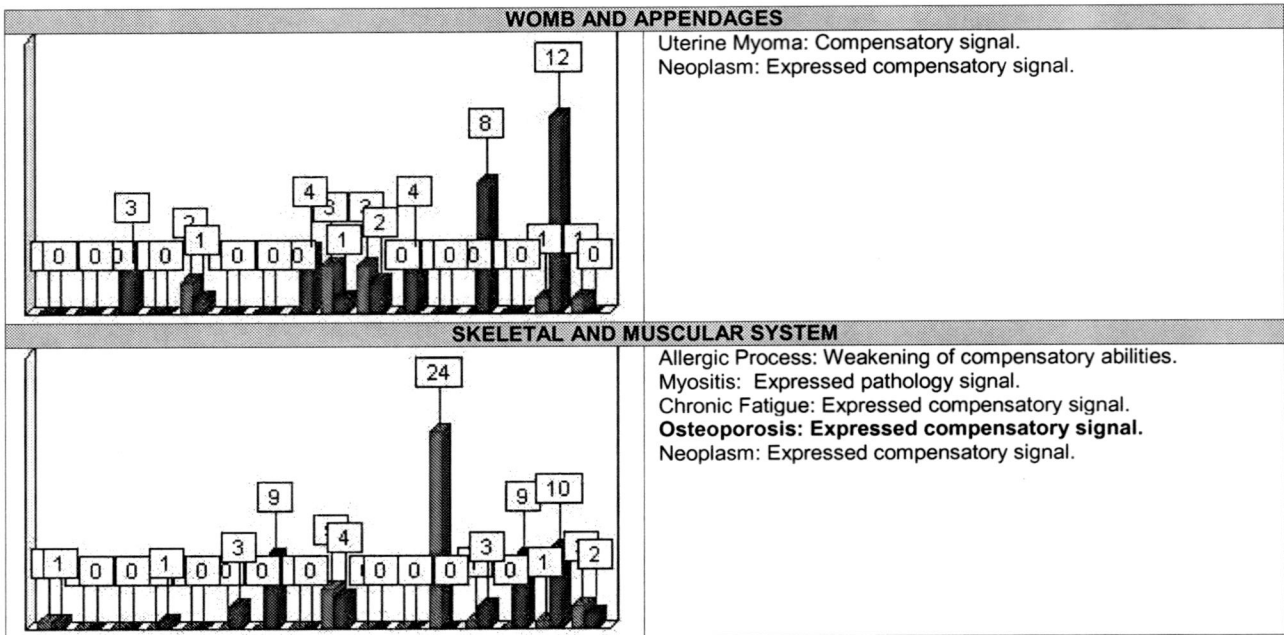

**WOMB AND APPENDAGES**

Uterine Myoma: Compensatory signal.
Neoplasm: Expressed compensatory signal.

**SKELETAL AND MUSCULAR SYSTEM**

Allergic Process: Weakening of compensatory abilities.
Myositis: Expressed pathology signal.
Chronic Fatigue: Expressed compensatory signal.
**Osteoporosis: Expressed compensatory signal.**
Neoplasm: Expressed compensatory signal.

## Discussion of Reported Results

Marginal indications of migraine 9 units pathology (below 10 units which is considered the symptomatic/presymptomatic threshold and also of impaired cerebral circulation and Arachnoiditis

Clearly significant indications of vertebral artery syndrome, spinal osteochondrosis, and osteoporosis, impaired spinal circulation and cardiac infarction which are consistent with impaired flow of arterial blood flow to the brain..

189

example 2: woman 59 years, Migraine

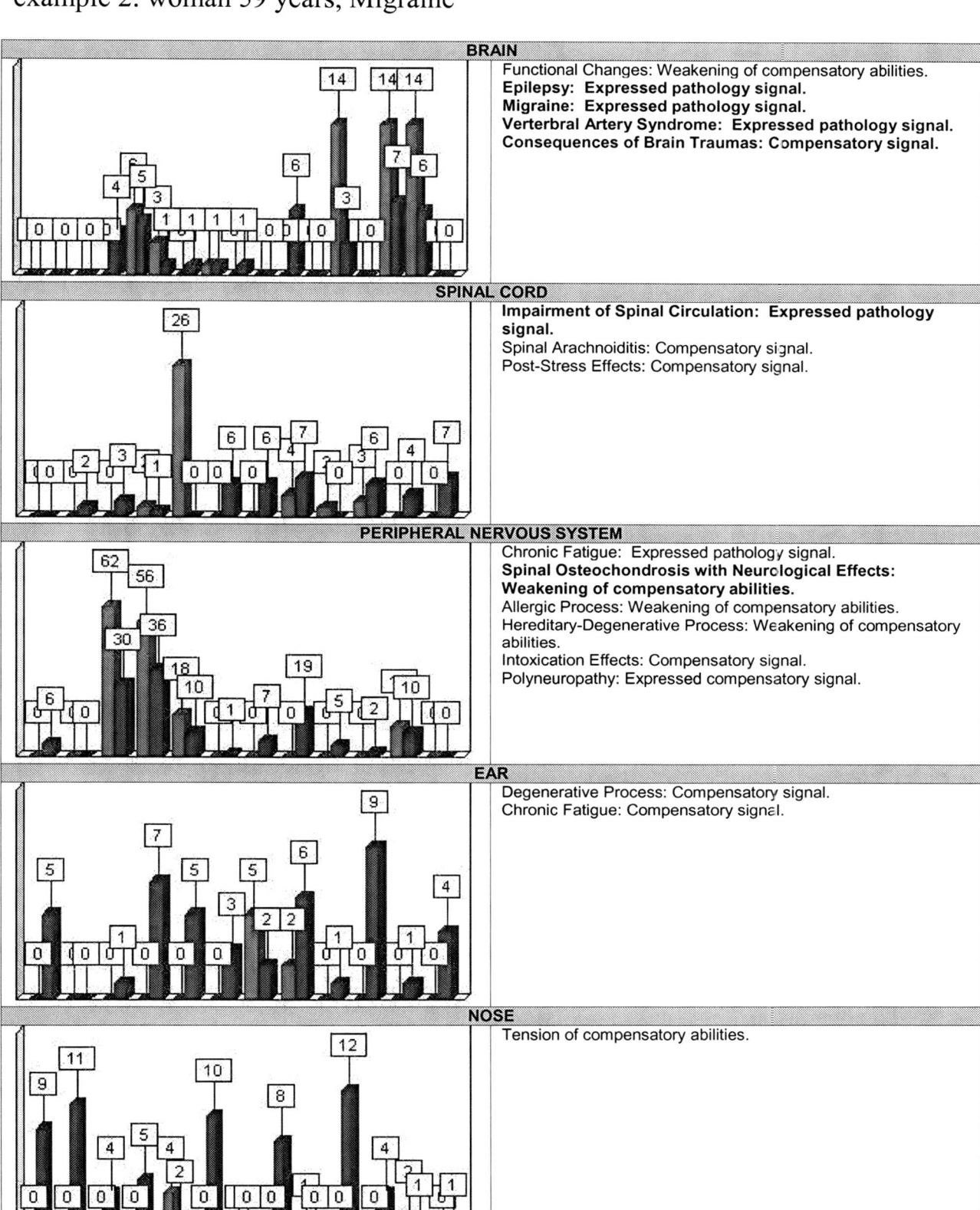

**BRAIN**

Functional Changes: Weakening of compensatory abilities.
**Epilepsy:  Expressed pathology signal.**
**Migraine:  Expressed pathology signal.**
**Verterbral Artery Syndrome:  Expressed pathology signal.**
**Consequences of Brain Traumas: Compensatory signal.**

**SPINAL CORD**

**Impairment of Spinal Circulation:  Expressed pathology signal.**
Spinal Arachnoiditis: Compensatory signal.
Post-Stress Effects: Compensatory signal.

**PERIPHERAL NERVOUS SYSTEM**

Chronic Fatigue:  Expressed pathology signal.
**Spinal Osteochondrosis with Neurological Effects: Weakening of compensatory abilities.**
Allergic Process: Weakening of compensatory abilities.
Hereditary-Degenerative Process: Weakening of compensatory abilities.
Intoxication Effects: Compensatory signal.
Polyneuropathy: Expressed compensatory signal.

**EAR**

Degenerative Process: Compensatory signal.
Chronic Fatigue: Compensatory signal.

**NOSE**

Tension of compensatory abilities.

190

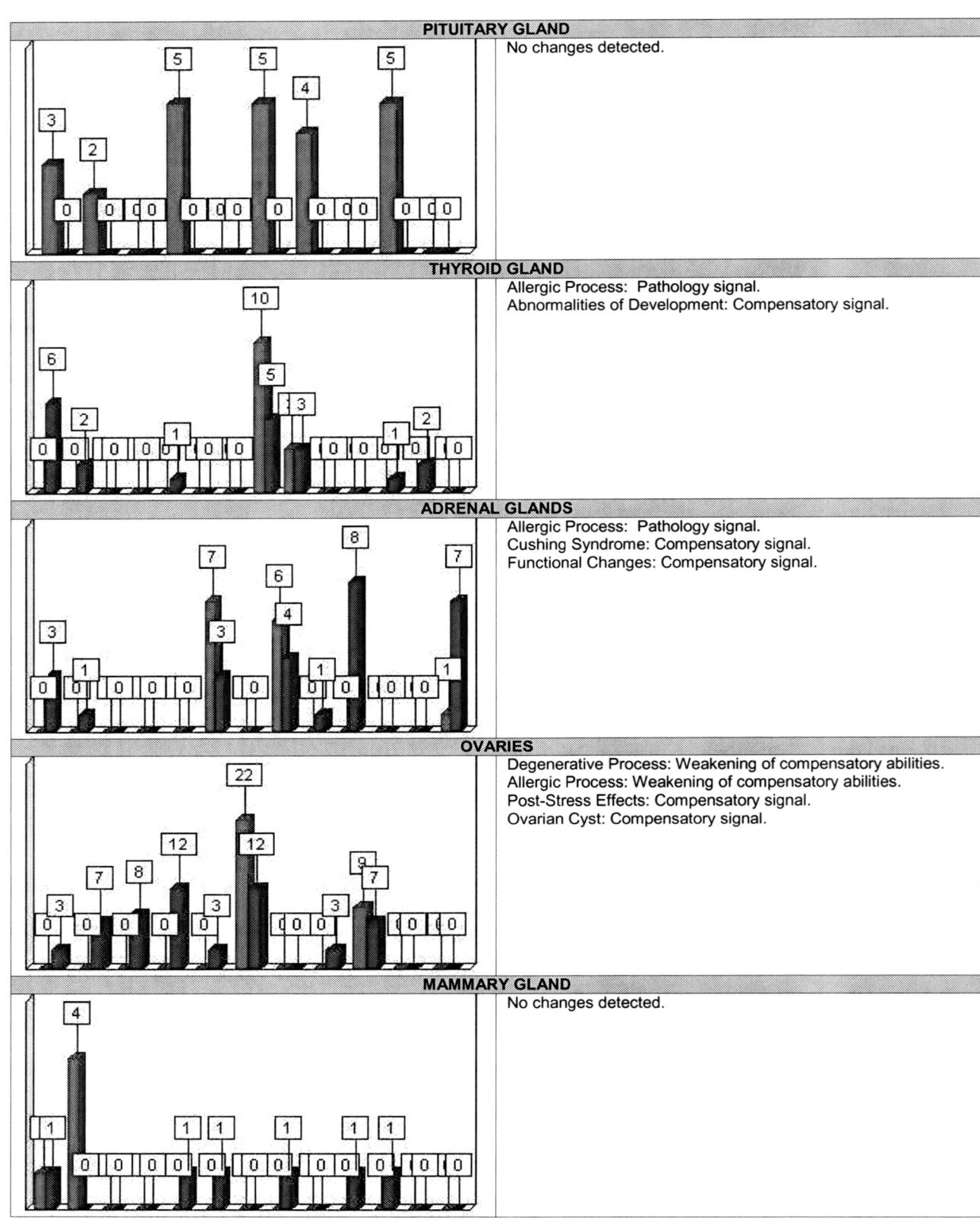

**PITUITARY GLAND**

No changes detected.

**THYROID GLAND**

Allergic Process: Pathology signal.
Abnormalities of Development: Compensatory signal.

**ADRENAL GLANDS**

Allergic Process: Pathology signal.
Cushing Syndrome: Compensatory signal.
Functional Changes: Compensatory signal.

**OVARIES**

Degenerative Process: Weakening of compensatory abilities.
Allergic Process: Weakening of compensatory abilities.
Post-Stress Effects: Compensatory signal.
Ovarian Cyst: Compensatory signal.

**MAMMARY GLAND**

No changes detected.

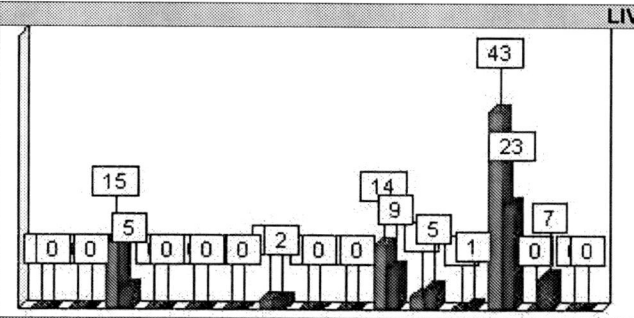

**LIVER**

Allergic Process: Expressed pathology signal.
Disruption of Bilirubin Metabolism: Weakening of compensatory abilities.
Liver Insufficiency: Weakening of compensatory abilities.
Neoplasm: Compensatory signal.

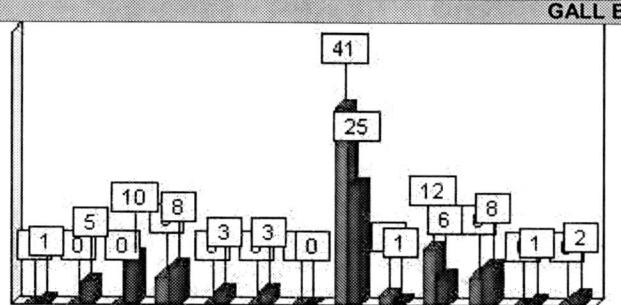

**GALL BLADDER**

Dyskinesia of Biliary Ducts and Gall Bladder: Weakening of compensatory abilities.
Chronic Fatigue: Pathology signal.
Post-Stress Effects: Compensatory signal.
Tissue Growth: Compensatory signal.
Cholangitis: Compensatory signal.

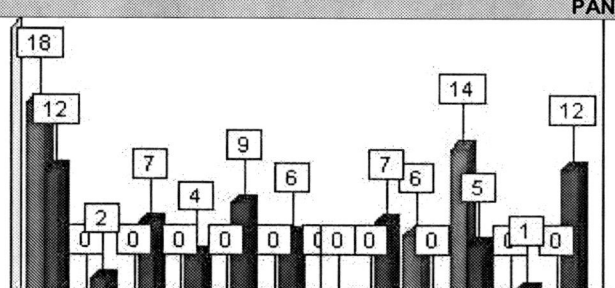

**PANCREAS**

Chronic Fatigue: Weakening of compensatory abilities.
**Pathology of Islands of Langerhans: Expressed pathology signal.**
Post-Stress Effects: Compensatory signal.
Age-Related Changes: Compensatory signal.
Functional Changes: Compensatory signal.
Abnormalities of Development: Compensatory signal.

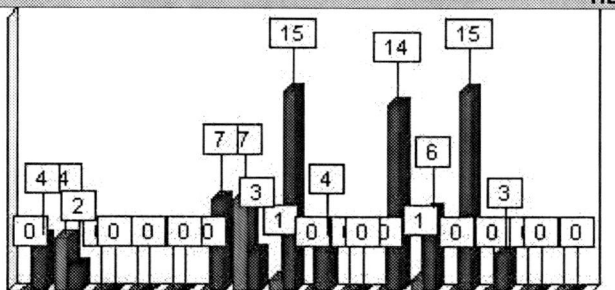

**HEART**

Chronic Fatigue: Pathology signal.
Cardiosclerosis: Compensatory signal.
Myocardial Dystrophy: Expressed compensatory signal.
Intoxication Effects: Expressed compensatory signal.
Cardiac Insufficiency: Compensatory signal.
Cardiac Myopathy: Expressed compensatory signal.

**BLOOD AND PERIPHERAL BLOOD VESSELS**

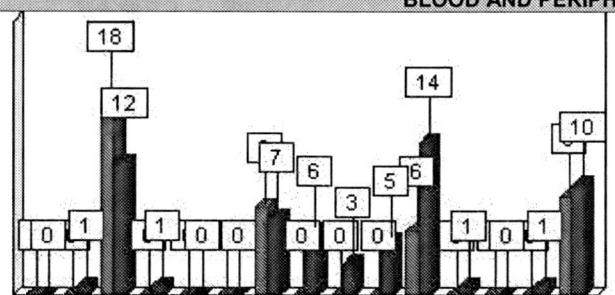

**Leukopenia: Weakening of compensatory abilities.**
**Haemorrhagic Vasculitis: Weakening of compensatory abilities.**
**Idiopathic Hypotension: Expressed compensatory signal.**
Post-Stress Effects: Compensatory signal.
Neoplasm: Compensatory signal.

192

## SPLEEN

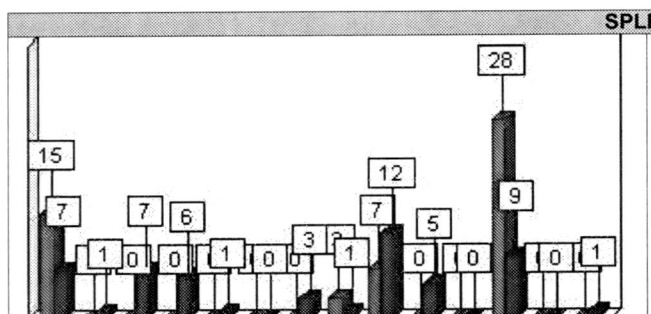

Chronic Fatigue: Expressed pathology signal.
Hyposplenism: Compensatory signal.
Chronic Staying Splenomegaly: Expressed pathology signal.
Splenomegaly: Compensatory signal.
Functional Changes: Compensatory signal.

## LUNGS AND BRONCHI

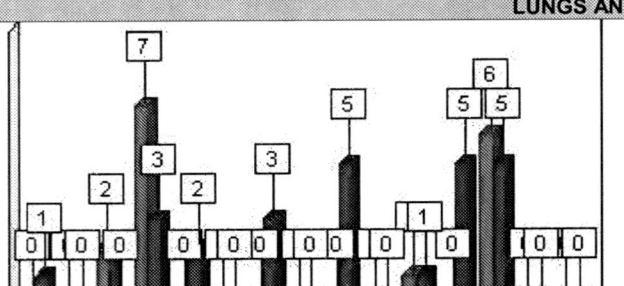

Bronchiectatic disease: Pathology signal.
Post-Stress Effects: Weakening of compensatory abilities.

## SKIN

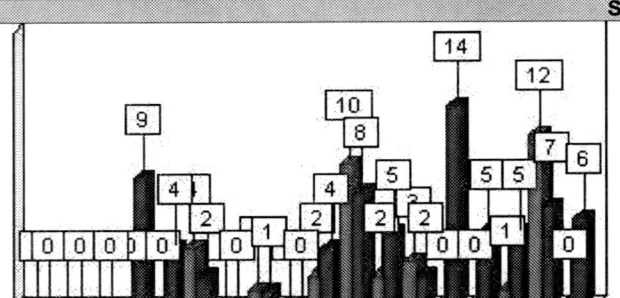

Eczema: Weakening of compensatory abilities.
Herpes: Weakening of compensatory abilities.
Neoplasm: Expressed compensatory signal.
Age-Related Changes: Compensatory signal.
Degenerative Process: Expressed compensatory signal.
Erythema: Compensatory signal.
Post-Stress Effects: Compensatory signal.
Intoxication Effects: Compensatory signal.

## OESOPHAGUS

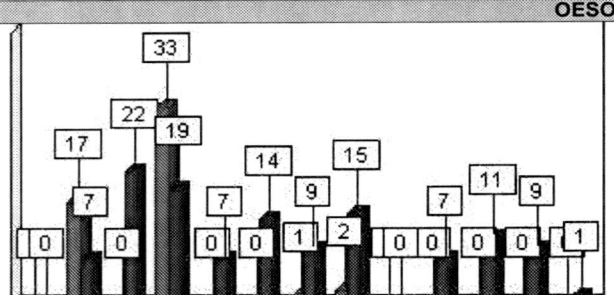

Degenerative Process: Expressed pathology signal.
Chronic Fatigue: Weakening of compensatory abilities.
Tension of compensatory abilities.

## STOMACH

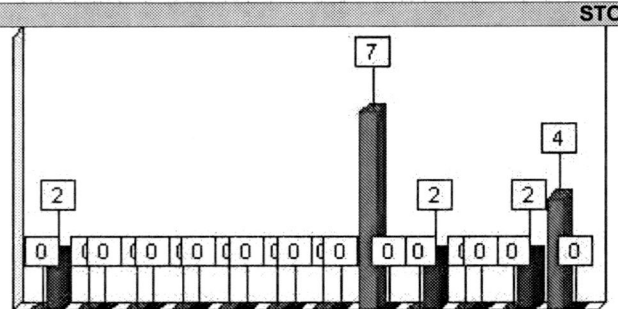

Ulcerative Disease: Pathology signal.

193

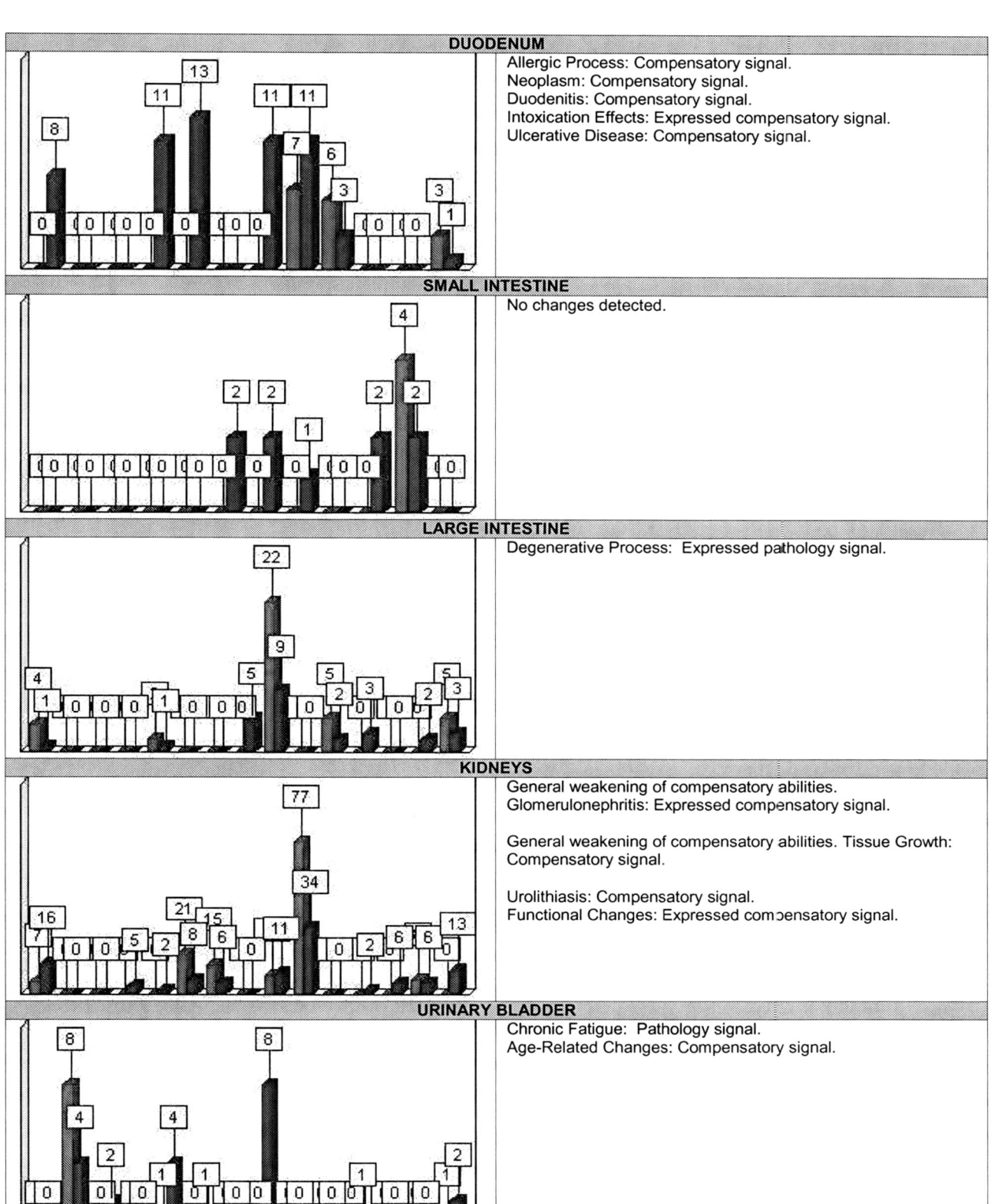

**DUODENUM**

Allergic Process: Compensatory signal.
Neoplasm: Compensatory signal.
Duodenitis: Compensatory signal.
Intoxication Effects: Expressed compensatory signal.
Ulcerative Disease: Compensatory signal.

**SMALL INTESTINE**

No changes detected.

**LARGE INTESTINE**

Degenerative Process: Expressed pathology signal.

**KIDNEYS**

General weakening of compensatory abilities.
Glomerulonephritis: Expressed compensatory signal.

General weakening of compensatory abilities. Tissue Growth: Compensatory signal.

Urolithiasis: Compensatory signal.
Functional Changes: Expressed compensatory signal.

**URINARY BLADDER**

Chronic Fatigue: Pathology signal.
Age-Related Changes: Compensatory signal.

194

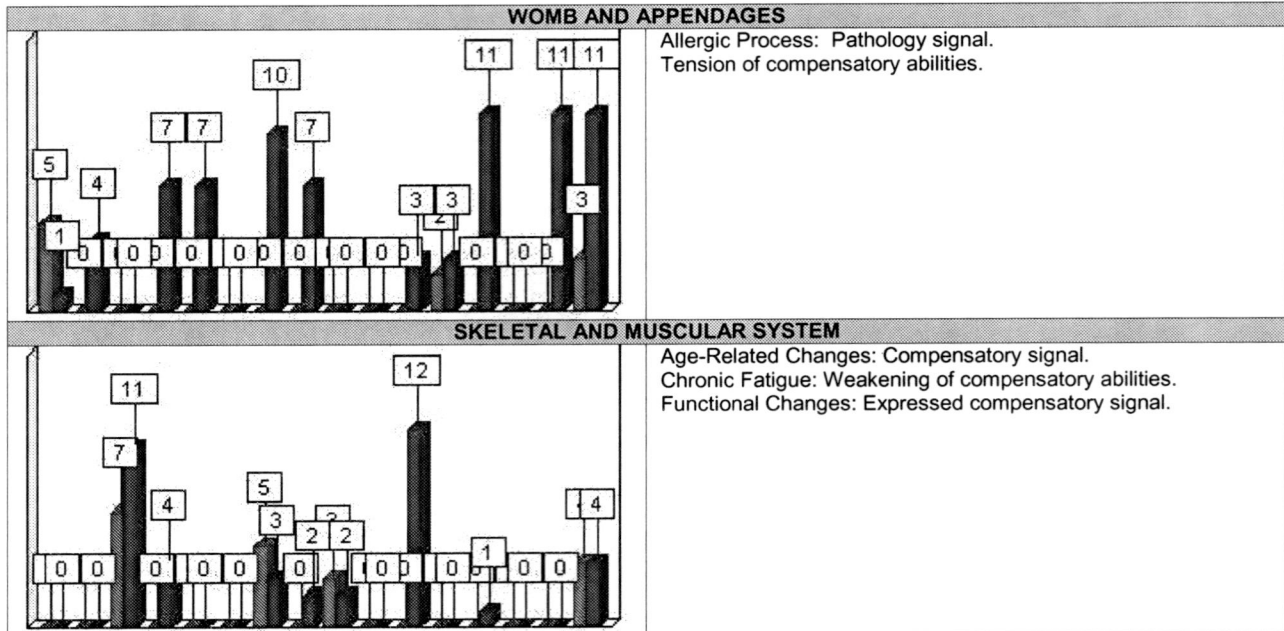

## Discussion of Reported Results

Clearly significant indications of impaired spinal circulation, spinal osteochondrosis, vertebral artery syndrome, migraine and also of clear indications of idiopathic hypotension, leukopenia and compensatory indications of cardiosclerosis, myocardial dystrophy and cardiac myopathy which support the hypothesis that the migraine attacks occur due to impaired flow of arterial blood to the brain.

## Observations

Like most therapeutic approaches or medications Virtual Scanning therapy depends on compliance to the prescription of 1-2 sessions per day, each session typically lasting 20 minutes. Patients with poor adherence to the therapy usually show the least consistent indications of improvement. The problem of adherence to the therapy appears to be the greatest encountered by practitioners.

Patients treated for Migraine have noted significant improvements to health manifesting as (1) longer periods free from migraine; (2) less intense migraines; (3) improved quality of sleep, mobility, energy, and demeanour; and (4) improved visual appearance - patients lose the 'dark circles under and around their eyes' often noted in migraine sufferers.

Improvements are also seen in indications of chronic or irreversible nature, which would limit or prevent progress e.g. illnesses, infections or injury (e.g. Lyme Disease; damage to the spine which affects blood-flow to the brain, etc).

For migraine itself, and results obtained using Virtual Scanning diagnosis and treatment:

The conclusions are consistent with observed phenomena and theories [8,9] e.g.

- Caffeine on its own is implicated as a trigger for migraine and headaches. It increases brain wave frequency, stimulates the heart and raises blood pressure.

- Caffeine (which is used as stimulant and to raise blood pressure) is sometimes used in combination with Aspirin (which has the effect of thinning the blood)

- Aspirin, on its own or in combination with another drug, has an ability to reduce the incidence of migraine. No explanation is known for why it should be more effective than paracetamol, an equivalent analgesic, except that aspirin's effect of thinning the blood and thereby making it easier for the heart to pump blood to the brain (see further reading: Aspirin).

- Research into treatment of Patent Foramen Ovale (PFO) in some migraine sufferers [10] concludes that the occurrence of migraines is stimulated by events associated with low blood pressure in or to the brain.

- Stress which causes constriction of blood vessels in the heart [14] and the arterial system with consequent increase in blood pressure etc., is one of the most common precipitating factors [10,11,12].

- Those who see auras before migraine onset have increased risk of stroke (TIA), heart attack and of dying from cardiovascular disease [15]. This clearly associates migraine, stroke and blood supply [16].

From the available statistics (Roses, GSK [13]) it appears that MIGRAINE type medications are, at best, only circa 50% effective in alleviating the symptoms of migraine. By contrast Virtual Scanning appears able to reduce their frequency and severity and even prevent their occurrence in a far higher percentage of sufferers.

This may seem less surprising when we recall that Migraine is responsive to other similar but less sophisticated types of therapy, including various kinds of photic stimulation [17,18], neurofeedback, biofeedback [19,20,21] and related technologies [22-29].

## Conclusions

Migraine results from a combination of factors affecting the brain's blood-supply i.e. the ability of the heart to pump blood, quality including thickness of the blood, the volume of blood in the system (hence one possible cause being blood loss during menstruation), the ability of the blood vessels to pump arterial blood and the associated effect of patent foramen ovale (hole-in-the-heart), and any issues which could impair the flow of blood to the brain (e.g. spondylosis, vertebral artery syndrome, osteochondrosis, etc).

Virtual Scanning appears able to alleviate the fundamental cause(s) of the condition. It appears to be more effective in the treatment of migraines of stress-related origin i.e. those related to the dysfunction of the body's physiological systems, and less effective for those due to physical injury or deterioration.

## 4.4 Virtual Scanning: Assessment and Treatment of Dyslexia

Dyslexia is disorder which manifests in ways which impair writing, reading, learning, concentration, memory and behaviour. It is not due to any single factor although there are clearly instances where dyslexia runs in the family and both parents and children have the defect. Other environmental influences affect the neural development of the individual and hence their ability to concentrate, memorise, read, learn and on their balance, co-ordination and writing.

Whilst dyslexia is undoubtedly a difficulty for those which have this condition it must not be overlooked that this condition occurs in even the most intelligent of people. There are many who have learned to overcome this disability and who have gone on in their lives to be highly successful sportsmen and businessmen therefore it is important to recognise that these people have been able to compensate for the disability of dyslexia throughout their lives by the development of other positive life factors. So dyslexia is often associated with achievement (of those who have been able to compensate for this impediment) as well as underachievement.

In common with most other medical and psychological conditions it is necessary to address the fundamental cause of the condition as well as its symptoms.

The synchronisation of component parts of the brain affects our intelligence, health and our behaviour from childhood and throughout our adult lives. This affects overall brain function and is reliant upon the production of hormones (HGH et al) and related biochemicals. These affect the production of neurons and synapse formation in the brain. The greater the number of neurons, axons and of synapse formation the greater our physical and mental capabilities however, if these are incorrectly connected and/or synchronized for various reasons, this may/will lead to problems of neural processing including dyslexia and related conditions.

If the regulatory programme which is responsible for the physiological systems in our body is in some way desynchronized (perhaps due to stress-effects during early childhood) this will affect the absorption of nutrients and the levels of the various and necessary biochemical components in the body and/or brain. If these are deficient perhaps as a result of diet or stress the structure of the brain may not be adequately developed and able to support the development of neural pathways. As a result various neural disorders related to the poor regulation of our physiology can arise e.g. including dyslexia, dyspraxia, sleeping disorders, poor memory, balance and co-ordination problems, and perhaps also a number of other related disorders including attention deficit hyperactivity disorder.

This explanation is supported in many cases that giving a dyslexic child a supplement with omega-3 fish oils does have positive but limited effects, but this does not explain why it is not able to effect a cure or why a person with above average intelligence and other capabilities could suffer from dyslexia.

Both effects can be explained by considering that the desynchronisation of neural processing arising from the effects listed earlier in this article would affect (a) the physical construction of nerve structures, (b) the subsequent development of the neural pathways, (c) the speed of processing data within the neural pathways e.g. in which the data in the left hemisphere of the brain appears to be processed at a different rate from the right hemisphere of the brain and vice versa, (d) the flow of blood to the brain and hence of the occurrence of inner-ear defects, infection, etc.

The nature of dyslexia is therefore related to the adverse influences which suppress the brain's development and function irrespective of their origin e.g. by stress effects due to the effects of vaccines, antibiotics, infections, or of environmental circumstances.

Undoubtedly it has a biochemical basis. All aspects of our psychology as well as our physiology have a fundamental biochemical basis.

Examples of Successful Treatments using Virtual Scanning Colour Therapy

- A girl, 10 yo. The first indications of changed behaviour was evident within the first month. The first indications of improved writing (distinct) and reading were indicated by the third consultation. Whereas before her reading age was 2 years behind her calendar age of 10 years, her school end of term reported a stunning leap in her reading ability. Her reading ability was reassessed as being equivalent to a 14yo. Her writing has improved although there are indications of errors in spelling. Her first examination results at her new school are 9 grades 1 & 2, and 2 grade 3's.

- Another parent, a complementary health practitioner, of a young man in his early 20's reported: 'his short term memory has improved, he is more out-going in his personality, he no longer moves his lips when he reads, he is more communicative and initiates more conversations, he is more physically coordinated in his movements, his verbal responses are quicker and more confident'.

- A male 19yo university student commented after the first module of therapy of 'phenomenally improved concentration'. His mother, well respected in Special Educational Needs circles was delighted with her son's progress. Whereas before he had a 10-15 minutes span of attention, following therapy he was now able to concentrate for periods of 2-3 hours and was more organized.

- A girl 10 yo was identified with colitis and anaemia. The mother was recommended to change her daughter's diet from a heavily vegetarian diet to include protein and in particular red meat. Within 2 months the parent noted that her daughter has much less abdominal pain and that her daughter's behaviour and concentration had noticeably improved. These were confirmed by Virtual Scanning results. The parent commented of improvements in her daughter's reading and writing. Her end of term result reported much improved levels of concentration.

example 3: girl 11 years, Dyslexic

| BRAIN | |
|---|---|
| 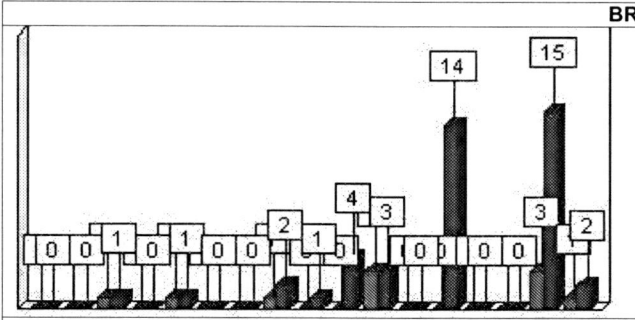 | Epilepsy: Expressed compensatory signal.<br>**Verterbral Artery Syndrome: Expressed compensatory signal.** |
| SPINAL CORD | |
| 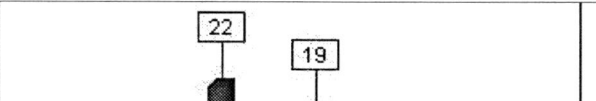 | Chronic Fatigue: Compensatory signal.<br>Intoxication Effects: Compensatory signal.<br>Allergic Process: Compensatory signal.<br>**Impairment of Spinal Circulation: Expressed compensatory signal.**<br>Abnormalities of Development: Expressed compensatory signal.<br>Post-Stress Effects: Compensatory signal. |
| PERIPHERAL NERVOUS SYSTEM | |
| 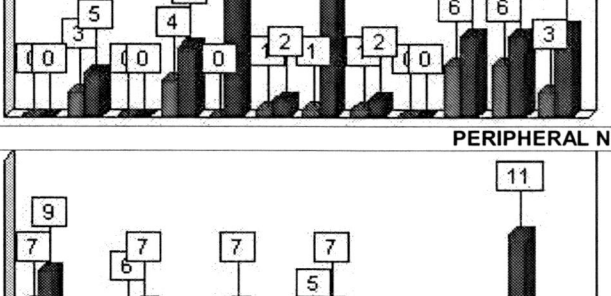 | Post-Stress Effects: Compensatory signal.<br>Chronic Fatigue: Compensatory signal.<br>Allergic Process: Compensatory signal.<br>Intoxication Effects: Compensatory signal.<br>Hereditary-Degenerative Process: Expressed compensatory signal. |
| EAR | |
| 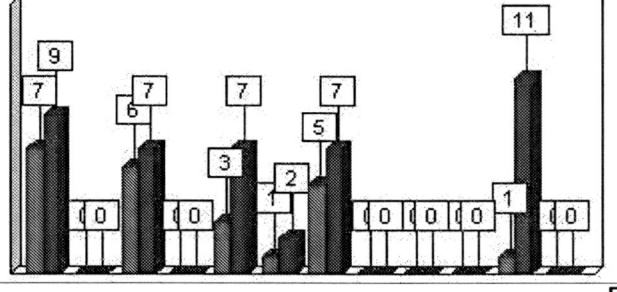 | **Inflammation of Middle Ear: Compensatory signal.**<br>**Otogenous Labyrinthitis: Compensatory signal.**<br>Chronic Fatigue: Compensatory signal.<br>**External Otitis: Compensatory signal.**<br>Abnormalities of Development: Compensatory signal. |
| NOSE | |
| 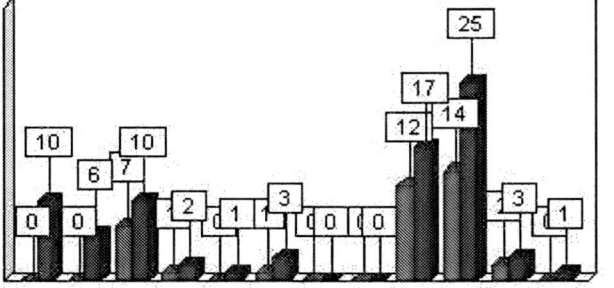 | Rhinitis: Compensatory signal.<br>Abnormalities of Development: Expressed compensatory signal.<br>Intoxication Effects: Compensatory signal.<br>Age-Related Changes: Expressed compensatory signal.<br>Functional Changes: Compensatory signal. |

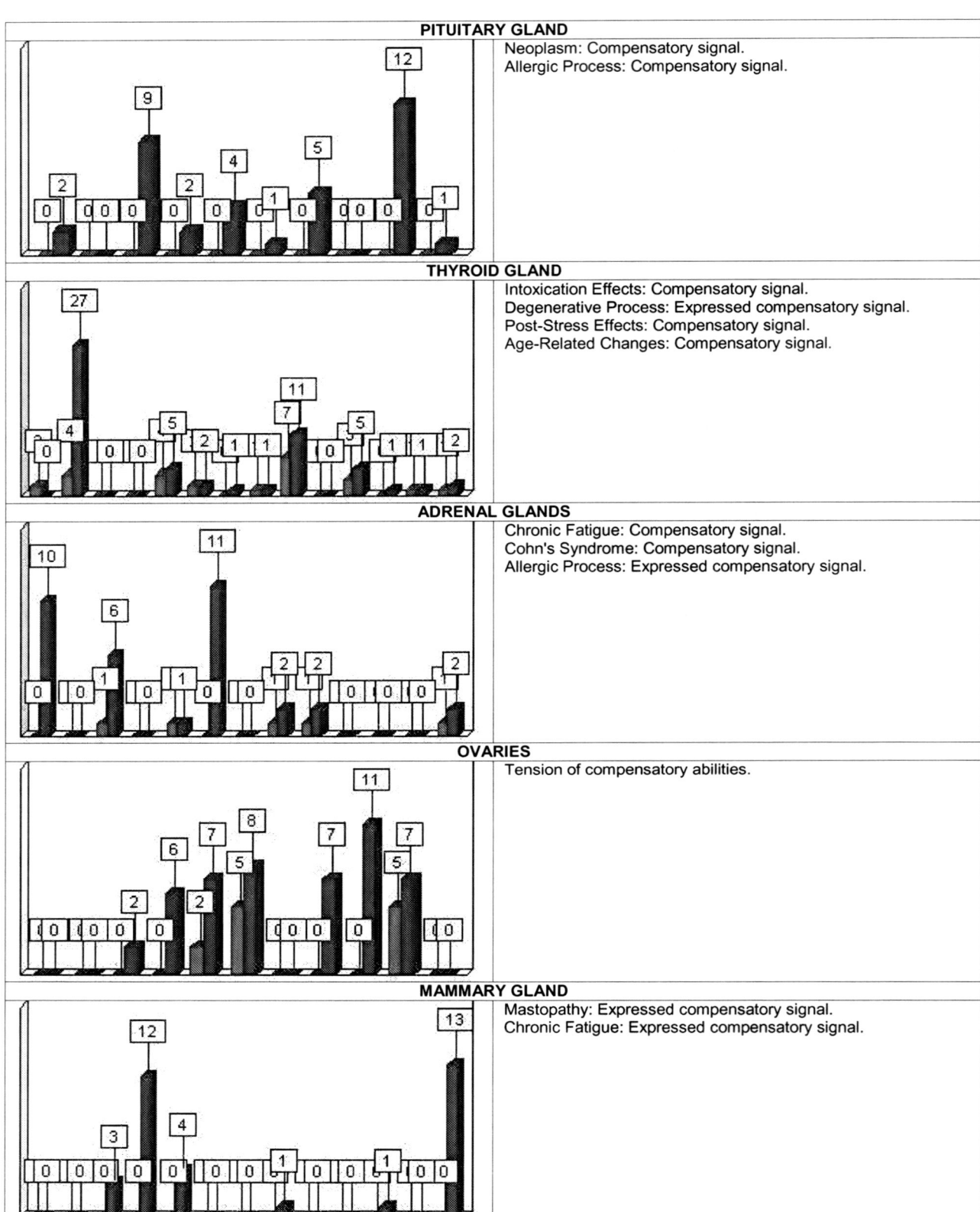

**PITUITARY GLAND**

Neoplasm: Compensatory signal.
Allergic Process: Compensatory signal.

**THYROID GLAND**

Intoxication Effects: Compensatory signal.
Degenerative Process: Expressed compensatory signal.
Post-Stress Effects: Compensatory signal.
Age-Related Changes: Compensatory signal.

**ADRENAL GLANDS**

Chronic Fatigue: Compensatory signal.
Cohn's Syndrome: Compensatory signal.
Allergic Process: Expressed compensatory signal.

**OVARIES**

Tension of compensatory abilities.

**MAMMARY GLAND**

Mastopathy: Expressed compensatory signal.
Chronic Fatigue: Expressed compensatory signal.

| LIVER | |
|---|---|
| 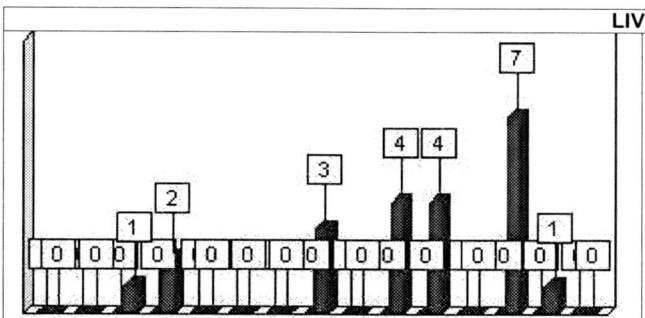 | Liver Insufficiency: Compensatory signal. |

| GALL BLADDER | |
|---|---|
| 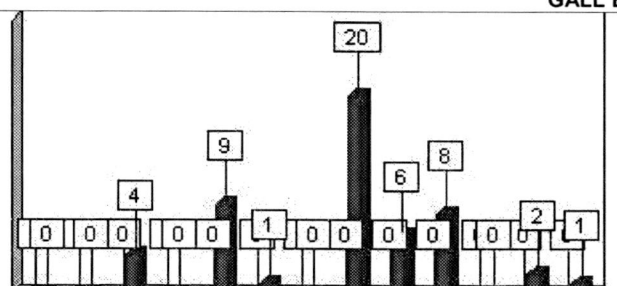 | Cholelithiasis: Compensatory signal.<br>Dyskinesia of Biliary Ducts and Gall Bladder: Expressed compensatory signal.<br>Allergic Process: Compensatory signal.<br>Chronic Fatigue: Compensatory signal. |

| PANCREAS | |
|---|---|
| 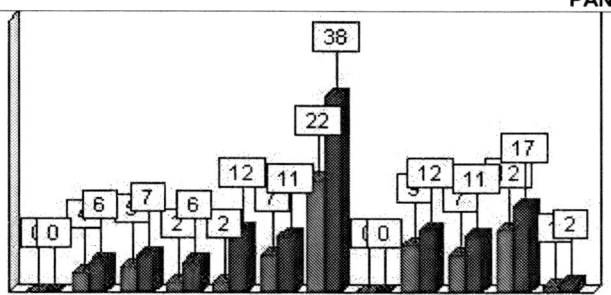 | General tension of compensatory abilities.<br>Intoxication Effects: Compensatory signal.<br>Post-Stress Effects: Compensatory signal.<br>Pancreatitis: Compensatory signal.<br>Age-Related Changes: Expressed compensatory signal. |

| HEART | |
|---|---|
| 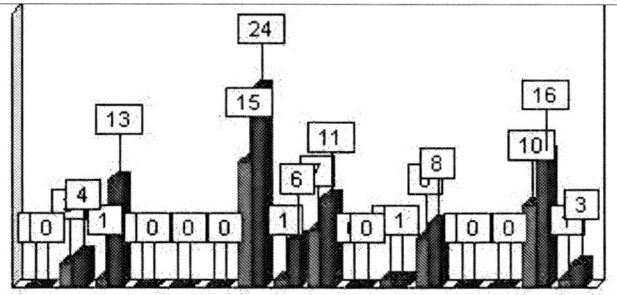 | **Chronic Fatigue: Compensatory signal.**<br>Abnormalities of Development: Compensatory signal.<br>**Cardiac Insufficiency: Compensatory signal.**<br>**Impairment of Cardiac Rhythm and Conduction: Compensatory signal.**<br>Angina Pectoris: Expressed compensatory signal.<br>Myocardial Dystrophy: Compensatory signal. |

| BLOOD AND PERIPHERAL BLOOD VESSELS | |
|---|---|
| 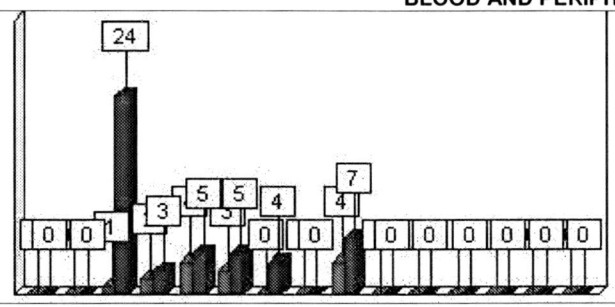 | Leukopenia: Expressed compensatory signal.<br>Hemorrhagic Diathesis: Compensatory signal.<br>Functional Changes: Compensatory signal.<br>Phlebitis and Thrombophlebitis: Compensatory signal. |

| **SPLEEN** | |
|---|---|
| 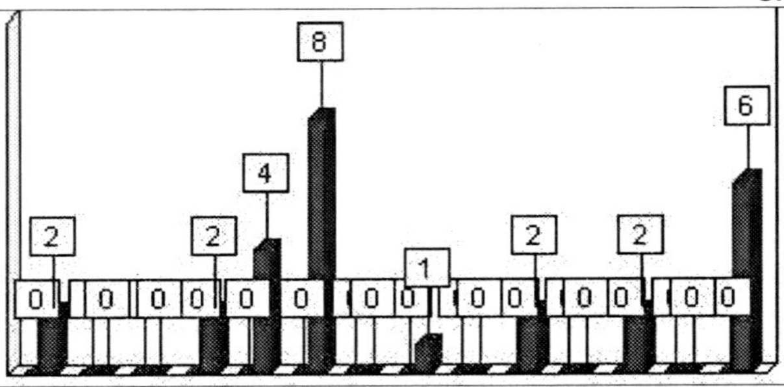 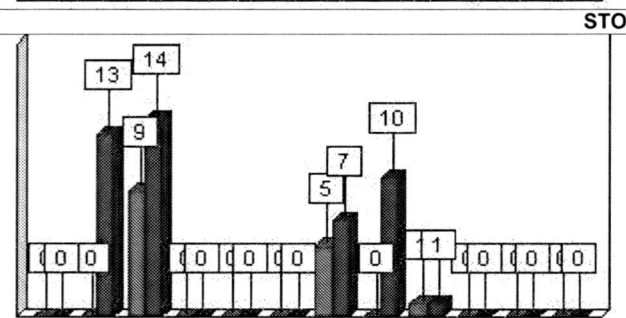 | Hypersplenism: Compensatory signal.<br>Tissue Growth: Compensatory signal. |

| **LUNGS AND BRONCHI** | |
|---|---|
| 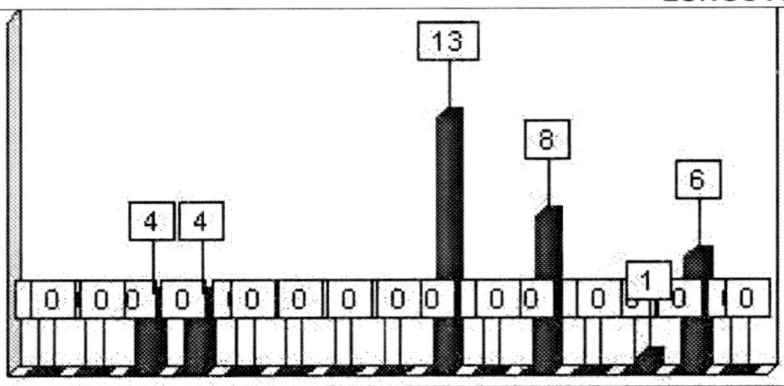 | Age-Related Changes: Expressed compensatory signal.<br>Chronic Fatigue: Compensatory signal.<br>Chronic Breathing Insufficiency: Compensatory signal. |

| **SKIN** | |
|---|---|
| 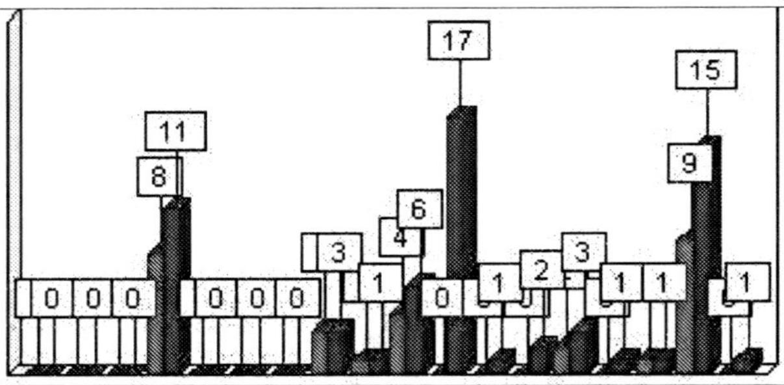 | Neoplasm: Compensatory signal.<br>Chronic Fatigue: Compensatory signal.<br>Herpes: Compensatory signal.<br>Eczema: Expressed compensatory signal. |

| **OESOPHAGUS** | |
|---|---|
| 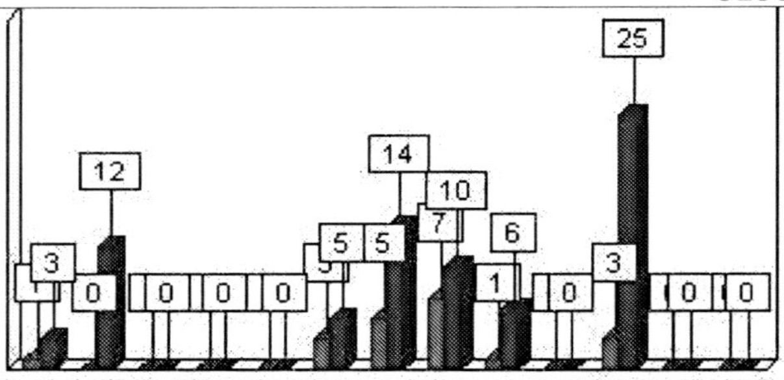 | Post-Stress Effects: Compensatory signal.<br>Degenerative Process: Expressed compensatory signal.<br>Allergic Process: Expressed compensatory signal.<br>Tissue Growth: Compensatory signal.<br>Neoplasm: Expressed compensatory signal. |

| **STOMACH** | |
|---|---|
| | Functional Changes: Compensatory signal.<br>Allergic Process: Expressed compensatory signal.<br>Post-Stress Effects: Compensatory signal.<br>Ulcerative Disease: Compensatory signal. |

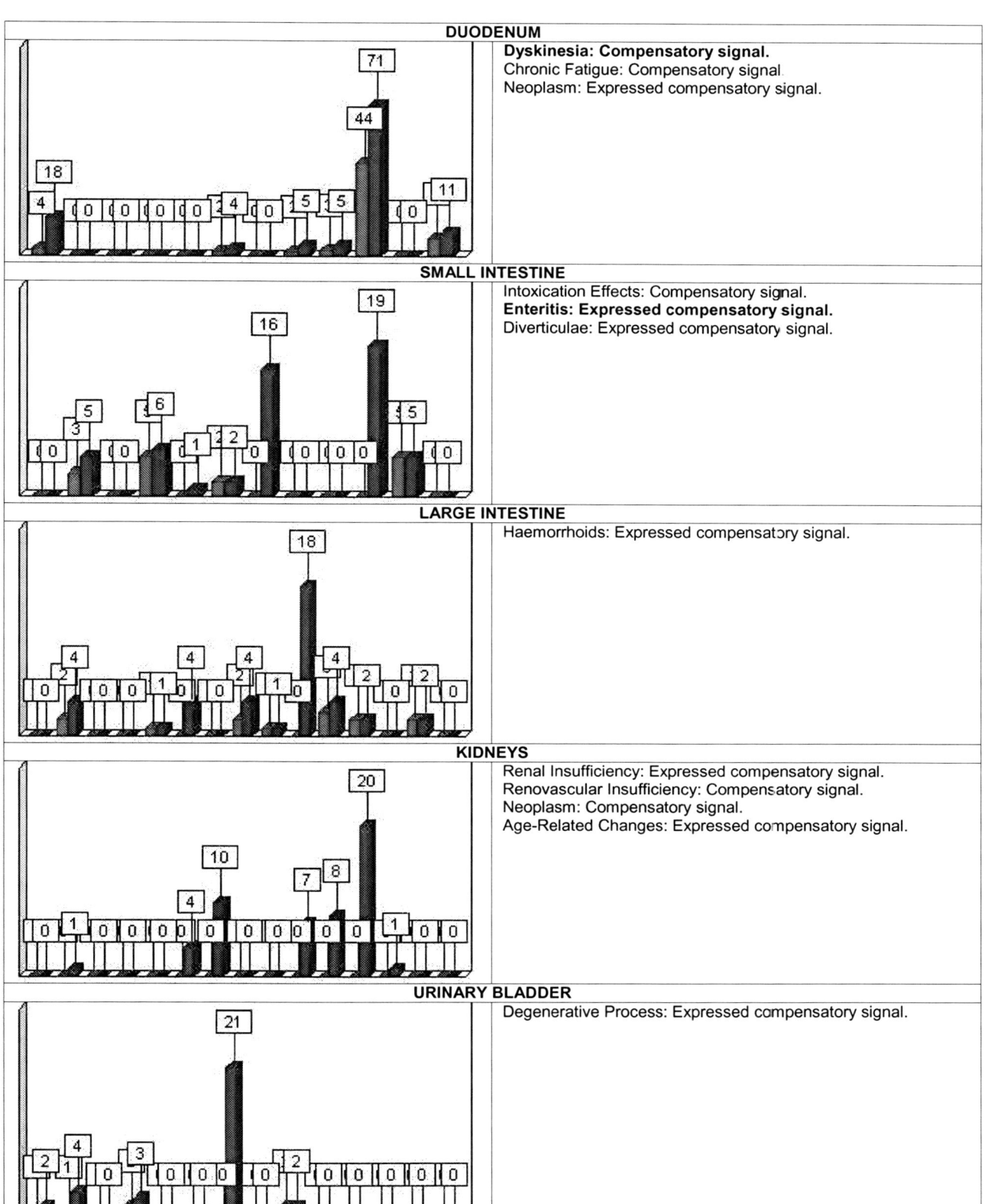

## DUODENUM

**Dyskinesia: Compensatory signal.**
Chronic Fatigue: Compensatory signal.
Neoplasm: Expressed compensatory signal.

## SMALL INTESTINE

Intoxication Effects: Compensatory signal.
**Enteritis: Expressed compensatory signal.**
Diverticulae: Expressed compensatory signal.

## LARGE INTESTINE

Haemorrhoids: Expressed compensatory signal.

## KIDNEYS

Renal Insufficiency: Expressed compensatory signal.
Renovascular Insufficiency: Compensatory signal.
Neoplasm: Compensatory signal.
Age-Related Changes: Expressed compensatory signal.

## URINARY BLADDER

Degenerative Process: Expressed compensatory signal.

204

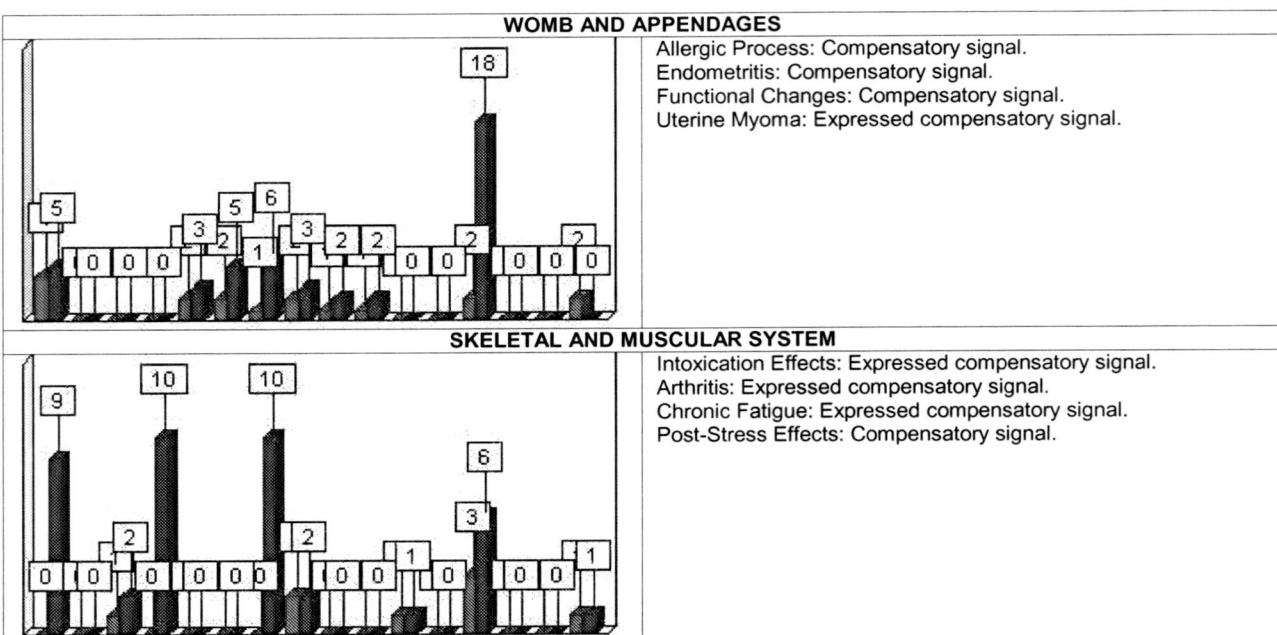

| WOMB AND APPENDAGES | |
|---|---|
| | Allergic Process: Compensatory signal.<br>Endometritis: Compensatory signal.<br>Functional Changes: Compensatory signal.<br>Uterine Myoma: Expressed compensatory signal. |

| SKELETAL AND MUSCULAR SYSTEM | |
|---|---|
| | Intoxication Effects: Expressed compensatory signal.<br>Arthritis: Expressed compensatory signal.<br>Chronic Fatigue: Expressed compensatory signal.<br>Post-Stress Effects: Compensatory signal. |

## Discussion of Reported Results

Virtual Scanning identifies a range of medical conditions (not necessarily the same for each dyslexic), clearly associated with **dyslexia**-type syndromes e.g.

- low blood pressure and poor quality of blood flow to the brain associated with improper function of the ears, inner-ear infection [72-73], balance disorders, poor memory, poor concentration, and coordination problems;

- otitis, otogenous labyrinthitis [81], cochlear neuritis, middle ear infection or inner ear infections, all conceivable consequencies of impaired brain blood flow which would affect the ability to hear, and to distinguish words or written text;

- spinal problems, perhaps due to inadequate levels of exercise [60-62], restricting the flow of blood to the brain, and hence affecting concentration and memory; and of impaired cerebral circulation, impaired spinal circulation, vertebral artery syndrome, spinal osteochondrosis, etc.

- weight problems, related to variable blood sugar and hence poor memory [53,55-58, 60-71], lack of fitness, and leukopenia (white blood cell count).

- digestive problems affecting nutrient absorption [41-45] and hence exerting negative influences on concentration, memory [53] and general function;

- poor physiological stability resulting in poor sleep patterns [54] perhaps resulting from too much television, inadequate quantity of sleep, poor absorption of nutrients, poor excretion, etc;

205

- too many soft drinks containing caffeine, high levels of sugar, phosphoric acid and aspartame [74-76].

    (a)    Caffeine [79] found/used in soft drinks, chocolate, tea and coffee, raises brain wave frequencies and gives a 'high'. It alters the brain waves and interferes with the body's natural rhythms and systems involved in processes of concentration and sleep.

            Some drinks containing high levels of caffeine have been banned in France and reformulated to have lower levels of caffeine in other countries.

    (b)    Aspartame [59] – a product manufactured by combining L-PhenylAlanine and L-Aspartic Acid – has a subtle influence, possibly affecting neurotransmitter levels in the brain, particularly phenylalanine.

    (c)    High levels of sugar inducing rapid changes in levels of blood insulin [101]

    (d)    High levels of phosphoric acid, quite apart from their destructive effects on the teeth, will inevitably affect digestive acidity and thus levels of both digestive flora and nutrient absorption thereby affecting the absorption and desorption of calcium [41-45, 75, 77-78] and other nutritional components

    (e)    In addition, many soft drinks, particularly Cola drinks, are associated with cravings, addictive and aggressive [80] behaviour.

- impaired blood flow may also result in eczema and other dermatological problems.

Recent thinking suggests that dyslexia has both genetic and psychosomatic components. In extreme cases, inherited genetic defects, are probably responsible for dyslexic symptoms. As can be seen from these examples there is evidence that stress in its various forms affects the regulatory processes and consequently organ function, health, ability to memorise, concentrate, co-ordinate and perform in the educational environment.

Similar observations apply to **autistic children**: (1) tests indicate levels of immune cells and proteins in their blood to be abnormal [30]; (2) clinical observations that high fever often temporarily alleviates autistic symptoms [31-33].

Further research supports the thesis that autistic spectrum disorders are related to physiological system dysfunction (such as abnormalities in hormone levels) [34]. In particular, disproportionately higher numbers of male children develop the condition; sleep patterns are often significantly disrupted [35-38]; breathing pattern disruption is also implicated in the development of autism [39-40]. A number of other medical conditions occur more frequently in those with autistism, adhd, etc – these include gastrointestinal and digestive disorders, problems with excretion including irregular stools, food allergies and food intolerances.

Dyslexia manifests as a broad range of symptoms presenting a multitude of problems for researchers who focus upon its SYMPTOMS. Defining symptoms of dyslexia include: (1) poor reading and writing, but others commonly associated with it include (2) poor physical coordination, memory, concentration, balance, hearing, etc.

The goal of any good theory would be to encompass *all* the symptoms and offer a coherent explanation fitting all the facts. Virtual Scanning technology enables us to offer plausible, systems-based explanations for all symptoms associated with dyslexia as developmental problems. These include:

- health related issues affecting abilities to function, such as

- poor memory;

- lack of concentration;

- hearing problems resulting in difficulty identifying words/speech;

- balance and coordination problems (and hence problems with writing);

- the symptoms of moving words when reading (otogenous labyrinthitis);

- the value of coloured lenses and other flashing light therapies in terms of the effects of colours and EEG frequency bands on the regulation of the 14 physiological systems.

## Conclusions

Virtual Scanning appears to explain all known symptoms and phenomena associated with dyslexia. This leads to insights connecting all such symptoms. The outcome is a technology which is able to identify and treat the main problems occurring in the dyslexic.

Initial results are highly encouraging although Virtual Scanning has not yet undergone evaluation programmes in the west such as clinical trials. All those treated have shown *some* form of improvement, if only in terms of decreases in Virtual Scanning's measures of pathology and compensation. Most encouragingly, NO child/person has proved unresponsive to Virtual Scanning therapy.

The best result obtained is of an 11yo girl who, in a six month period, progressed from a reading age two years below her calendar age to three years in advance of her calendar age. Other good results have been confirmed by letters and emails from parents.

Available information suggests that autistic spectrum disorders such as dyslexia, autism, aspergers syndrome, attention deficit disorder, etc; may be due to destabilisation of physiological systems regulating levels of biochemicals affecting sensory function e.g.

- Poor levels of white blood cells would be manifest through impaired immune system function as bacterial infection in the extremities i.e. skin, ears, throat, etc.

- Middle-ear dysfunction could be manifest as otogenous labyrinthitis thereby affecting the ability to read.

- Inner-ear and middle-ear problems would affect balance, hearing and vision.

- Adverse body acidity would affect the function of the endocrine system. This would be manifest as brittle bones [75-77], poor sleeping patterns, poor digestion, adverse absorption of minerals and vitamins, etc.

- Adverse absorption of iron (anaemia) would be manifest through impaired oxygen flow to the brain thereby reducing sensory function, memory and concentration.

- Poor sleeping patterns would affect the ability to regulate diet and satedness. This would subsequently be manifest as weight disorders.

- Poor brainwave stability exascerbated by stimulants decreases the ability to concentrate.

Is this so surprising when we consider that everything that we think and do results from biochemical change to our brain and body?

Further supportive evidence for this hypothesis can be obtained [46, 47] from other light-based systems used to treat dyslexia [98-100], and also from noted deficiencies in sensory perception and in particular of the hearing and vocal spectra: research indicates children with dyslexia to have deficiencies in their auditory spectra and that the use of artificially enhanced music can be used to treat their condition.

## 4.5    Assessment and Treatment of Chronic Fatigue Syndrome

Chronic Fatigue is defined as changes in physical, chemical and biological characteristics of tissues, resulting from stress, particularly psycho-emotional stress [88-92]. There is no evidence that it is caused by any specific causal factor including viral infection, the use of drugs, nutrition, etc.

It appears to be related to immunosuppression and the function of the central nervous system which is affected by stress. This affects the function of the hypothalamus and its relationship with the endocrine system leading to increased release of cortisol and other hormones. Cortisol and corticotrophin-releasing hormone (CRH), which are also produced during the activation of the HPA axis, influence the immune system and many other body systems.

Accordingly there is no test for Chronic Fatigue, Chronic Fatigue Syndrome (CFS) and Fibromyalgia (FM) and no standard therapy. Many people recover naturally over a period of up to 10 years although even after recovery most consider that their health remains at a dysfunctional level i.e. they have low levels of wellbeing.

Reviews of those with Chronic Fatigue, CFS and FM  assessed by Virtual Scanning reveals a number of features consistently appearing in those identified with this category of condition.

- The occurrence of low levels of compensatory signals in the endocrine glands of those suffering from CFS and FM

- The occurrence of significant *uncompensated* 'chronic fatigue' pathologies, in those suffering from 'chronic fatigue syndrome (CFS)'.

- The development of significant uncompensated chronic fatigue pathologies in the endocrine glands and digestive system in those suffering from 'chronic fatigue syndrome (CFS)'.

- In addition to the above, those with indications of Fibromyalgia (FM), show further significant pathologies in endocrine system organs e.g. pancreatic insufficiency, diabetes mellitus, etc.

n.b. 'Chronic Fatigue' - as defined by the test - is defined as the change in physical, chemical and biological characteristics of tissues, as a result of stress(es), including psycho-emotional stress(es).

example 4: girl, 13 years, 41 kgs, Chronic Fatigue, Dyslexic

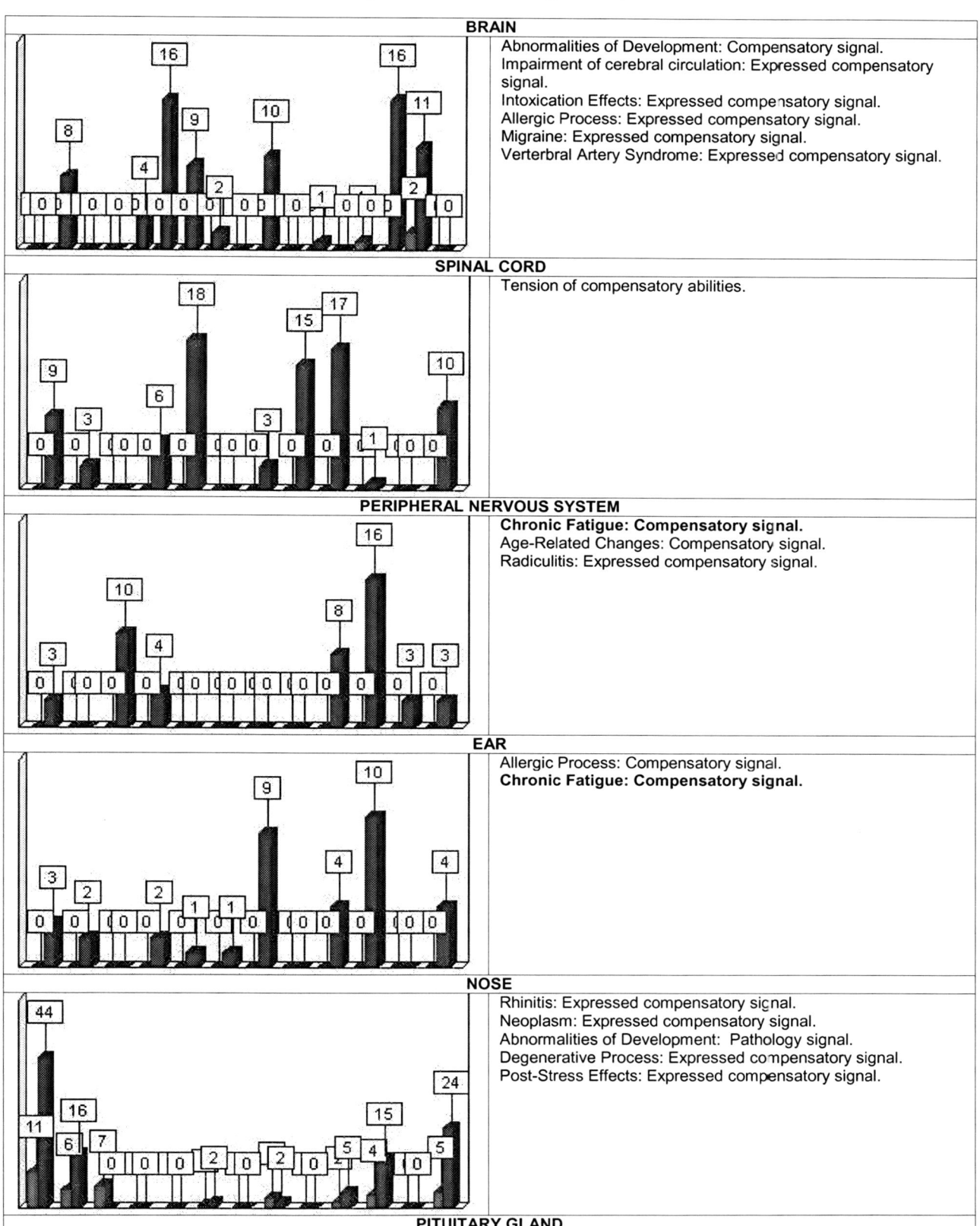

**BRAIN**

Abnormalities of Development: Compensatory signal.
Impairment of cerebral circulation: Expressed compensatory signal.
Intoxication Effects: Expressed compensatory signal.
Allergic Process: Expressed compensatory signal.
Migraine: Expressed compensatory signal.
Verterbral Artery Syndrome: Expressed compensatory signal.

**SPINAL CORD**

Tension of compensatory abilities.

**PERIPHERAL NERVOUS SYSTEM**

**Chronic Fatigue: Compensatory signal.**
Age-Related Changes: Compensatory signal.
Radiculitis: Expressed compensatory signal.

**EAR**

Allergic Process: Compensatory signal.
**Chronic Fatigue: Compensatory signal.**

**NOSE**

Rhinitis: Expressed compensatory signal.
Neoplasm: Expressed compensatory signal.
Abnormalities of Development: Pathology signal.
Degenerative Process: Expressed compensatory signal.
Post-Stress Effects: Expressed compensatory signal.

**PITUITARY GLAND**

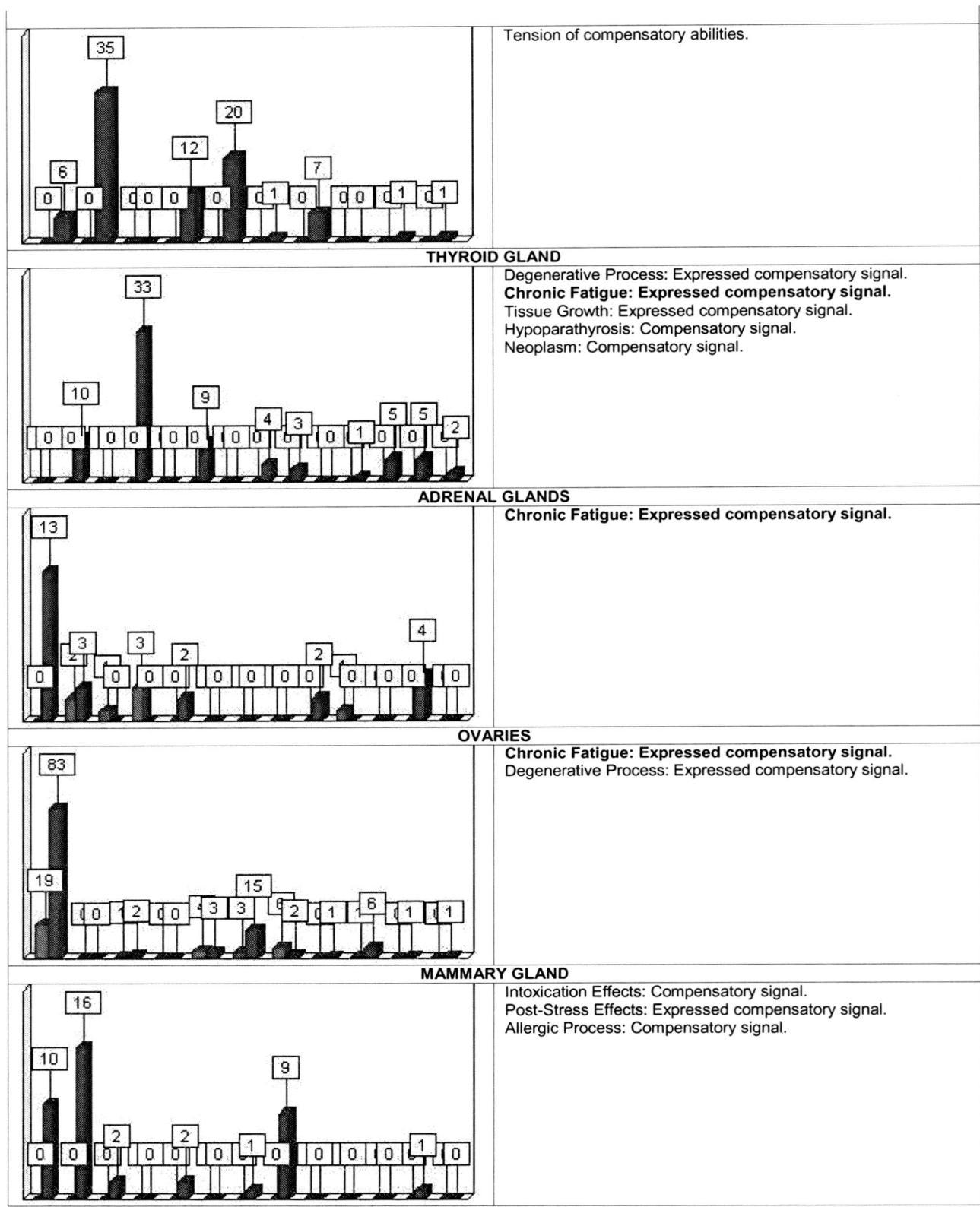

Tension of compensatory abilities.

**THYROID GLAND**

Degenerative Process: Expressed compensatory signal.
**Chronic Fatigue: Expressed compensatory signal.**
Tissue Growth: Expressed compensatory signal.
Hypoparathyrosis: Compensatory signal.
Neoplasm: Compensatory signal.

**ADRENAL GLANDS**

**Chronic Fatigue: Expressed compensatory signal.**

**OVARIES**

**Chronic Fatigue: Expressed compensatory signal.**
Degenerative Process: Expressed compensatory signal.

**MAMMARY GLAND**

Intoxication Effects: Compensatory signal.
Post-Stress Effects: Expressed compensatory signal.
Allergic Process: Compensatory signal.

211

## LIVER

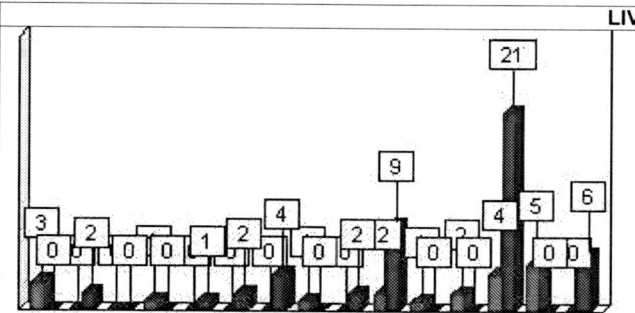

Neoplasm: Pathology signal.
Disruption of Bilirubin Metabolism: Expressed compensatory signal.
Liver Insufficiency: Expressed compensatory signal.
Post-Stress Effects: Compensatory signal.

## GALL BLADDER

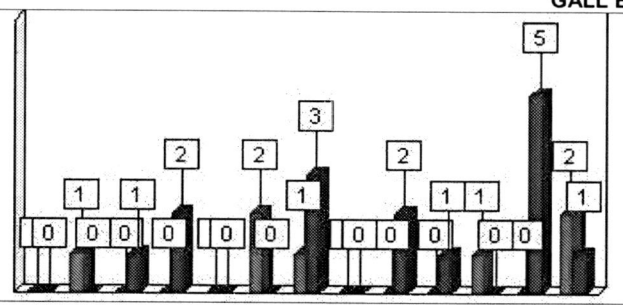

No changes detected.

## PANCREAS

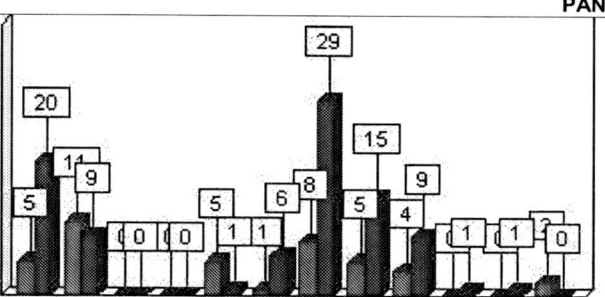

Intoxication Effects: Weakening of compensatory abilities.
Sclerotic Pancreatitis: Expressed compensatory signal.
**Chronic Fatigue: Expressed compensatory signal.**
Allergic Process: Compensatory signal.
Functional Changes: Expressed compensatory signal.
Degenerative Process: Compensatory signal.

## HEART

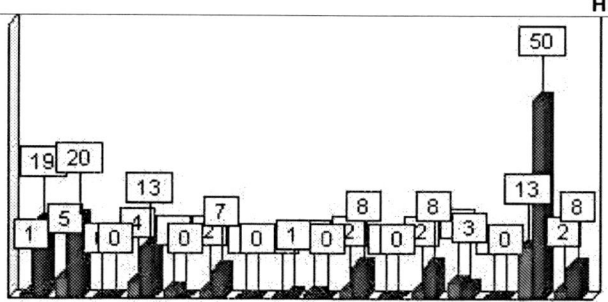

Functional Changes: Expressed compensatory signal.
**Impairment of Cardiac Rhythm and Conduction: Expressed compensatory signal.**
Tension of compensatory abilities.

## BLOOD AND PERIPHERAL BLOOD VESSELS

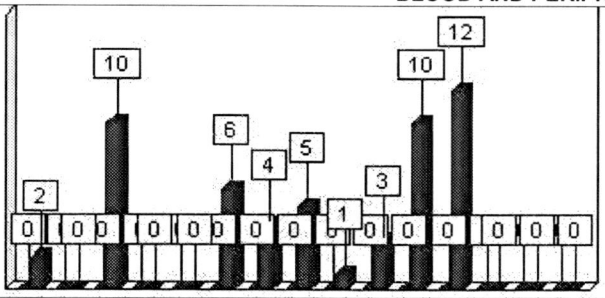

**Leukopenia: Expressed compensatory signal.**
Functional Changes: Compensatory signal.
Neoplasm: Compensatory signal.
**Idiopathic Hypotension: Expressed compensatory signal.**
Degenerative Process: Expressed compensatory signal.

212

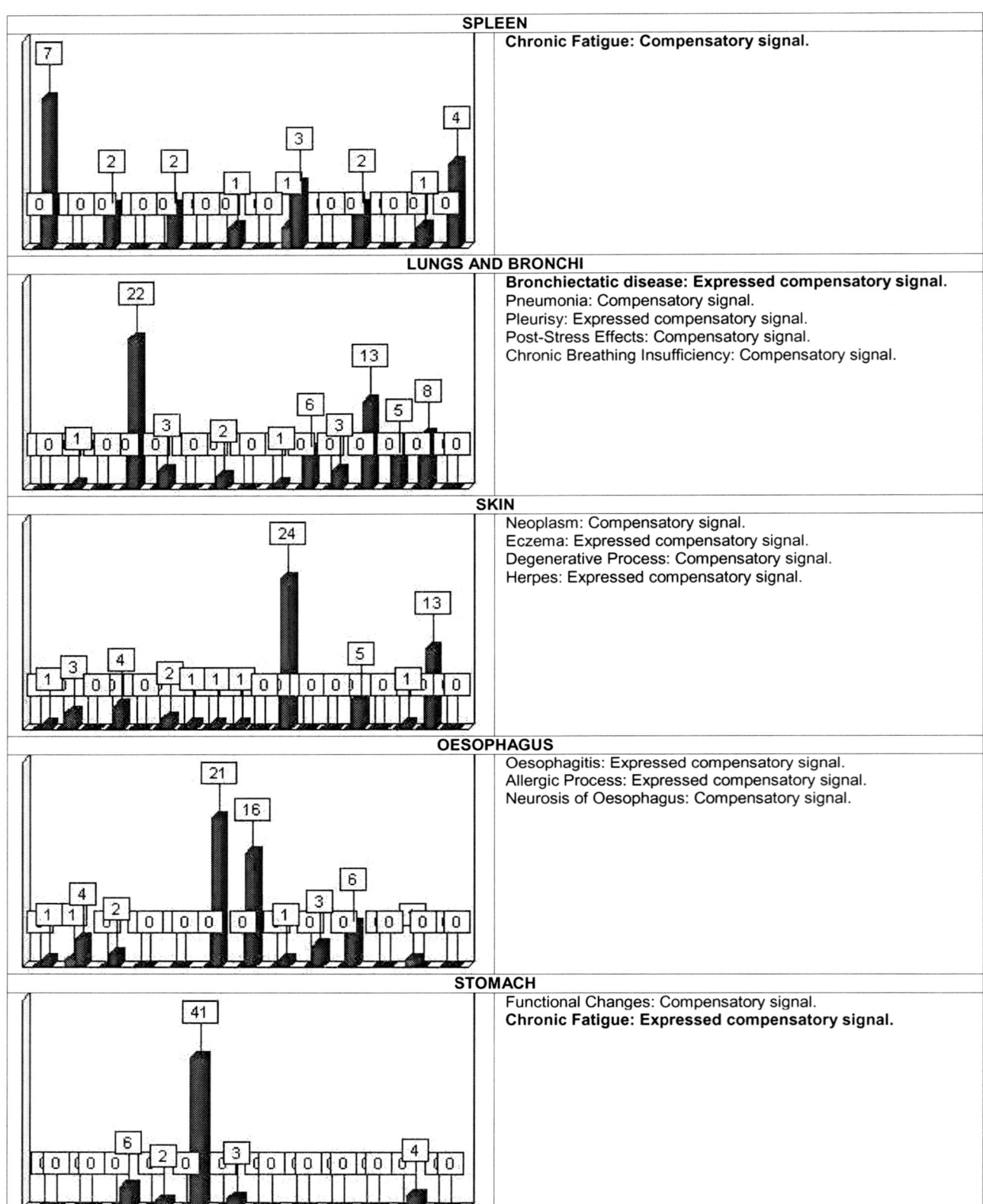

**SPLEEN**

Chronic Fatigue: Compensatory signal.

**LUNGS AND BRONCHI**

**Bronchiectatic disease: Expressed compensatory signal.**
Pneumonia: Compensatory signal.
Pleurisy: Expressed compensatory signal.
Post-Stress Effects: Compensatory signal.
Chronic Breathing Insufficiency: Compensatory signal.

**SKIN**

Neoplasm: Compensatory signal.
Eczema: Expressed compensatory signal.
Degenerative Process: Compensatory signal.
Herpes: Expressed compensatory signal.

**OESOPHAGUS**

Oesophagitis: Expressed compensatory signal.
Allergic Process: Expressed compensatory signal.
Neurosis of Oesophagus: Compensatory signal.

**STOMACH**

Functional Changes: Compensatory signal.
**Chronic Fatigue: Expressed compensatory signal.**

213

| DUODENUM | |
|---|---|
| 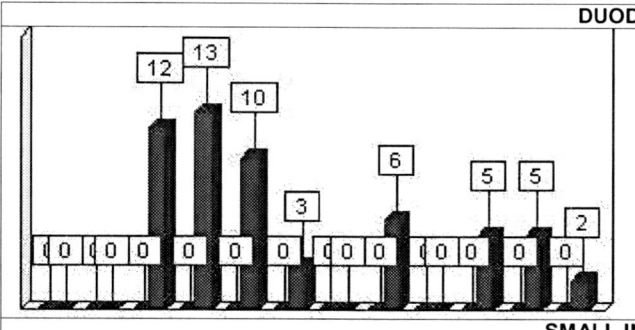 | Degenerative Process: Expressed compensatory signal. |
| | Duodenitis: Expressed compensatory signal. |
| | Intoxication Effects: Compensatory signal. |
| | Allergic Process: Compensatory signal. |

| SMALL INTESTINE | |
|---|---|
| 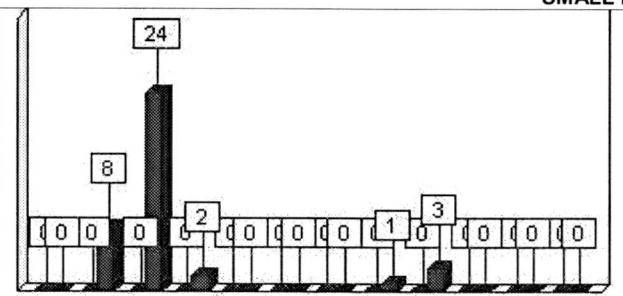 | Allergic Process: Compensatory signal. |
| | Dyskinesia: Expressed compensatory signal. |

| LARGE INTESTINE | |
|---|---|
| 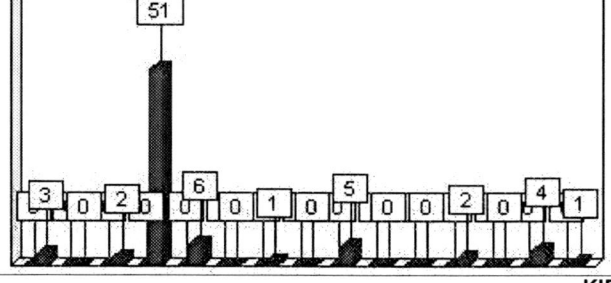 | Colitis: Expressed compensatory signal. |
| | **Chronic Fatigue: Compensatory signal.** |
| | Degenerative Process: Compensatory signal. |

| KIDNEYS | |
|---|---|
| 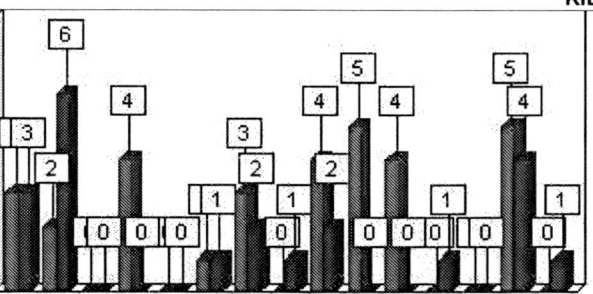 | Renovascular Insufficiency: Pathology signal. |
| | Allergic Process: Weakening of compensatory abilities. |
| | **Chronic Fatigue: Compensatory signal.** |

| URINARY BLADDER | |
|---|---|
| 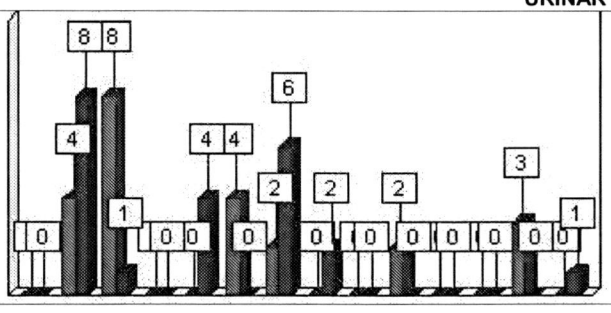 | Urolithiasis: Pathology signal. |
| | **Chronic Fatigue: Compensatory signal.** |
| | Degenerative Process: Compensatory signal. |

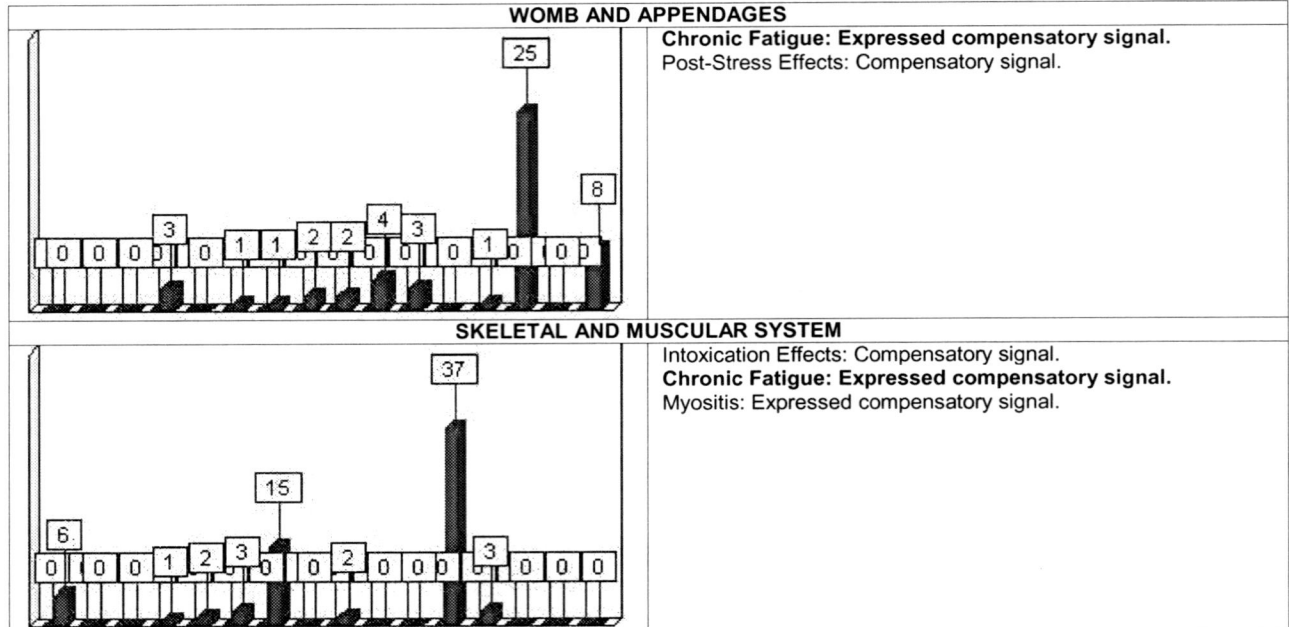

## Discussion of Reported Results

Note the presence of compensated indications (blue signals only) of 'Chronic Fatigue' in the endocrine system, the usual indication of 'chronic fatigue' in those who have not been diagnosed as having 'chronic fatigue syndrome'.

example 5: woman, 68 years/79kgs, Chronic Fatigue Syndrome

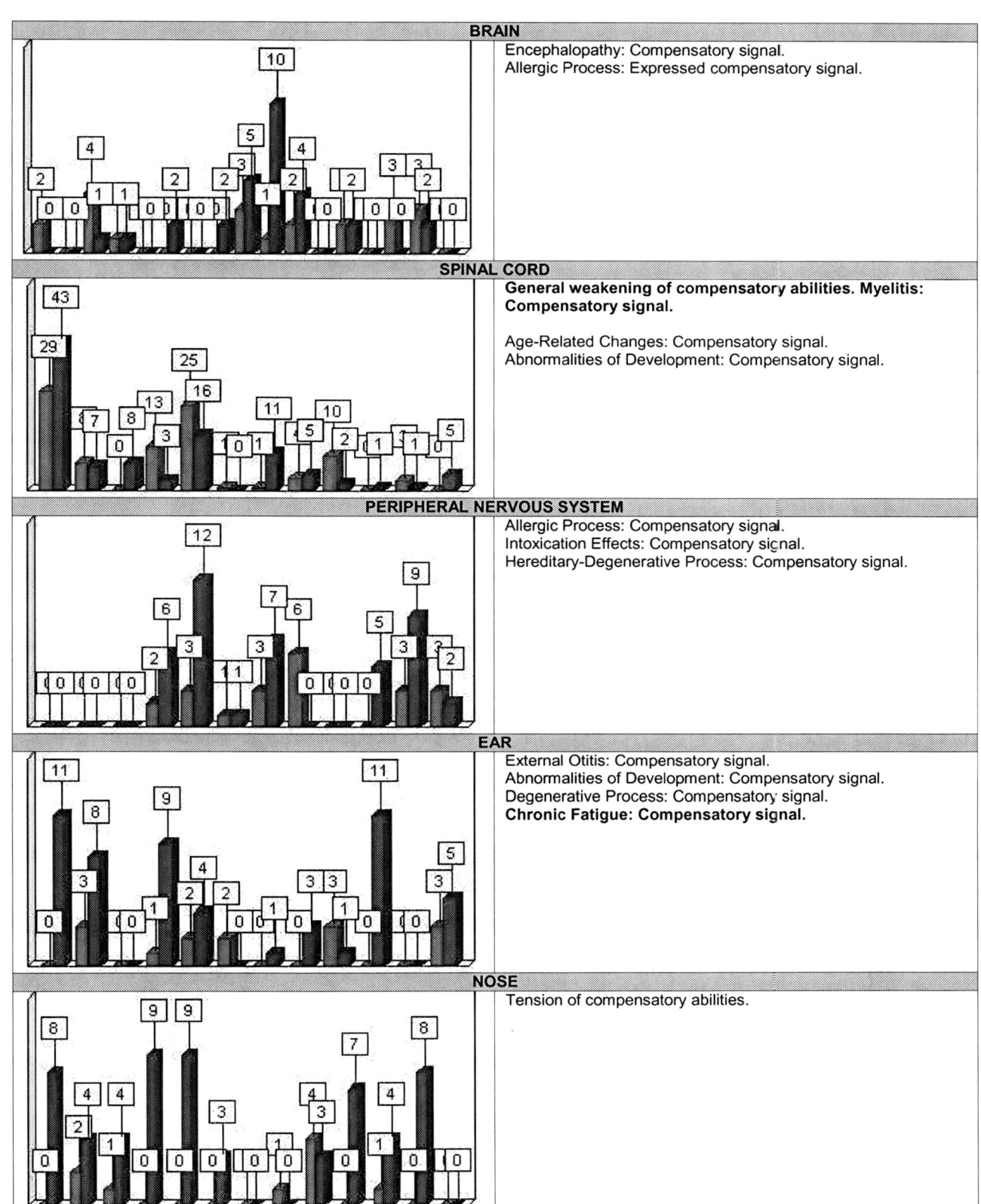

**BRAIN**

Encephalopathy: Compensatory signal.
Allergic Process: Expressed compensatory signal.

**SPINAL CORD**

**General weakening of compensatory abilities. Myelitis: Compensatory signal.**

Age-Related Changes: Compensatory signal.
Abnormalities of Development: Compensatory signal.

**PERIPHERAL NERVOUS SYSTEM**

Allergic Process: Compensatory signal.
Intoxication Effects: Compensatory signal.
Hereditary-Degenerative Process: Compensatory signal.

**EAR**

External Otitis: Compensatory signal.
Abnormalities of Development: Compensatory signal.
Degenerative Process: Compensatory signal.
**Chronic Fatigue: Compensatory signal.**

**NOSE**

Tension of compensatory abilities.

216

## PITUITARY GLAND

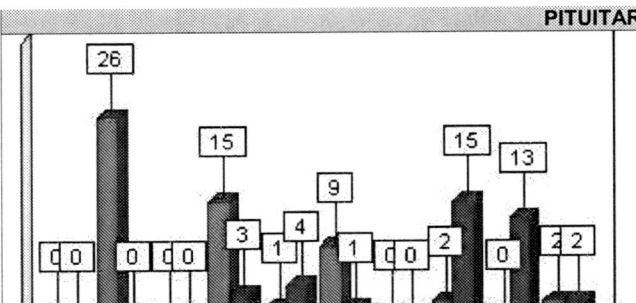

**Chronic Fatigue:  Expressed pathology signal.**
Functional Changes:  Expressed pathology signal.
Intoxication Effects:  Pathology signal.
Age-Related Changes: Expressed compensatory signal.
Allergic Process: Compensatory signal.

## THYROID GLAND

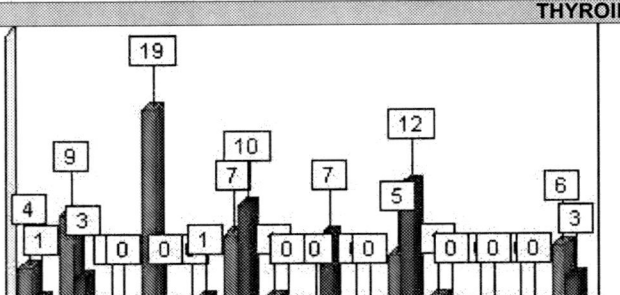

Degenerative Process:  Pathology signal.
**Chronic Fatigue:  Expressed pathology signal.**
Tissue Growth: Compensatory signal.
Functional Changes:  Pathology signal.
Allergic Process: Compensatory signal.
Thyroiditis: Expressed compensatory signal.

## ADRENAL GLANDS

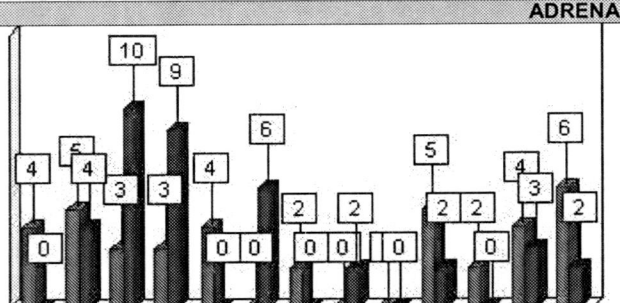

Cohn's Syndrome: Compensatory signal.
Abnormalities of Development: Compensatory signal.

## OVARIES

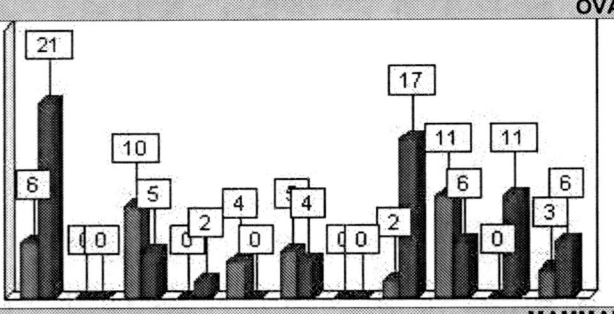

Post-Stress Effects:  Pathology signal.
Allergic Process: Weakening of compensatory abilities.
**Chronic Fatigue: Expressed compensatory signal.**
Neoplasm: Expressed compensatory signal.
Functional Changes: Compensatory signal.

## MAMMARY GLAND

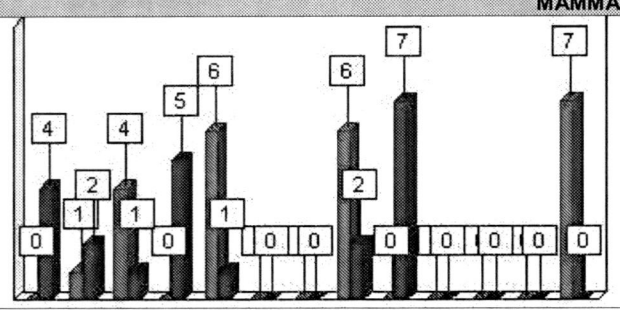

**Chronic Fatigue:  Pathology signal.**
Functional Changes: Compensatory signal.

217

## LIVER

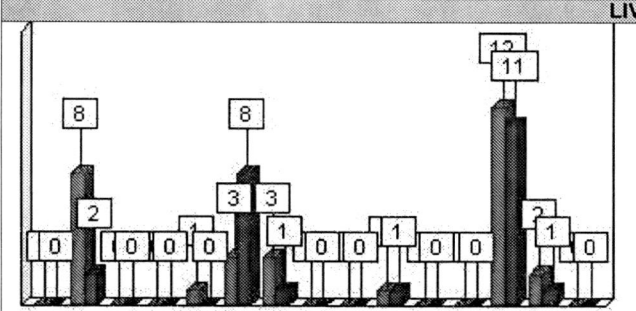

Age-Related Changes: Pathology signal.
Liver Insufficiency: Weakening of compensatory abilities.
Intoxication Effects: Compensatory signal.

## GALL BLADDER

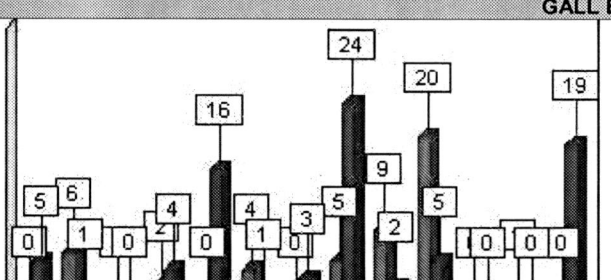

Allergic Process: Pathology signal.
**Chronic Fatigue: Expressed pathology signal.**
Cholelithiasis: Expressed compensatory signal.
Dyskinesia of Biliary Ducts and Gall Bladder: Expressed compensatory signal.
Age-Related Changes: Expressed compensatory signal.

## PANCREAS

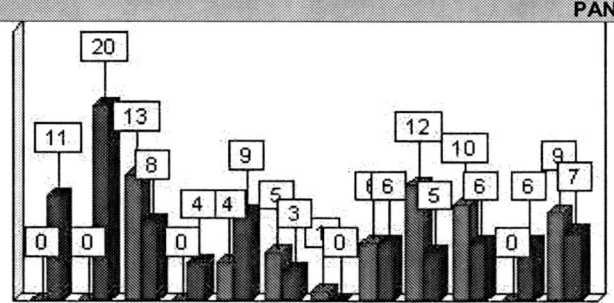

Post-Stress Effects: Weakening of compensatory abilities.
Degenerative Process: Pathology signal.
**Pathology of Islands of Langerhans: Weakening of compensatory abilities.**
Abnormalities of Development: Weakening of compensatory abilities.
**Chronic Fatigue: Compensatory signal.**
Intoxication Effects: Expressed compensatory signal.
Age-Related Changes: Compensatory signal.

## HEART

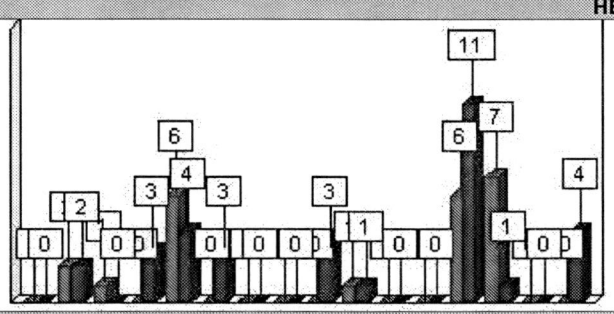

Cardiac Infarction: Weakening of compensatory abilities.
Cardiac Myopathy: Compensatory signal.
Age-Related Changes: Pathology signal.

## BLOOD AND PERIPHERAL BLOOD VESSELS

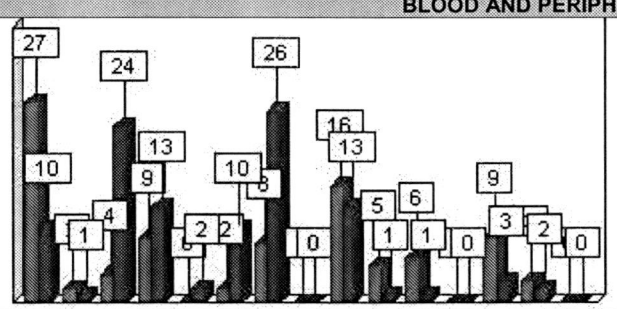

General weakening of compensatory abilities.
Allergic Process: Compensatory signal.

General weakening of compensatory abilities.
Haemorrhagic Vasculitis: Expressed compensatory signal.

Leukopenia: Expressed compensatory signal.
Functional Changes: Compensatory signal.

## SPLEEN

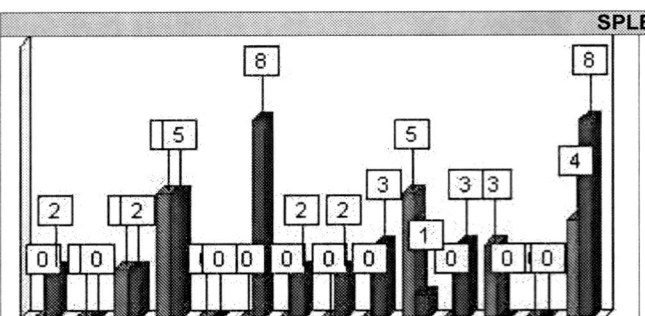

Hypersplenism: Compensatory signal.
Tissue Growth: Compensatory signal.

## LUNGS AND BRONCHI

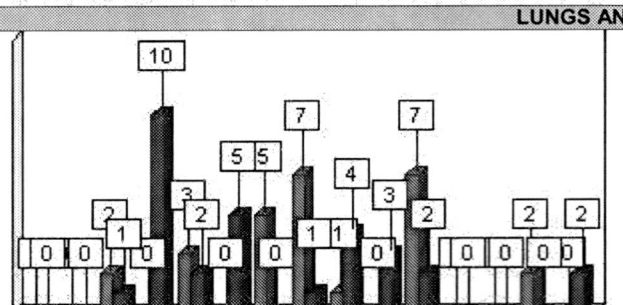

Neoplasm: Pathology signal.
**Chronic Fatigue: Pathology signal.**
Bronchiectatic disease: Compensatory signal.

## SKIN

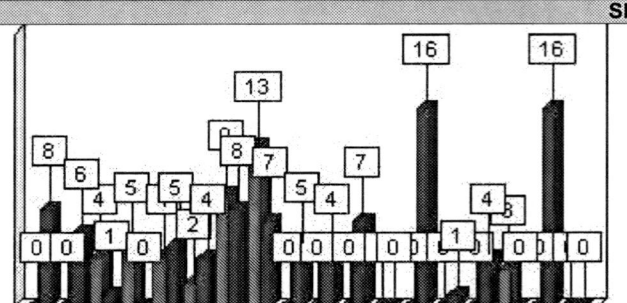

Neoplasm: Pathology signal.
Neurodermatitis: Weakening of compensatory abilities.
Allergic Process: Weakening of compensatory abilities.
Tension of compensatory abilities.

## OESOPHAGUS

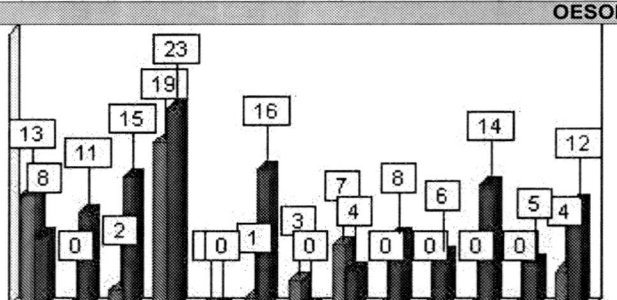

Functional Changes: Weakening of compensatory abilities.
**Chronic Fatigue: Compensatory signal.**
Post-Stress Effects: Weakening of compensatory abilities.
Tension of compensatory abilities.

## STOMACH

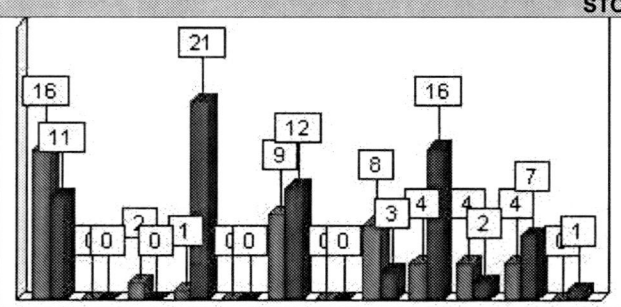

Age-Related Changes: Weakening of compensatory abilities.
Intoxication Effects: Compensatory signal.
Ulcerative Disease: Pathology signal.
Gastritis: Expressed compensatory signal.
Neoplasm: Expressed compensatory signal.
Degenerative Process: Compensatory signal.

| DUODENUM | |
|---|---|
| 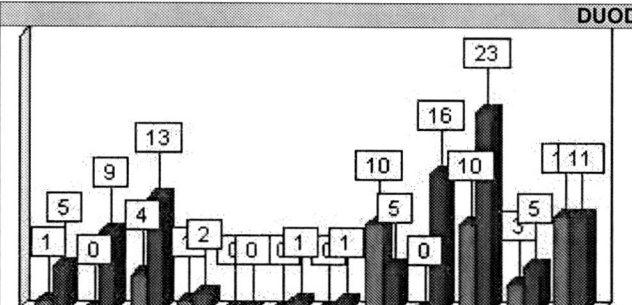 | Allergic Process:  Pathology signal.<br>Dyskinesia: Expressed compensatory signal.<br>**Chronic Fatigue: Compensated pathology condition.**<br>Abnormalities of Development: Compensatory signal.<br>Degenerative Process: Expressed compensatory signal.<br>Post-Stress Effects: Expressed compensatory signal. |

| SMALL INTESTINE | |
|---|---|
| 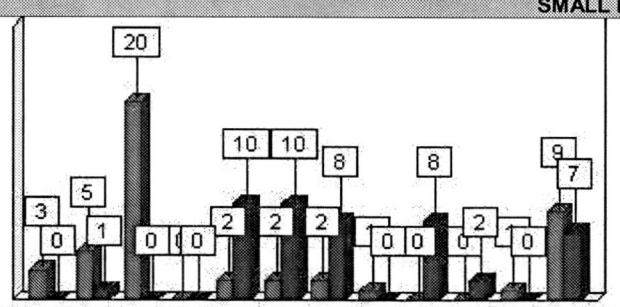 | Dyskinesia:  Expressed pathology signal.<br>Tissue Growth: Weakening of compensatory abilities.<br>Post-Stress Effects: Compensatory signal.<br>Abnormalities of Development: Compensatory signal.<br>Enteritis: Compensatory signal.<br>Degenerative Process: Compensatory signal. |

| LARGE INTESTINE | |
|---|---|
| 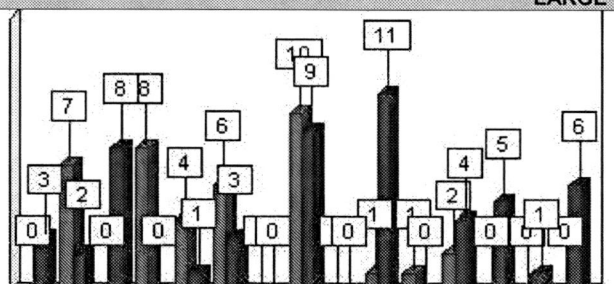 | Age-Related Changes:  Pathology signal.<br>Colitis:  Pathology signal.<br>Intoxication Effects:  Pathology signal.<br>Abnormalities of Development: Weakening of compensatory abilities.<br>Allergic Process: Compensatory signal.<br>Haemorrhoids: Expressed compensatory signal.<br>Post-Stress Effects: Compensatory signal. |

| KIDNEYS | |
|---|---|
| 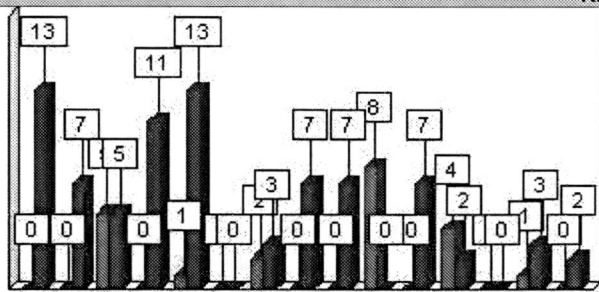 | Renovascular Insufficiency:  Pathology signal.<br>Tension of compensatory abilities. |

| URINARY BLADDER | |
|---|---|
| 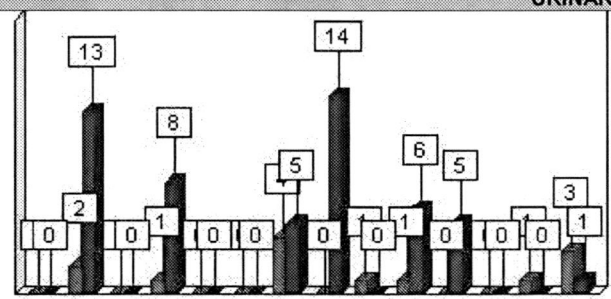 | **Chronic Fatigue: Expressed compensatory signal.**<br>Post-Stress Effects: Compensatory signal.<br>Age-Related Changes: Expressed compensatory signal.<br>Abnormalities of Development: Compensatory signal. |

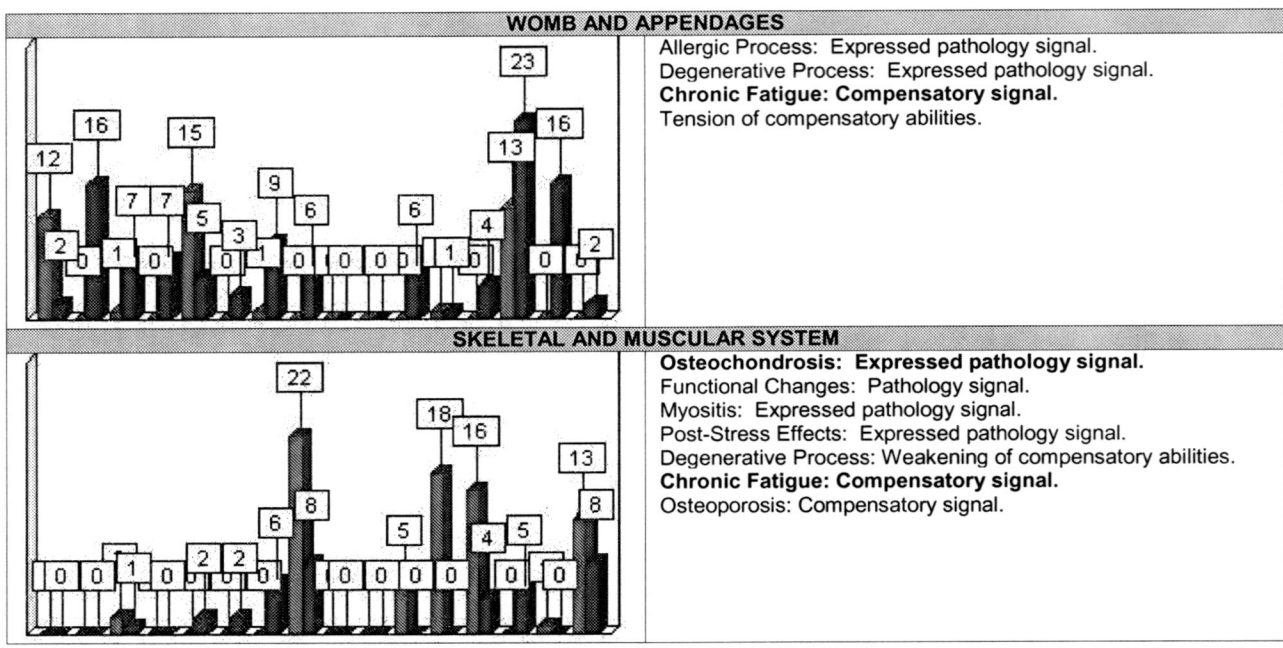

**WOMB AND APPENDAGES**

Allergic Process: Expressed pathology signal.
Degenerative Process: Expressed pathology signal.
**Chronic Fatigue: Compensatory signal.**
Tension of compensatory abilities.

**SKELETAL AND MUSCULAR SYSTEM**

**Osteochondrosis: Expressed pathology signal.**
Functional Changes: Pathology signal.
Myositis: Expressed pathology signal.
Post-Stress Effects: Expressed pathology signal.
Degenerative Process: Weakening of compensatory abilities.
**Chronic Fatigue: Compensatory signal.**
Osteoporosis: Compensatory signal.

## Discussion of Reported Results

In this case of Chronic Fatigue Syndrome, note the chronic fatigue signals throughout the body: particularly uncompensated (red) chronic fatigue signals from the endocrine system (thyroid & pituitary glands), compensated (blue and red) signals from the ovaries, womb, pancreas, and urinary bladder, and also in the digestive system (duodenum, gall bladder).

This is a typical profile of patients with Chronic Fatigue Syndrome.

221

example 6, male 39 years/96 kgs, Fibromyalgia

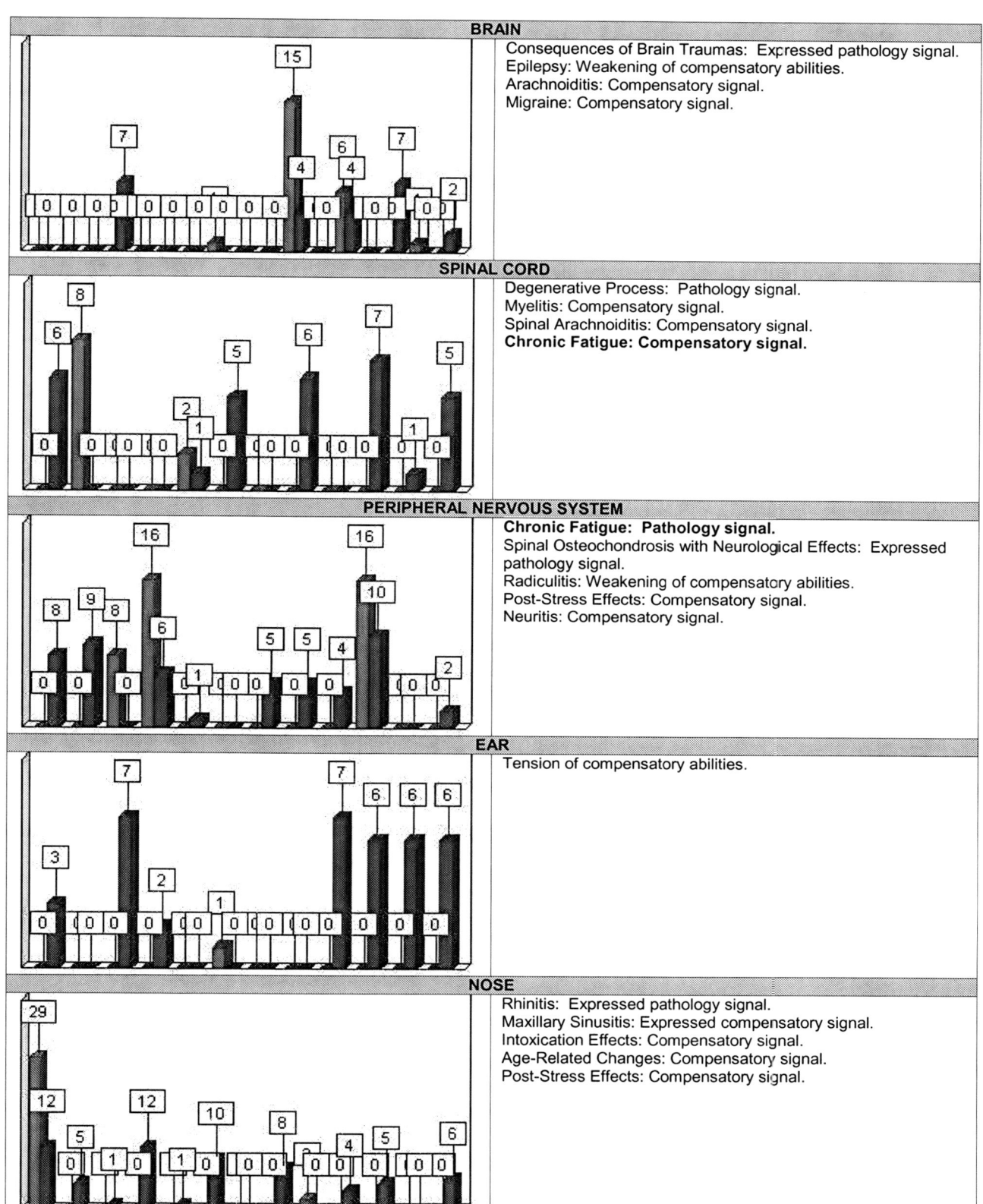

**BRAIN**

Consequences of Brain Traumas: Expressed pathology signal.
Epilepsy: Weakening of compensatory abilities.
Arachnoiditis: Compensatory signal.
Migraine: Compensatory signal.

**SPINAL CORD**

Degenerative Process: Pathology signal.
Myelitis: Compensatory signal.
Spinal Arachnoiditis: Compensatory signal.
**Chronic Fatigue: Compensatory signal.**

**PERIPHERAL NERVOUS SYSTEM**

**Chronic Fatigue: Pathology signal.**
Spinal Osteochondrosis with Neurological Effects: Expressed pathology signal.
Radiculitis: Weakening of compensatory abilities.
Post-Stress Effects: Compensatory signal.
Neuritis: Compensatory signal.

**EAR**

Tension of compensatory abilities.

**NOSE**

Rhinitis: Expressed pathology signal.
Maxillary Sinusitis: Expressed compensatory signal.
Intoxication Effects: Compensatory signal.
Age-Related Changes: Compensatory signal.
Post-Stress Effects: Compensatory signal.

222

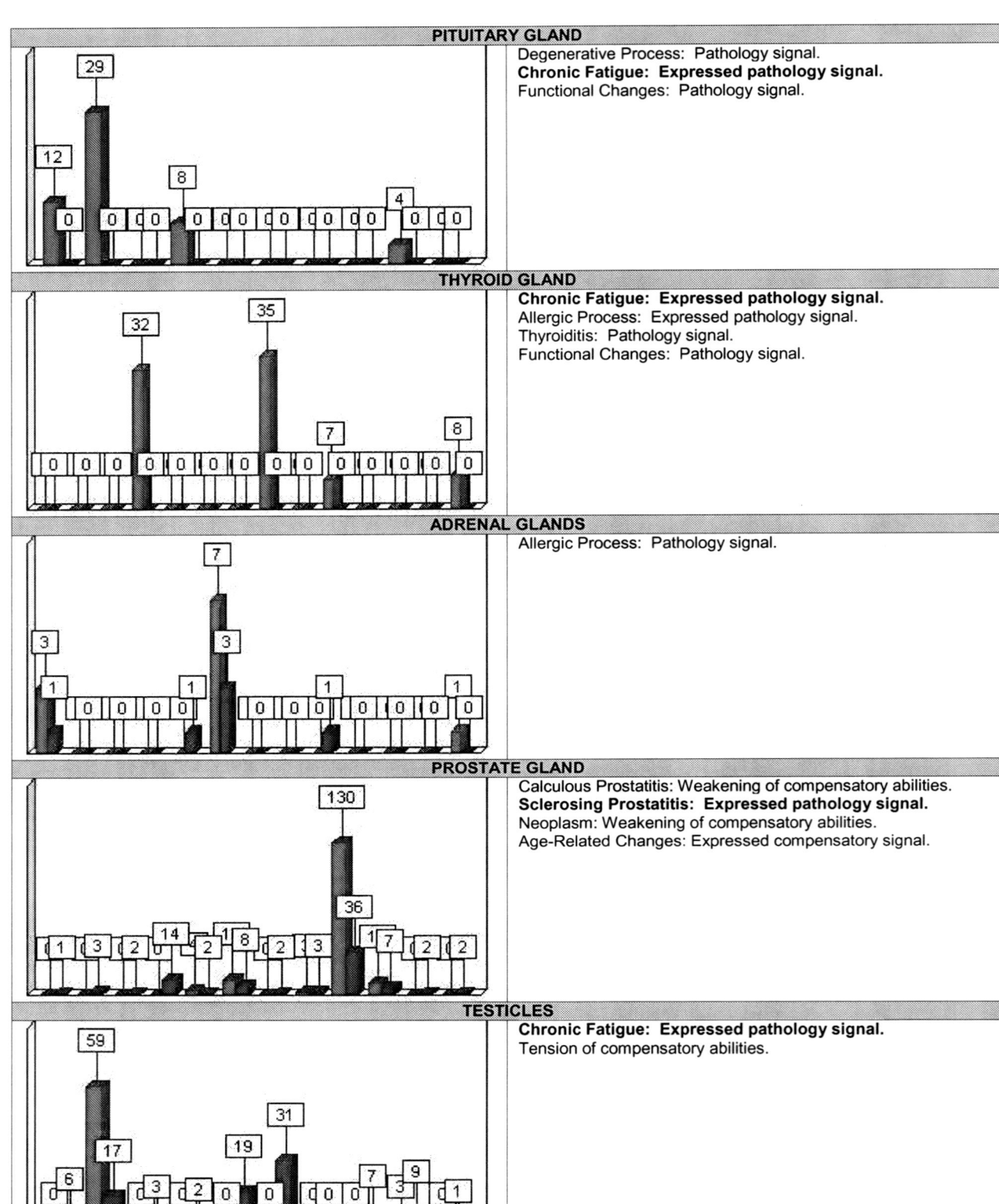

**PITUITARY GLAND**

Degenerative Process:  Pathology signal.
**Chronic Fatigue:  Expressed pathology signal.**
Functional Changes:  Pathology signal.

**THYROID GLAND**

**Chronic Fatigue:  Expressed pathology signal.**
Allergic Process:  Expressed pathology signal.
Thyroiditis:  Pathology signal.
Functional Changes:  Pathology signal.

**ADRENAL GLANDS**

Allergic Process:  Pathology signal.

**PROSTATE GLAND**

Calculous Prostatitis: Weakening of compensatory abilities.
**Sclerosing Prostatitis:  Expressed pathology signal.**
Neoplasm: Weakening of compensatory abilities.
Age-Related Changes: Expressed compensatory signal.

**TESTICLES**

**Chronic Fatigue:  Expressed pathology signal.**
Tension of compensatory abilities.

223

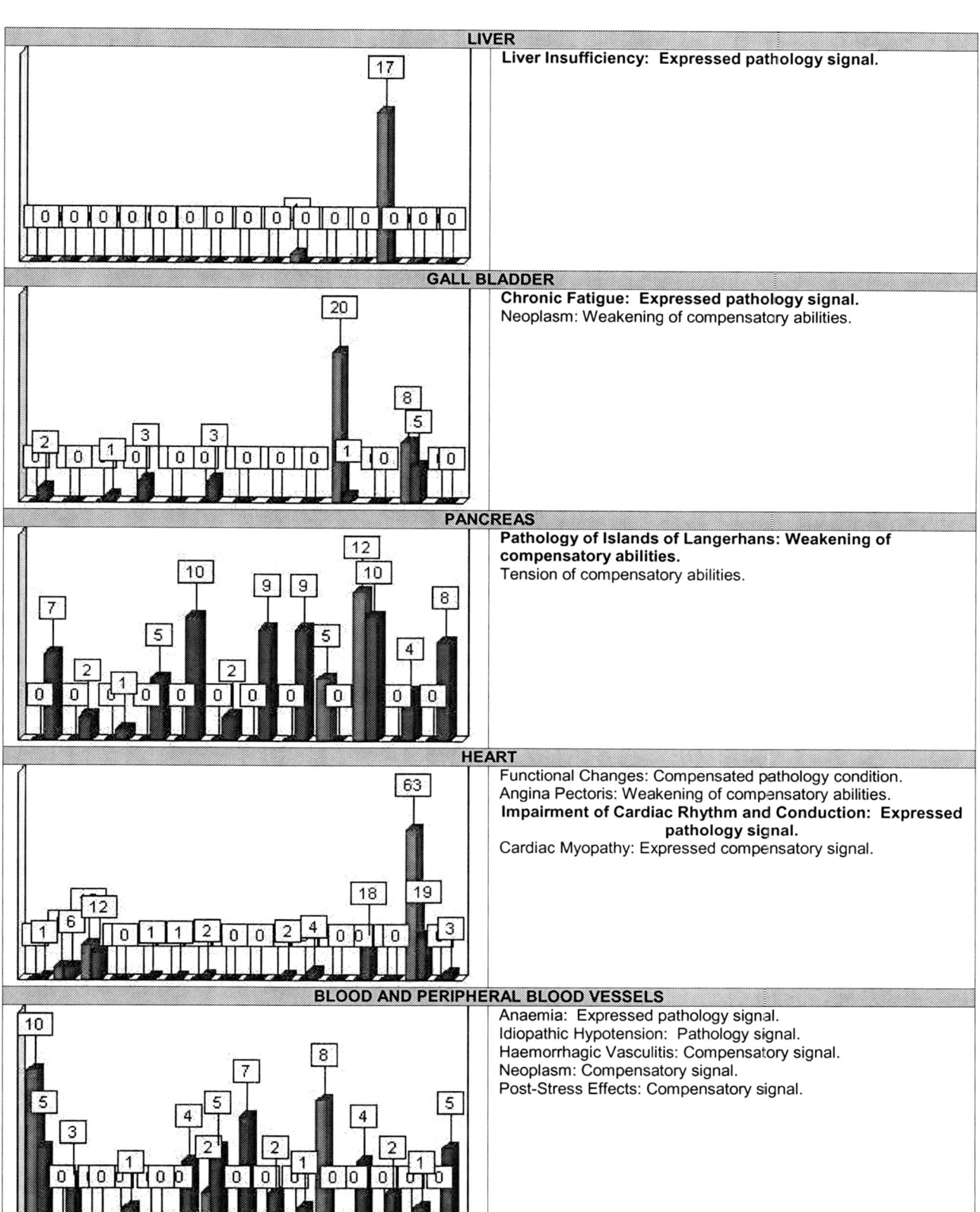

**LIVER**

Liver Insufficiency: **Expressed pathology signal.**

**GALL BLADDER**

**Chronic Fatigue: Expressed pathology signal.**
Neoplasm: Weakening of compensatory abilities.

**PANCREAS**

**Pathology of Islands of Langerhans: Weakening of compensatory abilities.**
Tension of compensatory abilities.

**HEART**

Functional Changes: Compensated pathology condition.
Angina Pectoris: Weakening of compensatory abilities.
**Impairment of Cardiac Rhythm and Conduction: Expressed pathology signal.**
Cardiac Myopathy: Expressed compensatory signal.

**BLOOD AND PERIPHERAL BLOOD VESSELS**

Anaemia: Expressed pathology signal.
Idiopathic Hypotension: Pathology signal.
Haemorrhagic Vasculitis: Compensatory signal.
Neoplasm: Compensatory signal.
Post-Stress Effects: Compensatory signal.

224

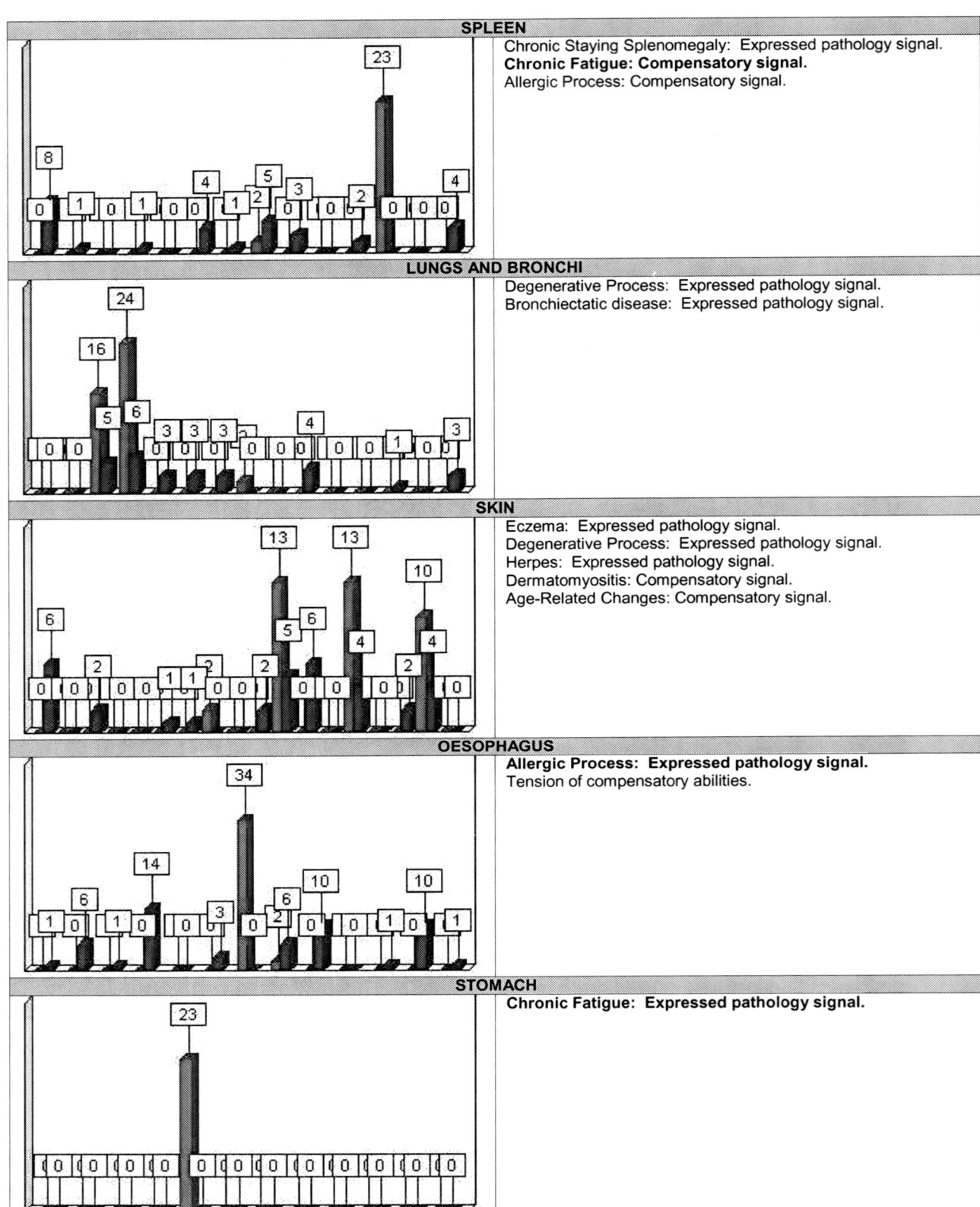

**SPLEEN**

Chronic Staying Splenomegaly: Expressed pathology signal.
**Chronic Fatigue: Compensatory signal.**
Allergic Process: Compensatory signal.

**LUNGS AND BRONCHI**

Degenerative Process: Expressed pathology signal.
Bronchiectatic disease: Expressed pathology signal.

**SKIN**

Eczema: Expressed pathology signal.
Degenerative Process: Expressed pathology signal.
Herpes: Expressed pathology signal.
Dermatomyositis: Compensatory signal.
Age-Related Changes: Compensatory signal.

**OESOPHAGUS**

**Allergic Process: Expressed pathology signal.**
Tension of compensatory abilities.

**STOMACH**

**Chronic Fatigue: Expressed pathology signal.**

225

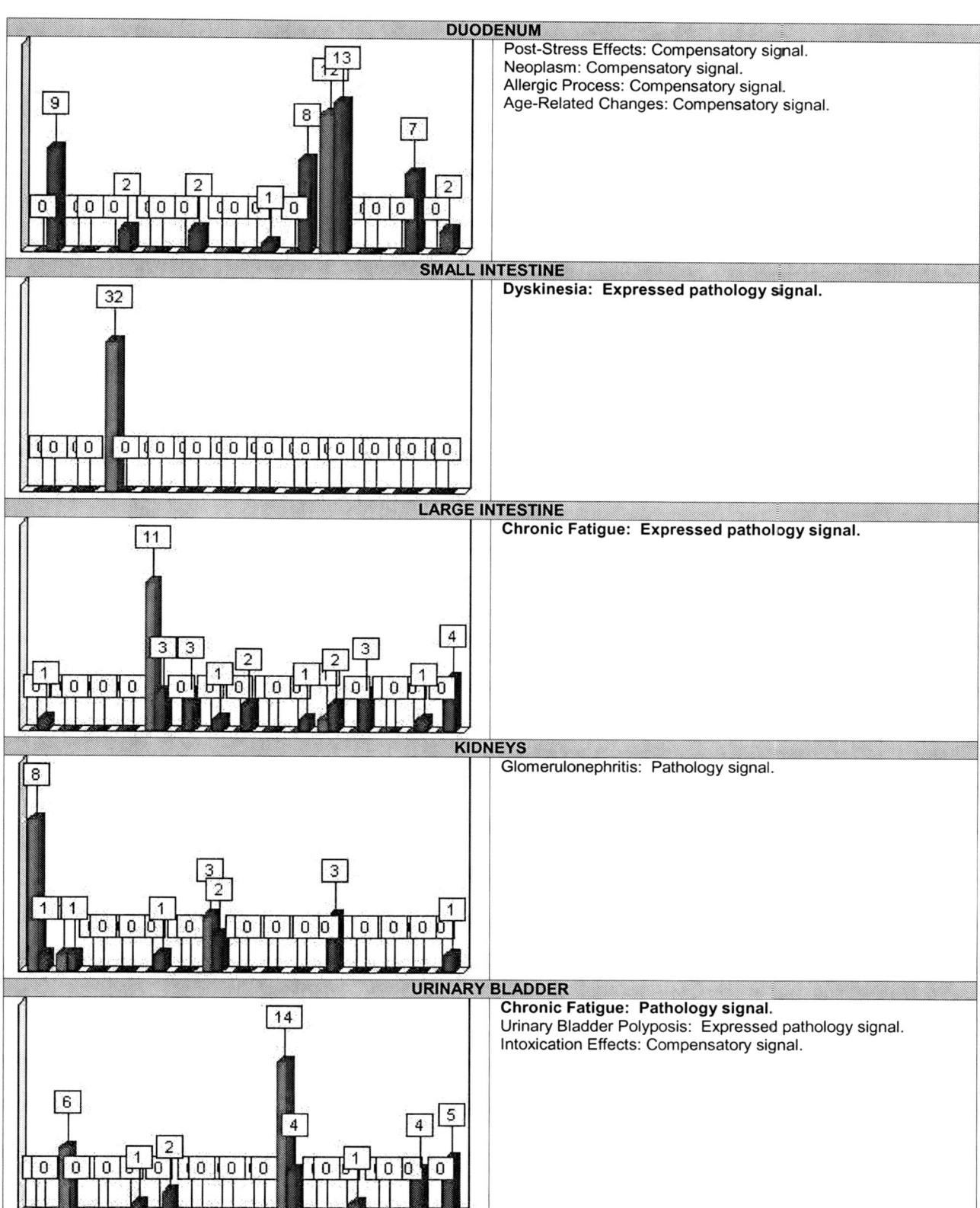

**DUODENUM**

Post-Stress Effects: Compensatory signal.
Neoplasm: Compensatory signal.
Allergic Process: Compensatory signal.
Age-Related Changes: Compensatory signal.

**SMALL INTESTINE**

**Dyskinesia: Expressed pathology signal.**

**LARGE INTESTINE**

**Chronic Fatigue: Expressed pathology signal.**

**KIDNEYS**

Glomerulonephritis: Pathology signal.

**URINARY BLADDER**

**Chronic Fatigue: Pathology signal.**
Urinary Bladder Polyposis: Expressed pathology signal.
Intoxication Effects: Compensatory signal.

226

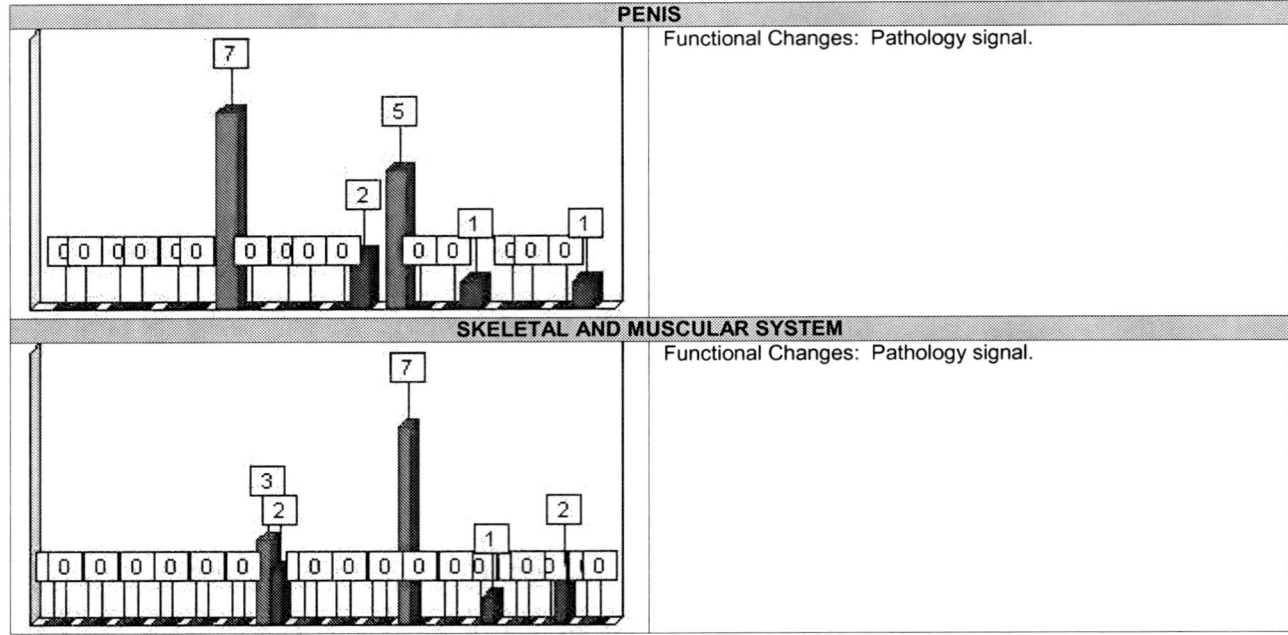

## Discussion of Reported Results

Fibromyalgia: note the strong, uncompensated chronic fatigue signals in the endocrine system (thyroid, pituitary, adrenals, testicles), with uncompensated signals from digestive system organs (pancreas, stomach, spleen, gall bladder, large intestine, urinary bladder) accompanied by indications of diabetes (pathology of islets of Langerhans), sclerosing pancreatitis, liver insufficiency and impaired cardiac rhythm and conduction.

This assessment appears to be typical of Fibromyalgia patients in which the minor indications of myelitis, myositis, neuritis and osteochondrosis contribute to the structural or muscular aches and pains which are typical of the condition.

## Observations & Conclusions

These examples illustrate how increasing degrees of chronic fatigue show up as increasing degrees of failure of the brain's regulatory function, which no longer provides the required level of compensation or immune system response.

Virtual Scanning may not have identified specific causes of the pathology/syndrome but it does identify its physiological effects on the body.

Virtual Scanning version 7G health assessments of fibromyalgia patients often indicate destabilised Sleeping Patterns, which is consistent with current medical findings 48,49. The muscular aches and pains and other medical symptoms of fibromyalgia appears likely to be the consequences of stress including impaired sleeping patterns, associated with dysfunction of the endocrine glands, which subsequently affect the stability of the other physiological systems and associated organs including, in particular, the pituitary gland and to a lesser extent the thyroid gland.

These conclusions are consistent with findings 49 that almost half of those with fibromyalgia have disturbed delta sleep patterns, which, as outlined in earlier chapters, is intimately involved in the regulation of the body's 14 physiological systems. Such disturbed sleeping patterns would progressively manifest from the earliest stages of chronic fatigue. This seems to be followed by various possible sequences of side-effects arising from destabilisation of other systems and organs.

The further consequences of the above are the dysregulation of the digestive system leading to mineral and vitamin deficiencies which leads to dysfunction of the pancreas and hence to degenerative conditions such as osteoporosis.

Such complicating pathologies include lowered immune system function, deteriorating cognition and memory, etc; all recognised associated symptoms of Chronic Fatigue Syndrome (CFS), eventually manifesting as Fibromyalgia. Progressive development of the condition may also be accompanied by impaired cardiac function and circulatory disturbances consistent with the findings by previous researchers [50-52]

## 4.6      Virtual Scanning: Assessment and Treatment of IBS [97]

Irritable bowel syndrome is a digestive disorder which we recognise through symptoms such as stomach cramps, abdominal pain, bloating, and diarrhea. It causes discomfort and distress but does not appear to harm the intestines or to lead to serious disease. It can be controlled to some extent by diet, stress management, and medications.

Up to 20% of the adult population experiences at some stage in their lives IBS-type symptoms. This makes it one of the most common disorders diagnosed by doctors. It occurs more commonly in women and it begins before the age of 35 in about 50% of the population.

There are no recognised tests for IBS and there is no cure but many options are available to treat the symptoms.

Medications include supplements or laxatives for constipation or medicines to decrease diarrhea, such as Lomotil or loperamide (Imodium). Antispasmodic medications help to control colon muscle spasms and reduce abdominal pain.

The following example illustrates how Virtual Scanning can be used to diagnose the precise effect of IBS upon the digestive system

example 7: woman 23 years, 39 kgs, Irritable Bowel Syndrome

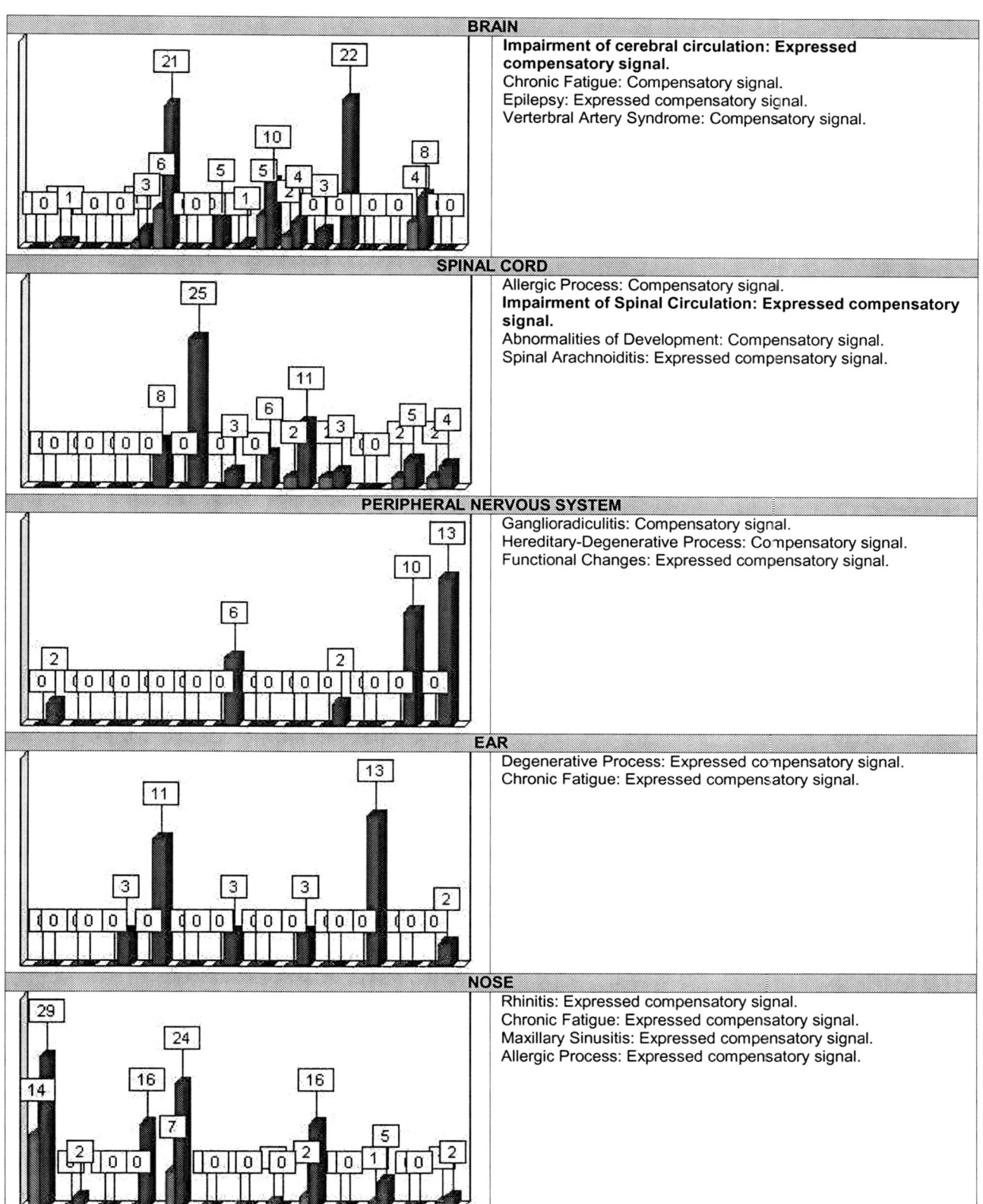

**BRAIN**

**Impairment of cerebral circulation: Expressed compensatory signal.**
Chronic Fatigue: Compensatory signal.
Epilepsy: Expressed compensatory signal.
Verterbral Artery Syndrome: Compensatory signal.

**SPINAL CORD**

Allergic Process: Compensatory signal.
**Impairment of Spinal Circulation: Expressed compensatory signal.**
Abnormalities of Development: Compensatory signal.
Spinal Arachnoiditis: Expressed compensatory signal.

**PERIPHERAL NERVOUS SYSTEM**

Ganglioradiculitis: Compensatory signal.
Hereditary-Degenerative Process: Compensatory signal.
Functional Changes: Expressed compensatory signal.

**EAR**

Degenerative Process: Expressed compensatory signal.
Chronic Fatigue: Expressed compensatory signal.

**NOSE**

Rhinitis: Expressed compensatory signal.
Chronic Fatigue: Expressed compensatory signal.
Maxillary Sinusitis: Expressed compensatory signal.
Allergic Process: Expressed compensatory signal.

230

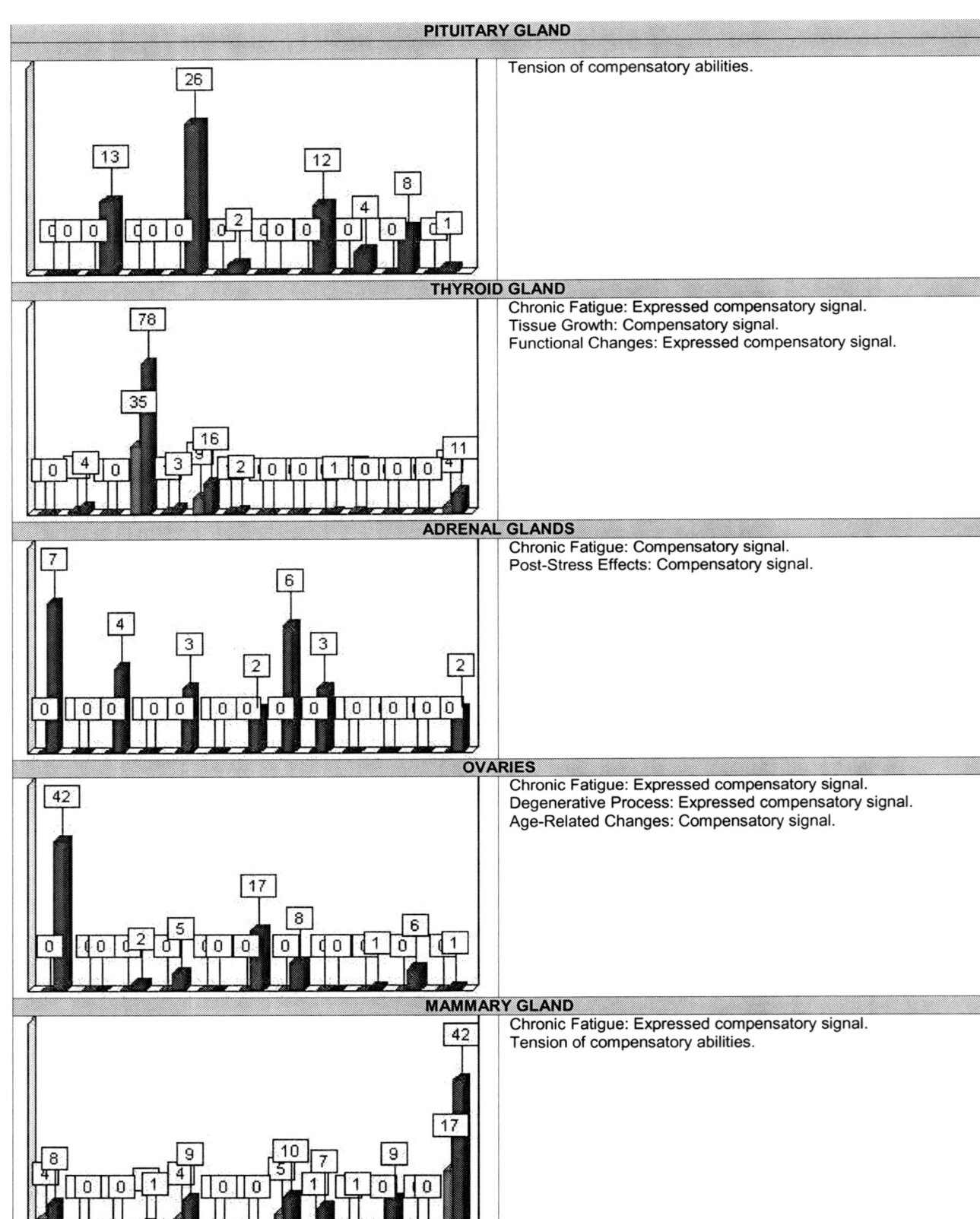

**PITUITARY GLAND**

Tension of compensatory abilities.

**THYROID GLAND**

Chronic Fatigue: Expressed compensatory signal.
Tissue Growth: Compensatory signal.
Functional Changes: Expressed compensatory signal.

**ADRENAL GLANDS**

Chronic Fatigue: Compensatory signal.
Post-Stress Effects: Compensatory signal.

**OVARIES**

Chronic Fatigue: Expressed compensatory signal.
Degenerative Process: Expressed compensatory signal.
Age-Related Changes: Compensatory signal.

**MAMMARY GLAND**

Chronic Fatigue: Expressed compensatory signal.
Tension of compensatory abilities.

231

## LIVER

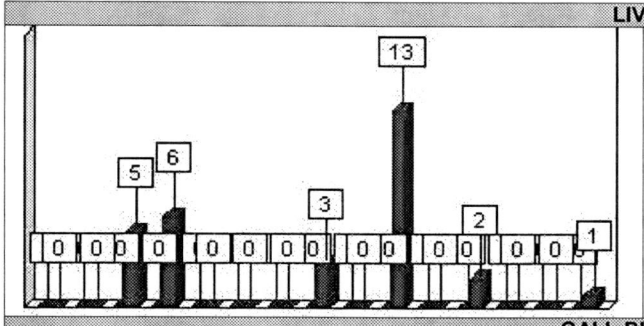

Allergic Process: Compensatory signal.
Hepatocirrhosis: Compensatory signal.
Disruption of Bilirubin Metabolism: Expressed compensatory signal.

## GALL BLADDER

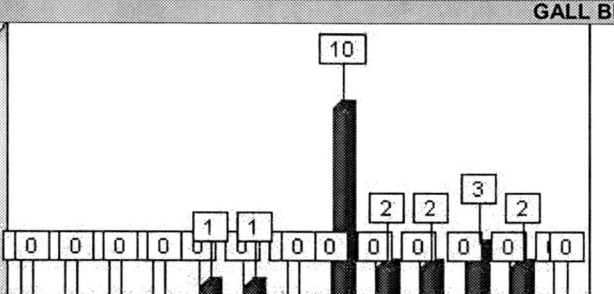

**Dyskinesia of Biliary Ducts and Gall Bladder: Compensatory signal.**

## PANCREAS

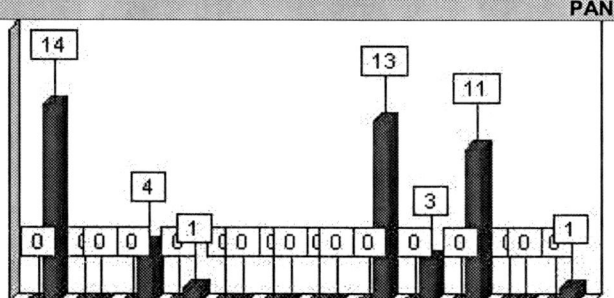

Chronic Fatigue: Expressed compensatory signal.
Functional Changes: Expressed compensatory signal.
Pathology of Islands of Langerhans: Expressed compensatory signal.

## HEART

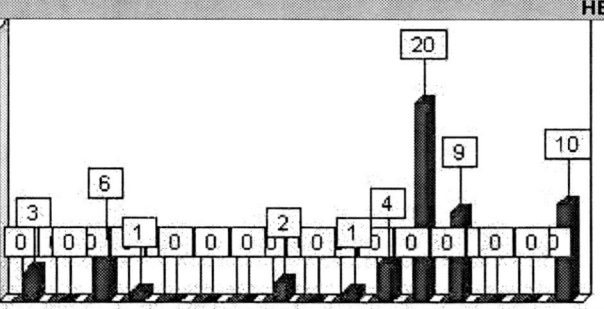

Cardiac Insufficiency: Expressed compensatory signal.
Cardiac Myopathy: Expressed compensatory signal.

Allergic Process: Expressed compensatory signal.
Abnormalities of Development: Compensatory signal.

## BLOOD AND PERIPHERAL BLOOD VESSELS

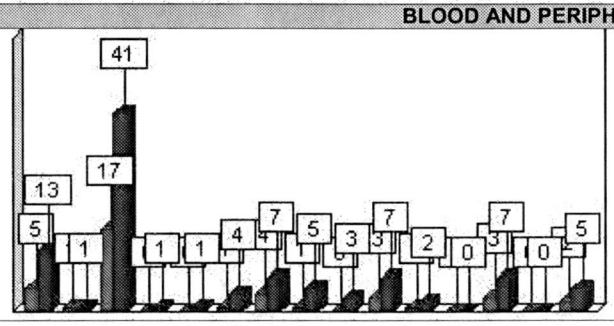

Anaemia: Expressed compensatory signal.
**Leukopenia: Expressed compensatory signal.**
Haemorrhagic Vasculitis: Compensatory signal.
Neoplasm: Compensatory signal.
Chronic Fatigue: Compensatory signal.
Hypertonia: Compensatory signal.
Post-Stress Effects: Compensatory signal.

232

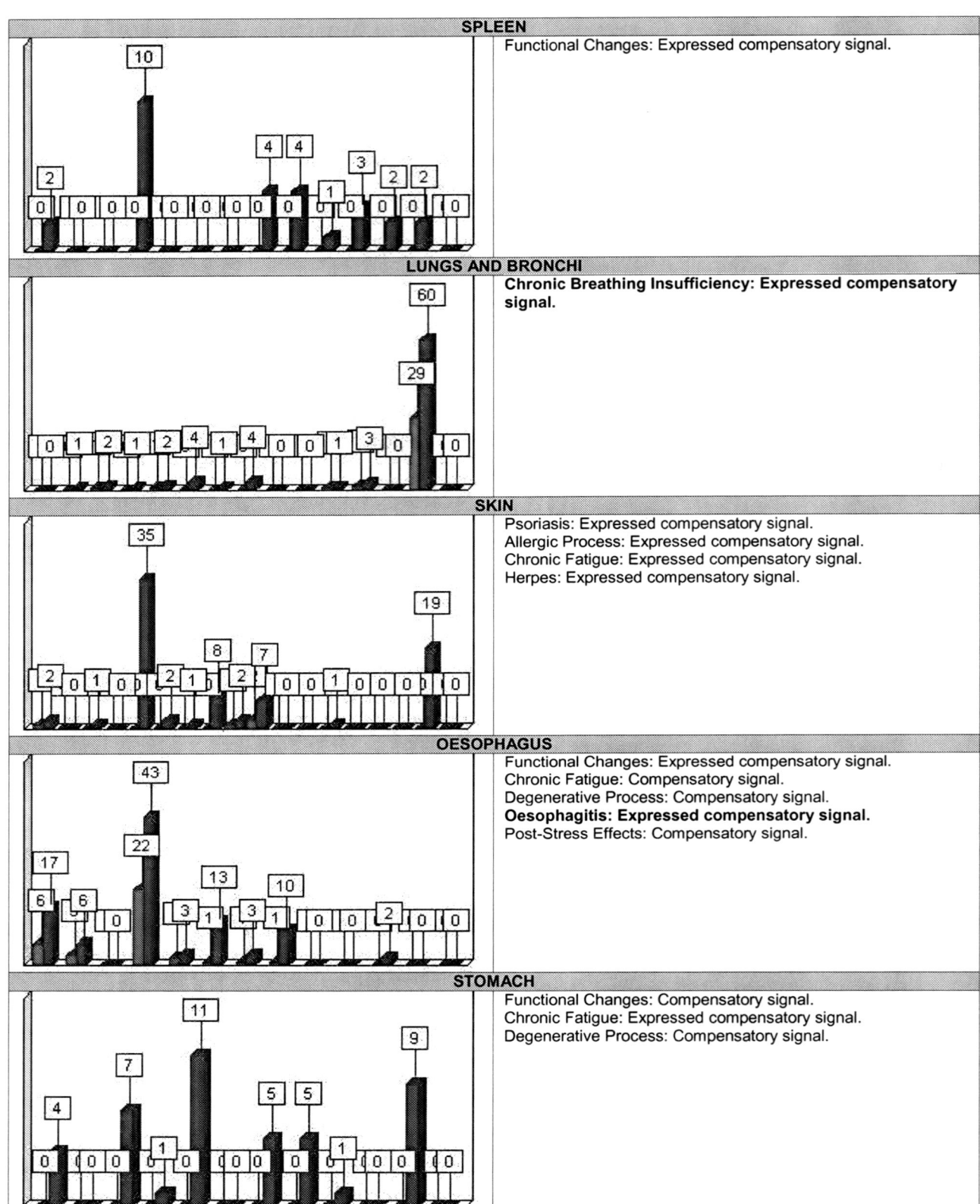

**SPLEEN**

Functional Changes: Expressed compensatory signal.

**LUNGS AND BRONCHI**

**Chronic Breathing Insufficiency: Expressed compensatory signal.**

**SKIN**

Psoriasis: Expressed compensatory signal.
Allergic Process: Expressed compensatory signal.
Chronic Fatigue: Expressed compensatory signal.
Herpes: Expressed compensatory signal.

**OESOPHAGUS**

Functional Changes: Expressed compensatory signal.
Chronic Fatigue: Compensatory signal.
Degenerative Process: Compensatory signal.
**Oesophagitis: Expressed compensatory signal.**
Post-Stress Effects: Compensatory signal.

**STOMACH**

Functional Changes: Compensatory signal.
Chronic Fatigue: Expressed compensatory signal.
Degenerative Process: Compensatory signal.

233

## DUODENUM

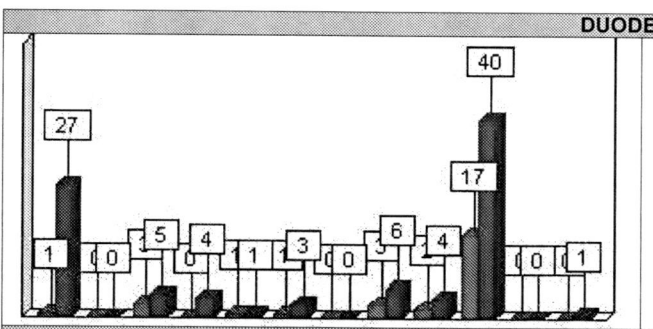

**Dyskinesia: Expressed compensatory signal.**
Neoplasm: Expressed compensatory signal.
Allergic Process: Compensatory signal.

## SMALL INTESTINE

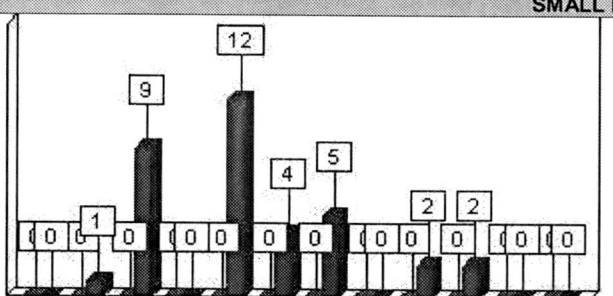

**Dyskinesia: Compensatory signal.**
Post-Stress Effects: Expressed compensatory signal.

## LARGE INTESTINE

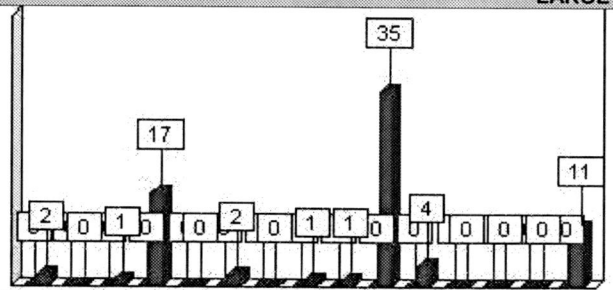

**Colitis: Expressed compensatory signal.**
Hemorrhoids: Expressed compensatory signal.
Post-Stress Effects: Expressed compensatory signal.

## KIDNEYS

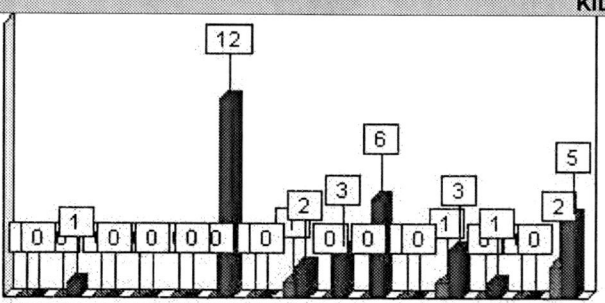

Degenerative Process: Expressed compensatory signal.
Renovascular Insufficiency: Compensatory signal.
Functional Changes: Compensatory signal.

## URINARY BLADDER

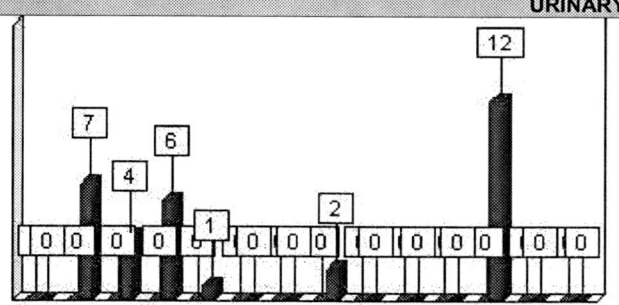

Chronic Fatigue: Compensatory signal.
Post-Stress Effects: Compensatory signal.
**Urethral Infections: Expressed compensatory signal.**

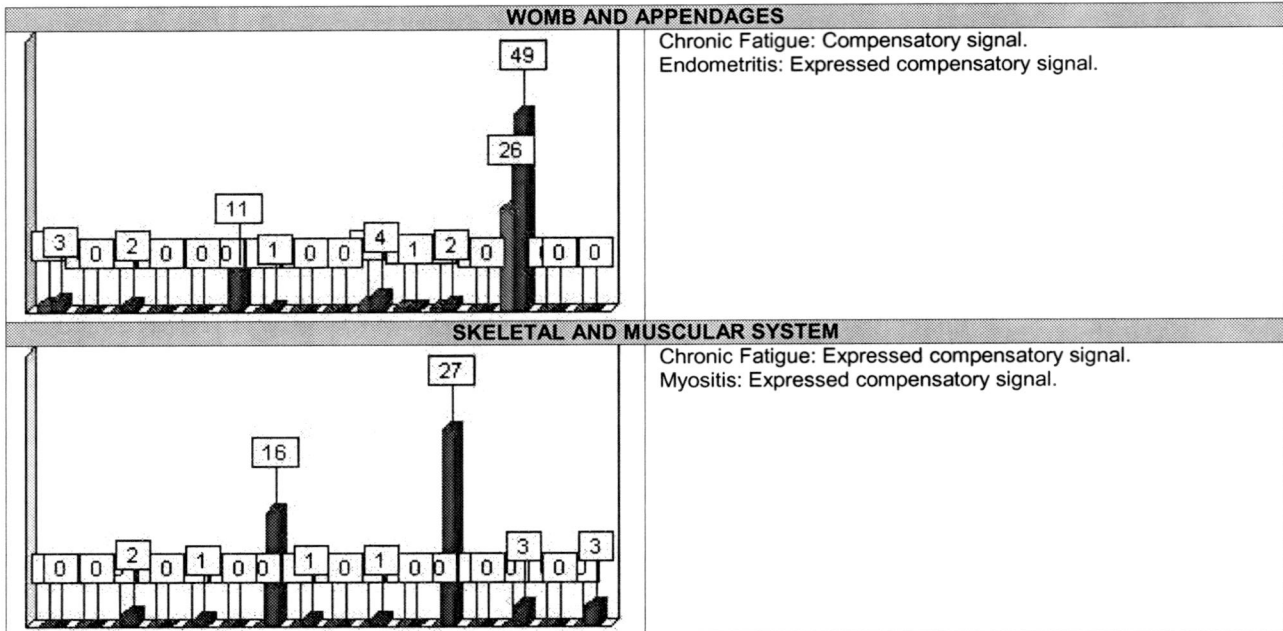

**WOMB AND APPENDAGES**

Chronic Fatigue: Compensatory signal.
Endometritis: Expressed compensatory signal.

**SKELETAL AND MUSCULAR SYSTEM**

Chronic Fatigue: Expressed compensatory signal.
Myositis: Expressed compensatory signal.

## Discussion of Reported Results

The above example of a woman 23 years, 39 kgs with a history of congenital heart disease and irritable bowel clearly illustrates the ability of Virtual Scanning to diagnose irregular function (Dyskinesia) of the Gall Bladder, Duodenum and Small Intestine.

These are accompanied by clear indications of Oesophagitis, Colitis and Urethral infections.

The current indications are mainly compensated (blue signals) which indicate that this condition is currently in remission but likely to reoccur under the influence of stressors.

## 4.7    Virtual Scanning: Assessment and Treatment of STROKE

A 'stroke' can occur when the normal supply of blood to your brain or to parts of your brain is interrupted. If the cells of the brain do not get a constant supply of oxygen from the blood, the cells in the affected area may become damaged or die.

A person's susceptibility to migraine is increasingly considered to be indicative of their pre-disposition to stroke.

The neural blood supply is provided by four main arteries which divide into smaller arteries. The amount of damage inflicted on the brain and the location of the damage depends on the artery affected.

Strokes are the leading cause of disability in the UK, and the third most common cause of death.

In general a person's susceptibility to stroke is based upon their lifestyle. This includes diet, exercise, alcoholic consumption, and other factors which affect the ability to pump oxygenated blood to the brain.

There are few commercially viable techniques which can be used to determine a person's predisposition to stroke.

The following example illustrates how Virtual Scanning can be used to diagnose the effect of stroke on a person. The person has to be able to complete the cognitive test. Later results (examples 14-21) illustrate the ability to diagnose the health of the heart, blood and peripheral vessels, etc and hence to determine a person's predisposition to stroke.

example 8: male, 60 years: Stroke

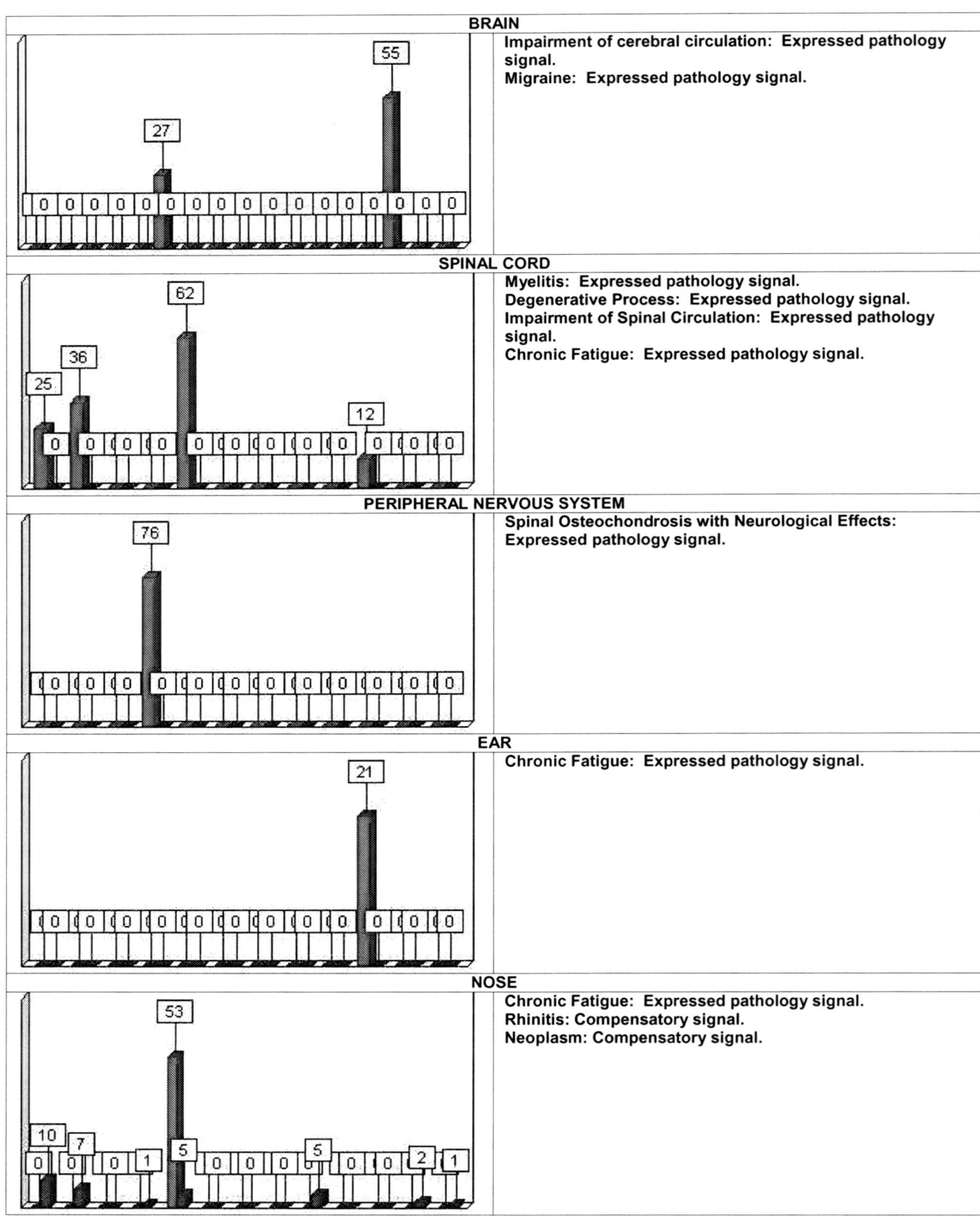

**BRAIN**

Impairment of cerebral circulation: Expressed pathology signal.
Migraine: Expressed pathology signal.

**SPINAL CORD**

Myelitis: Expressed pathology signal.
Degenerative Process: Expressed pathology signal.
Impairment of Spinal Circulation: Expressed pathology signal.
Chronic Fatigue: Expressed pathology signal.

**PERIPHERAL NERVOUS SYSTEM**

Spinal Osteochondrosis with Neurological Effects: Expressed pathology signal.

**EAR**

Chronic Fatigue: Expressed pathology signal.

**NOSE**

Chronic Fatigue: Expressed pathology signal.
Rhinitis: Compensatory signal.
Neoplasm: Compensatory signal.

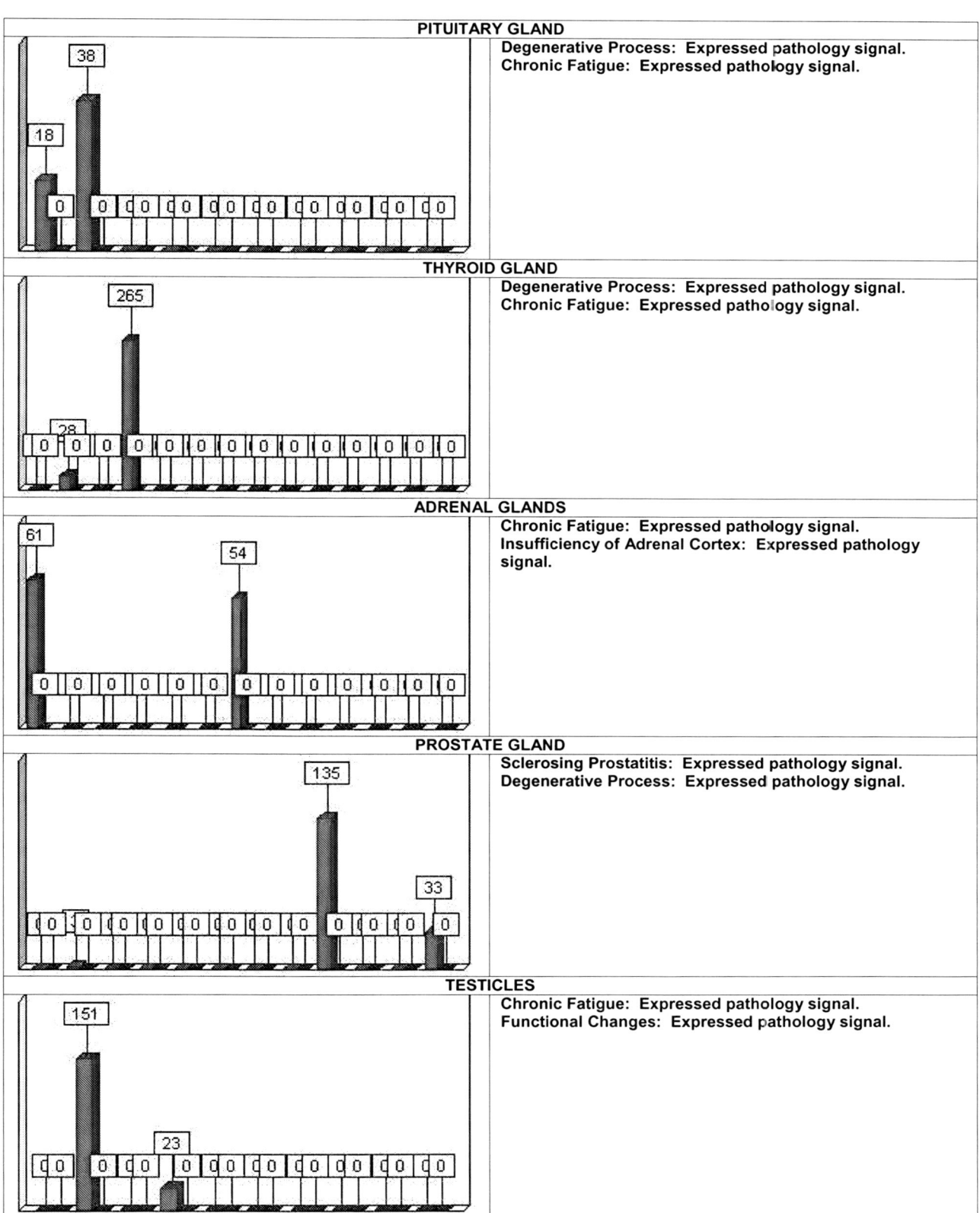

**PITUITARY GLAND**

Degenerative Process: Expressed pathology signal.
Chronic Fatigue: Expressed pathology signal.

**THYROID GLAND**

Degenerative Process: Expressed pathology signal.
Chronic Fatigue: Expressed pathology signal.

**ADRENAL GLANDS**

Chronic Fatigue: Expressed pathology signal.
Insufficiency of Adrenal Cortex: Expressed pathology signal.

**PROSTATE GLAND**

Sclerosing Prostatitis: Expressed pathology signal.
Degenerative Process: Expressed pathology signal.

**TESTICLES**

Chronic Fatigue: Expressed pathology signal.
Functional Changes: Expressed pathology signal.

238

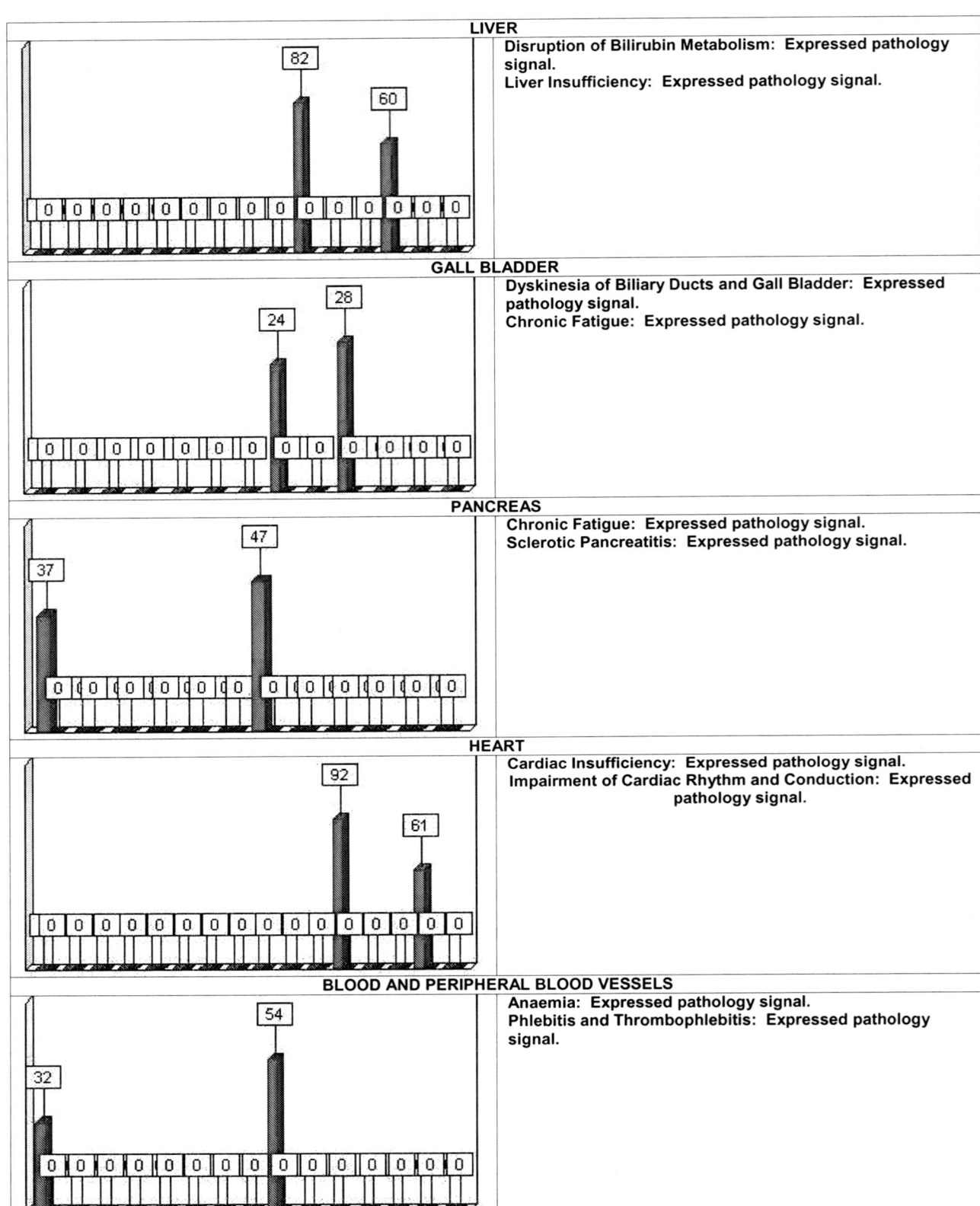

**LIVER**

Disruption of Bilirubin Metabolism: Expressed pathology signal.
Liver Insufficiency: Expressed pathology signal.

**GALL BLADDER**

Dyskinesia of Biliary Ducts and Gall Bladder: Expressed pathology signal.
Chronic Fatigue: Expressed pathology signal.

**PANCREAS**

Chronic Fatigue: Expressed pathology signal.
Sclerotic Pancreatitis: Expressed pathology signal.

**HEART**

Cardiac Insufficiency: Expressed pathology signal.
Impairment of Cardiac Rhythm and Conduction: Expressed pathology signal.

**BLOOD AND PERIPHERAL BLOOD VESSELS**

Anaemia: Expressed pathology signal.
Phlebitis and Thrombophlebitis: Expressed pathology signal.

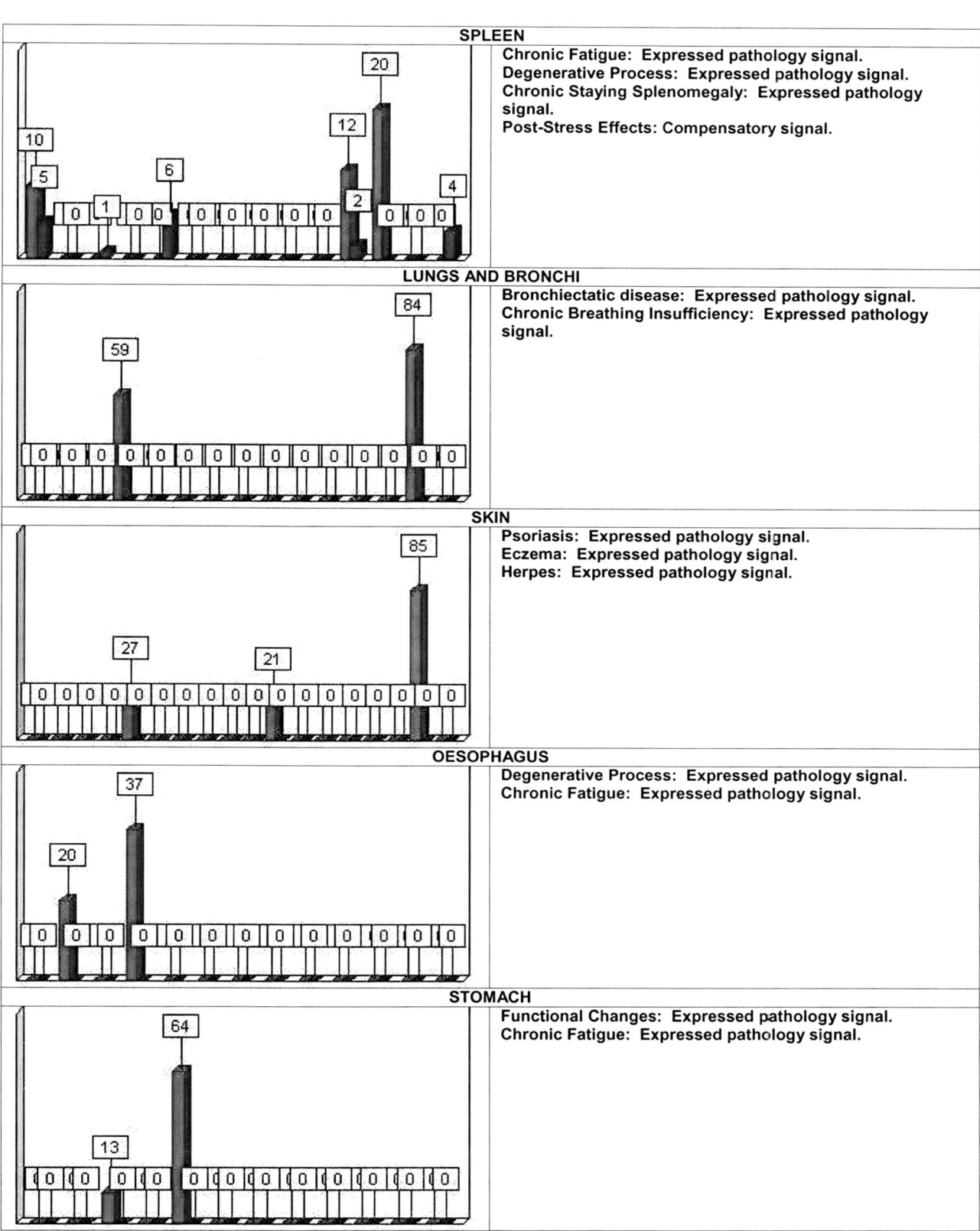

**SPLEEN**

Chronic Fatigue:  Expressed pathology signal.
Degenerative Process:  Expressed pathology signal.
Chronic Staying Splenomegaly:  Expressed pathology signal.
Post-Stress Effects:  Compensatory signal.

**LUNGS AND BRONCHI**

Bronchiectatic disease:  Expressed pathology signal.
Chronic Breathing Insufficiency:  Expressed pathology signal.

**SKIN**

Psoriasis:  Expressed pathology signal.
Eczema:  Expressed pathology signal.
Herpes:  Expressed pathology signal.

**OESOPHAGUS**

Degenerative Process:  Expressed pathology signal.
Chronic Fatigue:  Expressed pathology signal.

**STOMACH**

Functional Changes:  Expressed pathology signal.
Chronic Fatigue:  Expressed pathology signal.

240

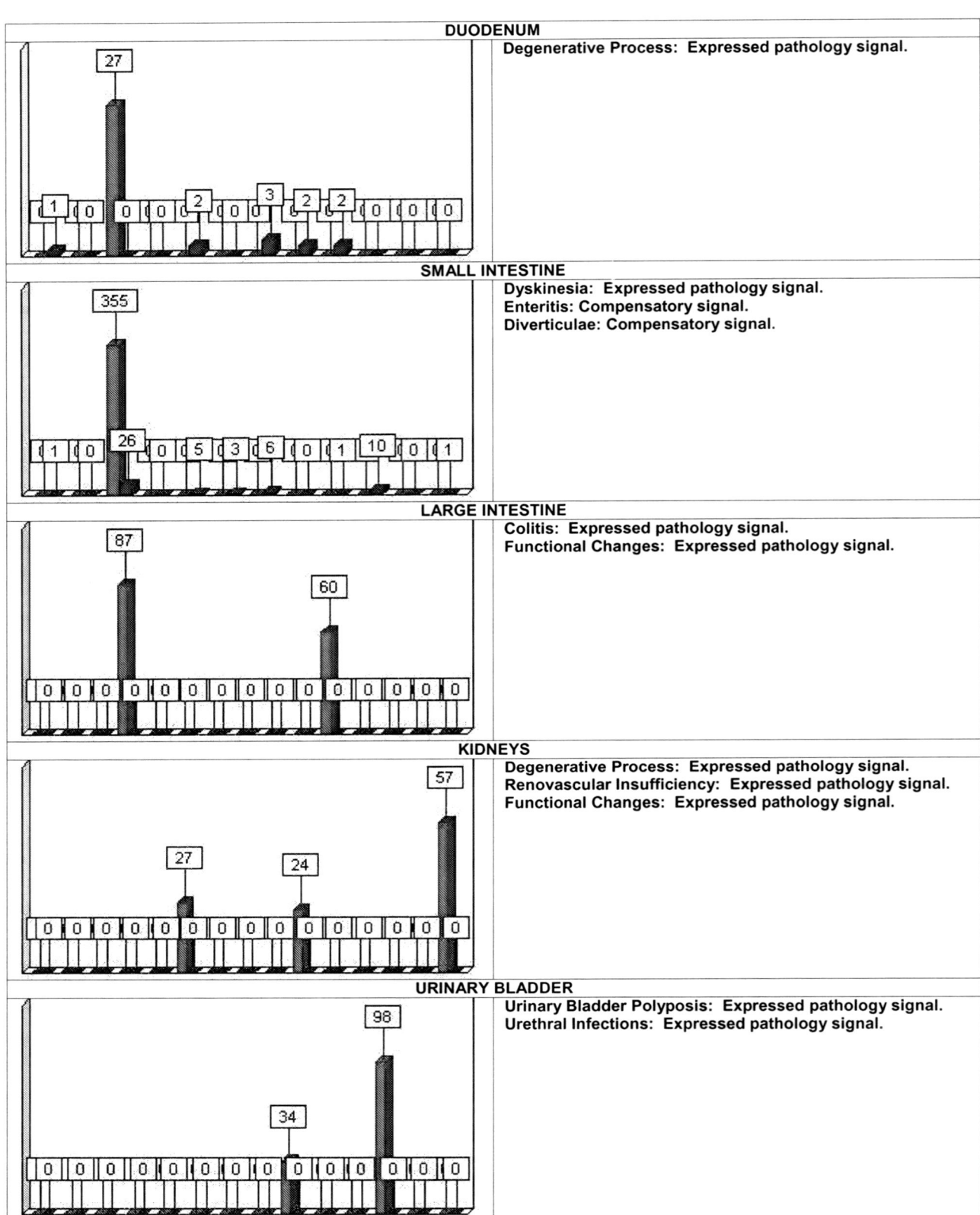

**DUODENUM**

Degenerative Process: Expressed pathology signal.

**SMALL INTESTINE**

Dyskinesia: Expressed pathology signal.
Enteritis: Compensatory signal.
Diverticulae: Compensatory signal.

**LARGE INTESTINE**

Colitis: Expressed pathology signal.
Functional Changes: Expressed pathology signal.

**KIDNEYS**

Degenerative Process: Expressed pathology signal.
Renovascular Insufficiency: Expressed pathology signal.
Functional Changes: Expressed pathology signal.

**URINARY BLADDER**

Urinary Bladder Polyposis: Expressed pathology signal.
Urethral Infections: Expressed pathology signal.

241

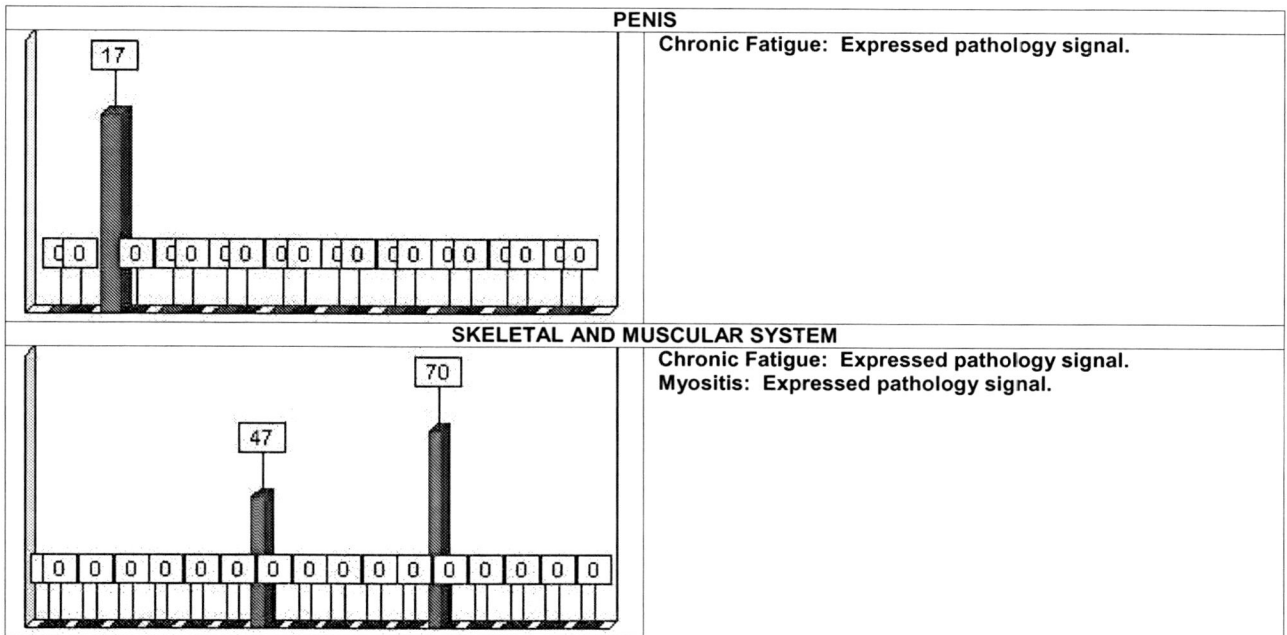

| PENIS | |
|---|---|
| 17 ... | Chronic Fatigue: Expressed pathology signal. |
| SKELETAL AND MUSCULAR SYSTEM | |
| 47 ... 70 ... | Chronic Fatigue: Expressed pathology signal.<br>Myositis: Expressed pathology signal. |

## Discussion of Reported Results

This case study of a male stroke victim, aged 60 years, with a history of being a heavy smoker, identifies extensive failure of brain function, in terms of zero compensatory signals to body organs (denoted by the absence of blue signals).

12 months previously, the patient suffered a stroke which completely paralysed his left side and semi-paralysed his right side. Despite receiving regular massage and his brain being alert, his physiological function deteriorated steadily. Virtual Scanning Health Assessment helps to explain why this occurred: since his brain was unable to transmit the required compensatory signals to the body organs, their quality of physiological function progressively degenerated – their functioning is interdependent, and the quality of functioning of each depends critically on the functioning of others, which are required to influence their ongoing function in response to changing conditions of the external and internal environments.

## 4.8  Assessment of ULCERATIVE DISEASE

example 9: Patient with ulcerative disease:

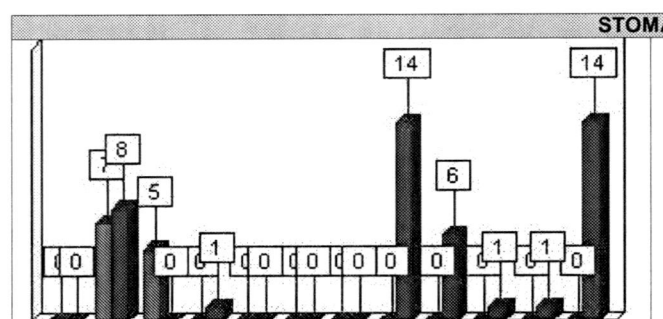

**STOMACH**

Allergic Process: Compensatory signal.
**Ulcerative Disease: Expressed compensatory signal.**
Neoplasm: Compensatory signal.
Tissue Growth: Expressed compensatory signal.

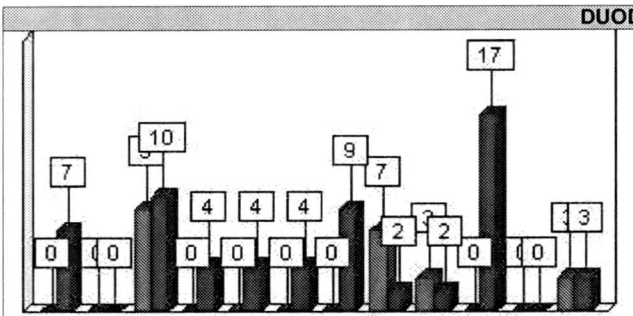

**DUODENUM**

Degenerative Process: Compensatory signal.
Allergic Process:  Pathology signal.
Neoplasm: Compensatory signal.
**Ulcerative Disease: Compensatory signal.**
Dyskinesia: Expressed compensatory signal.

## 4.9  Assessment of DIABETES

example 10: Patient with diabetes:

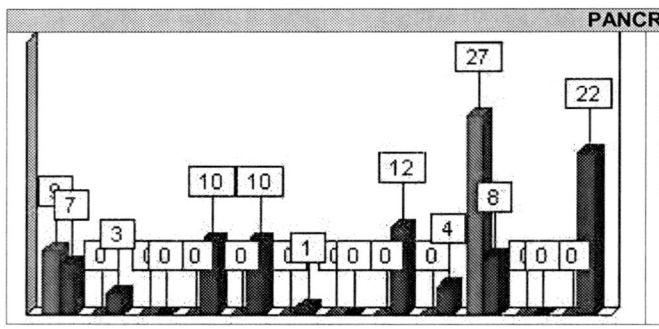

**PANCREAS**

Chronic Fatigue: Weakening of compensatory abilities.
**8/27  Pathology of Islands of Langerhans:  Expressed pathology signal.**
Pancreatitis: Compensatory signal.
Age-Related Changes: Compensatory signal.
Functional Changes: Expressed compensatory signal.
Abnormalities of Development: Expressed compensatory signal.

## 4.10 Assessment of BREATHING DISORDER

example 11: Patient with Breathing Disorder:

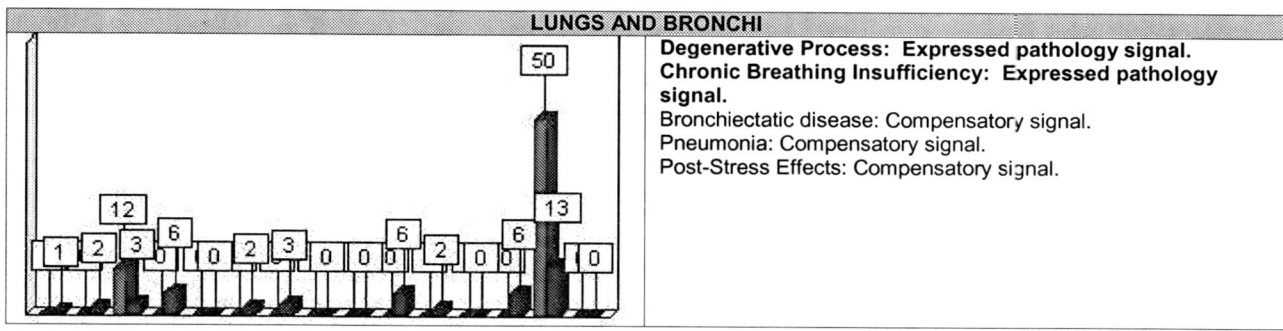

**LUNGS AND BRONCHI**

**Degenerative Process: Expressed pathology signal.**
**Chronic Breathing Insufficiency: Expressed pathology signal.**
Bronchiectatic disease: Compensatory signal.
Pneumonia: Compensatory signal.
Post-Stress Effects: Compensatory signal.

## 4.11 Health assessment of a Professional footballer

example 12: male, 21 yrs, history of leg fractures.

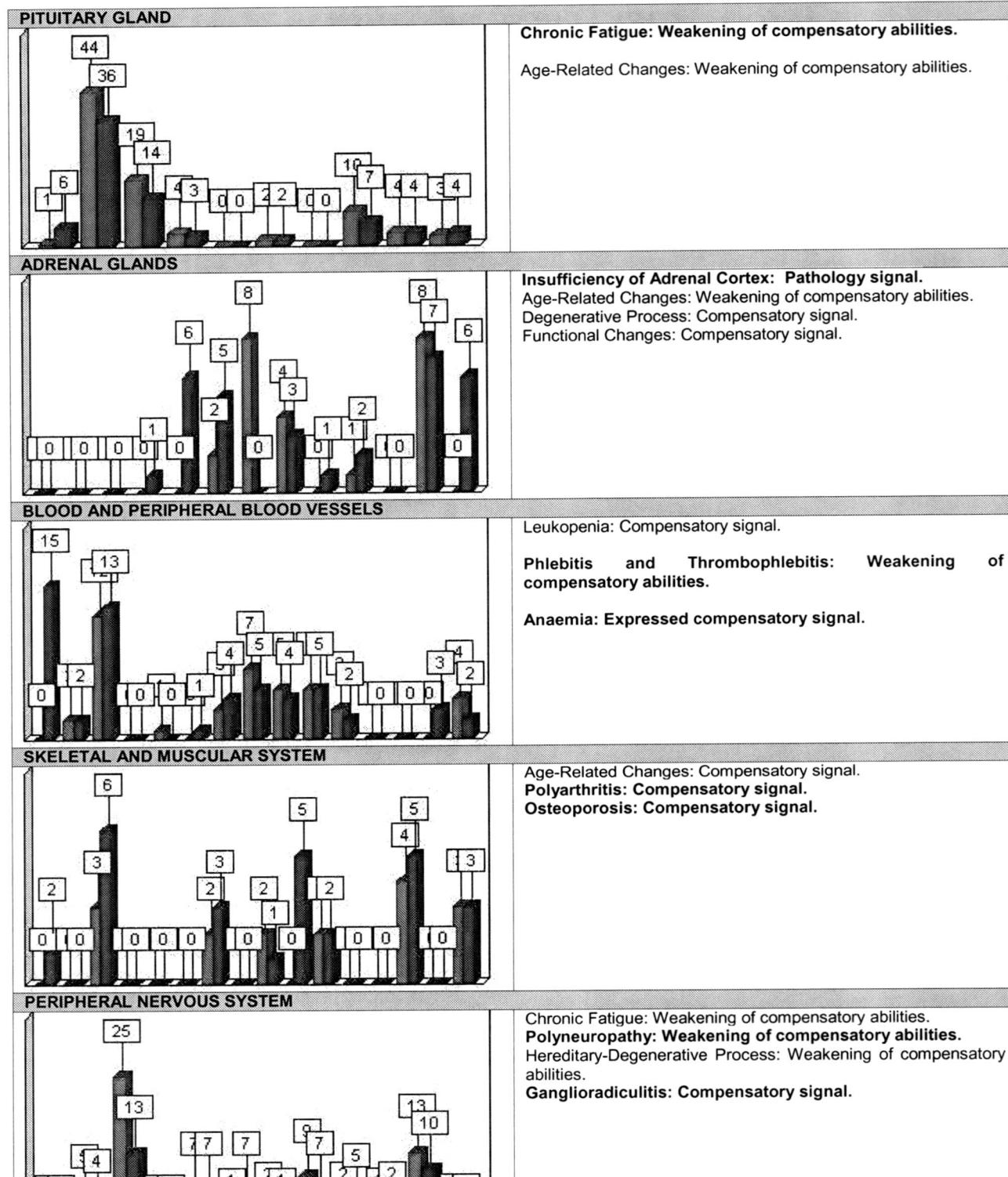

**PITUITARY GLAND**

Chronic Fatigue: **Weakening of compensatory abilities.**

Age-Related Changes: Weakening of compensatory abilities.

**ADRENAL GLANDS**

**Insufficiency of Adrenal Cortex: Pathology signal.**
Age-Related Changes: Weakening of compensatory abilities.
Degenerative Process: Compensatory signal.
Functional Changes: Compensatory signal.

**BLOOD AND PERIPHERAL BLOOD VESSELS**

Leukopenia: Compensatory signal.

**Phlebitis and Thrombophlebitis: Weakening of compensatory abilities.**

**Anaemia: Expressed compensatory signal.**

**SKELETAL AND MUSCULAR SYSTEM**

Age-Related Changes: Compensatory signal.
**Polyarthritis: Compensatory signal.**
**Osteoporosis: Compensatory signal.**

**PERIPHERAL NERVOUS SYSTEM**

Chronic Fatigue: Weakening of compensatory abilities.
**Polyneuropathy: Weakening of compensatory abilities.**
Hereditary-Degenerative Process: Weakening of compensatory abilities.
**Ganglioradiculitis: Compensatory signal.**

245

## 4.12  Assessment of DEPRESSION

example 13: woman, 46 years, 55 kgs, depression:

## BRAIN

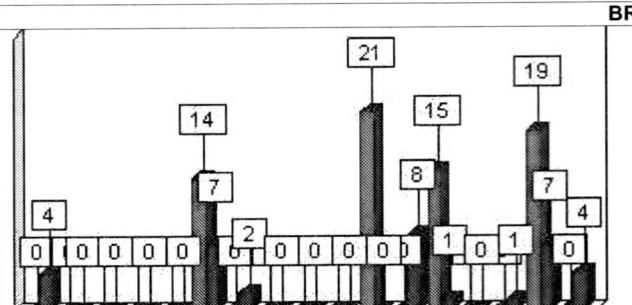

**Impairment of cerebral circulation: Expressed pathology signal.**
**Consequences of Brain Traumas: Expressed pathology signal.**
**Epilepsy: Expressed pathology signal.**
**Verterbral Artery Syndrome: Expressed pathology signal.**
Growth of new cells: Compensatory signal.

## SPINAL CORD

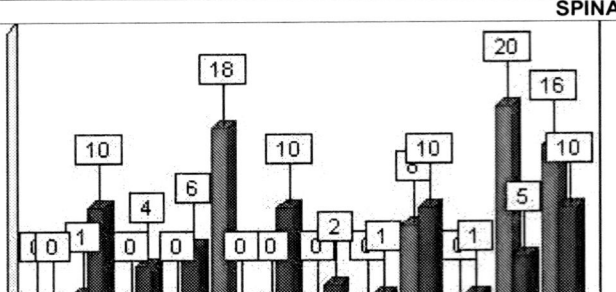

**Impairment of Spinal Circulation: Expressed pathology signal.**
**Functional Changes: Compensatory signal.**
**Intoxication Effects: Expressed pathology signal.**
**Post-Stress Effects: Weakening of compensatory abilities.**
**Degenerative Process: Compensatory signal.**
**Allergic Process: Compensatory signal.**
**Neoplasm: Compensatory signal.**

## PERIPHERAL NERVOUS SYSTEM

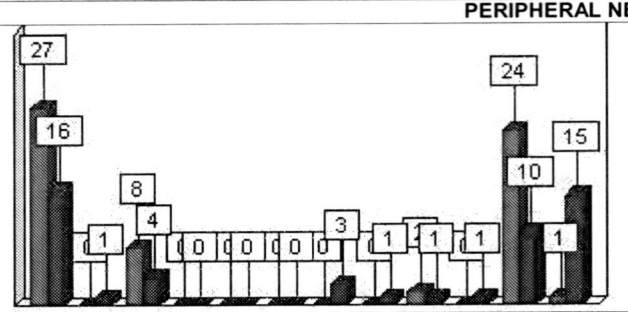

**Post-Stress Effects: Weakening of compensatory abilities.**
**Chronic Fatigue: Pathology signal.**
**Hereditary-Degenerative Process: Expressed pathology signal.**
**Functional Changes: Expressed compensatory signal.**

## EAR

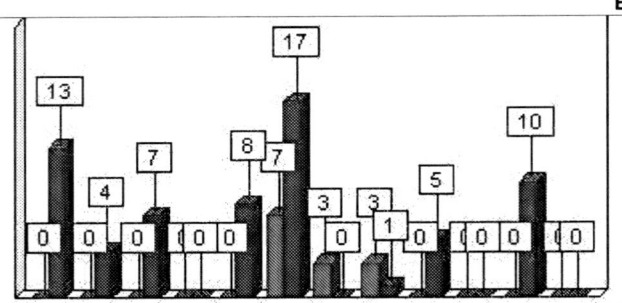

**Cochlear Neuritis: Expressed compensatory signal.**
External Otitis: Expressed compensatory signal.
Inflammation of Middle Ear: Compensatory signal.
Age-Related Changes: Compensatory signal.
Intoxication Effects: Compensatory signal.

## NOSE

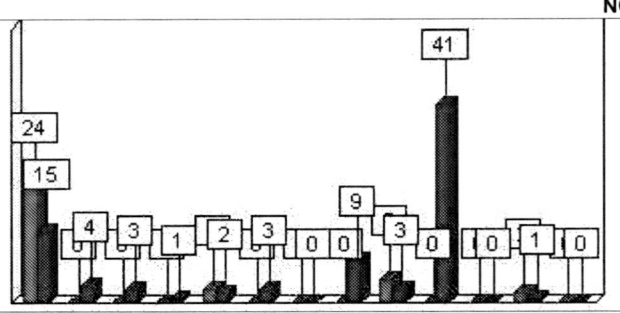

**Rhinitis: Weakening of compensatory abilities.**
Age-Related Changes: Compensatory signal.
Frontitis: Expressed compensatory signal.

## PITUITARY GLAND

247

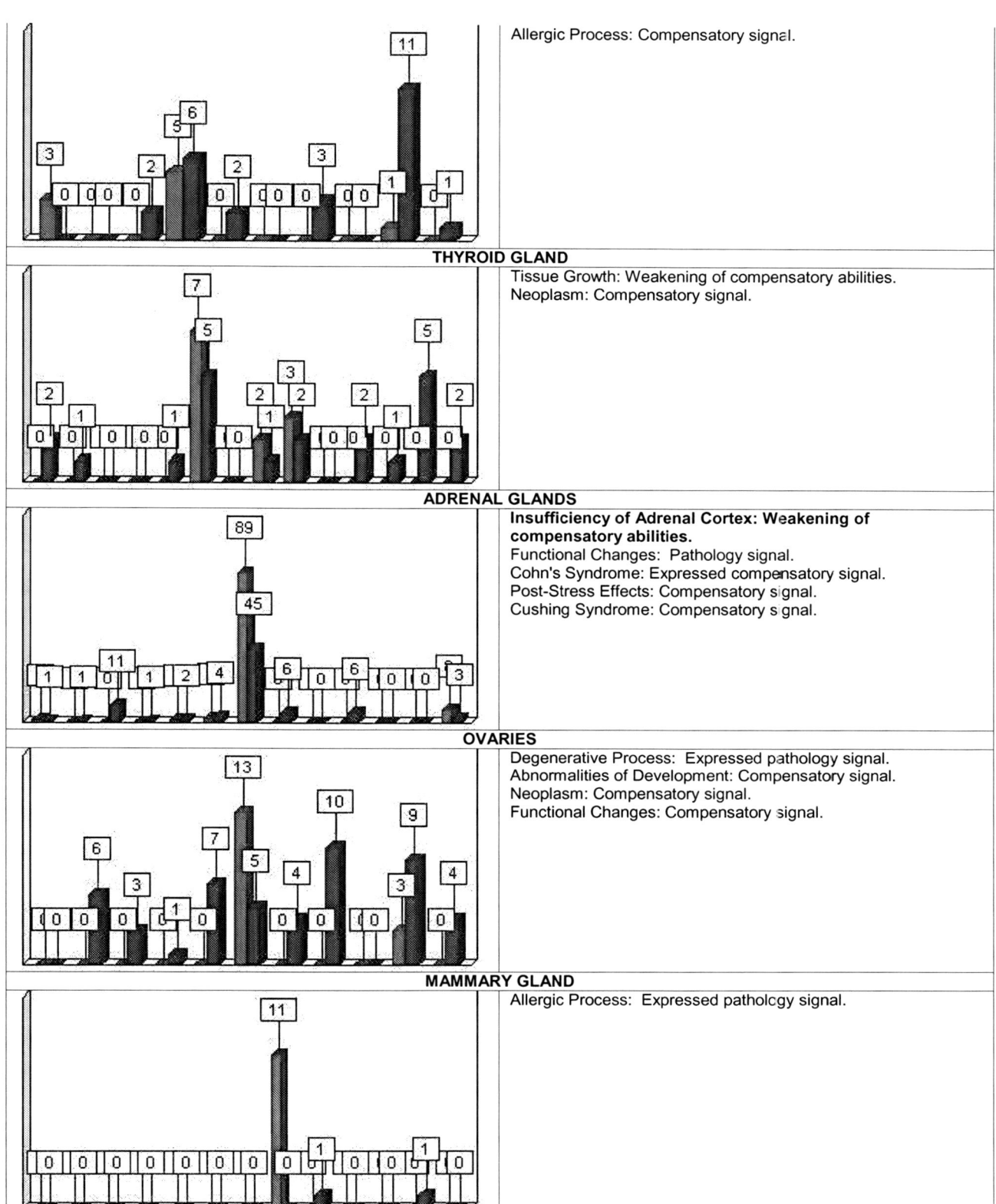

Allergic Process: Compensatory signal.

**THYROID GLAND**

Tissue Growth: Weakening of compensatory abilities.
Neoplasm: Compensatory signal.

**ADRENAL GLANDS**

**Insufficiency of Adrenal Cortex: Weakening of compensatory abilities.**
Functional Changes: Pathology signal.
Cohn's Syndrome: Expressed compensatory signal.
Post-Stress Effects: Compensatory signal.
Cushing Syndrome: Compensatory signal.

**OVARIES**

Degenerative Process: Expressed pathology signal.
Abnormalities of Development: Compensatory signal.
Neoplasm: Compensatory signal.
Functional Changes: Compensatory signal.

**MAMMARY GLAND**

Allergic Process: Expressed pathology signal.

248

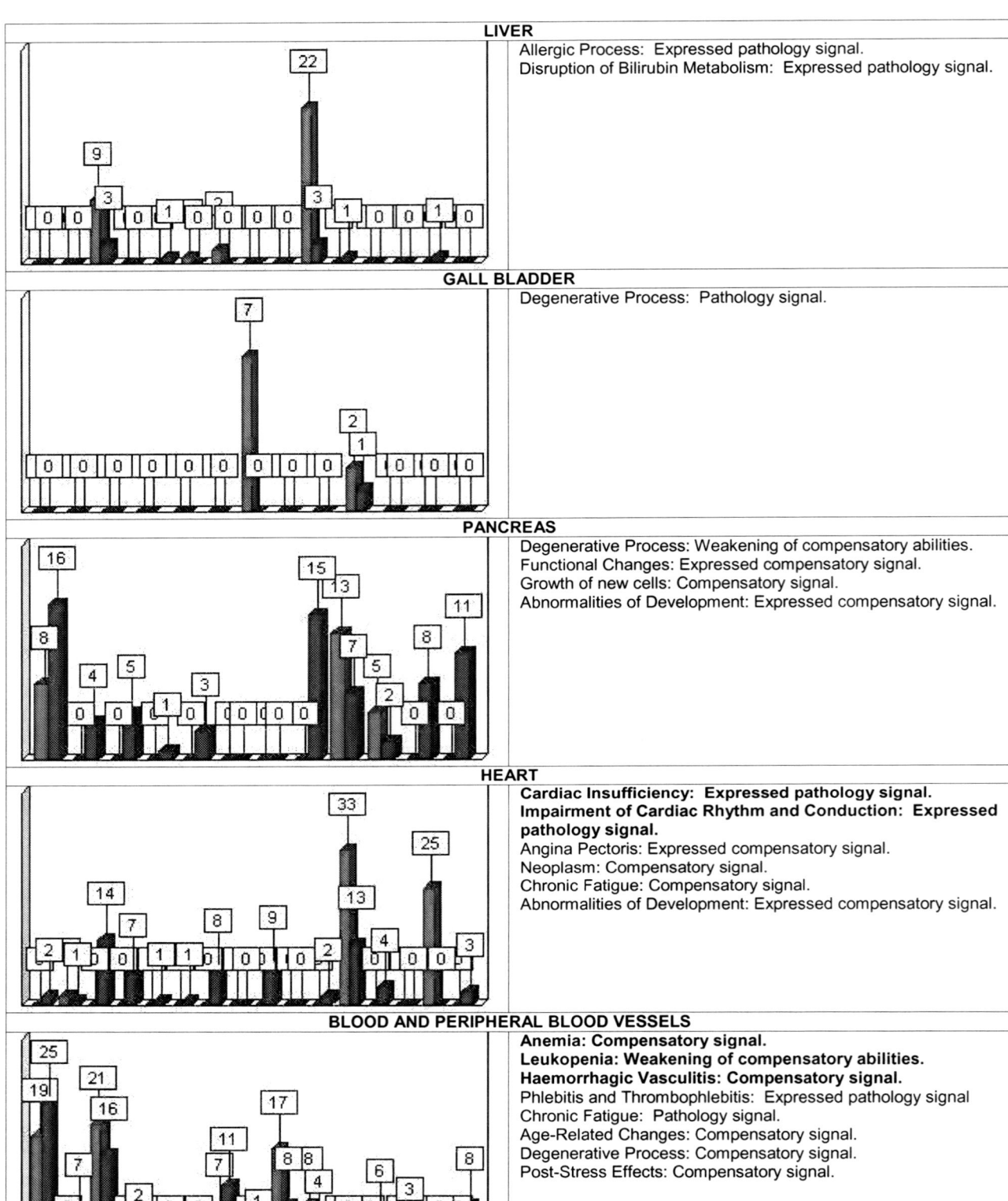

**LIVER**

Allergic Process: Expressed pathology signal.
Disruption of Bilirubin Metabolism: Expressed pathology signal.

**GALL BLADDER**

Degenerative Process: Pathology signal.

**PANCREAS**

Degenerative Process: Weakening of compensatory abilities.
Functional Changes: Expressed compensatory signal.
Growth of new cells: Compensatory signal.
Abnormalities of Development: Expressed compensatory signal.

**HEART**

**Cardiac Insufficiency: Expressed pathology signal.**
**Impairment of Cardiac Rhythm and Conduction: Expressed pathology signal.**
Angina Pectoris: Expressed compensatory signal.
Neoplasm: Compensatory signal.
Chronic Fatigue: Compensatory signal.
Abnormalities of Development: Expressed compensatory signal.

**BLOOD AND PERIPHERAL BLOOD VESSELS**

**Anemia: Compensatory signal.**
**Leukopenia: Weakening of compensatory abilities.**
**Haemorrhagic Vasculitis: Compensatory signal.**
Phlebitis and Thrombophlebitis: Expressed pathology signal
Chronic Fatigue: Pathology signal.
Age-Related Changes: Compensatory signal.
Degenerative Process: Compensatory signal.
Post-Stress Effects: Compensatory signal.

249

## SPLEEN

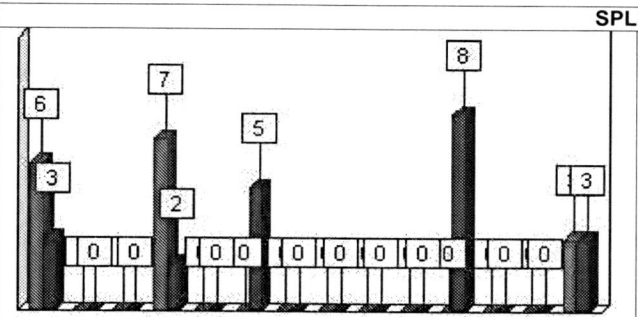

Chronic Fatigue: Pathology signal.
Functional Changes: Pathology signal.
Hypersplenism: Compensatory signal.
Degenerative Process: Compensatory signal.

## LUNGS AND BRONCHI

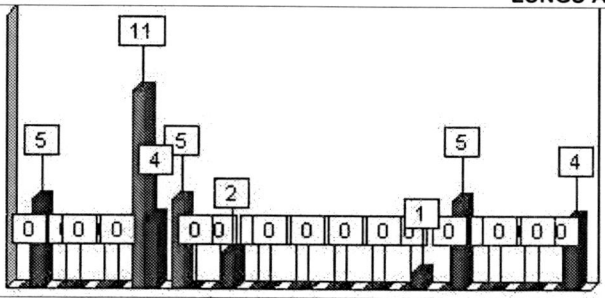

Bronchiectatic disease: Expressed pathology signal.
Allergic Process: Pathology signal.
Bronchitis: Compensatory signal.
Pleurisy: Compensatory signal.

## SKIN

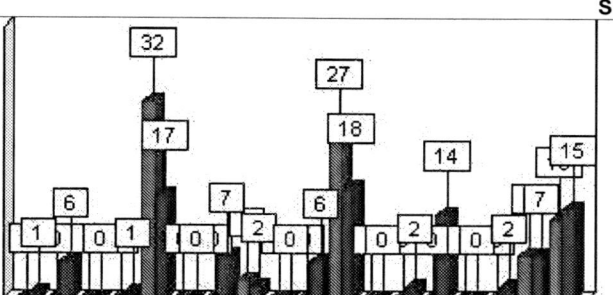

**Psoriasis: Weakening of compensatory abilities.**
**Eczema: Weakening of compensatory abilities.**
Herpes: Compensated pathology condition.
Intoxication Effects: Compensatory signal.
Abnormalities of Development: Compensatory signal.
Neurodermatitis: Expressed compensatory signal.
Chronic Fatigue: Compensatory signal.
Degenerative Process: Expressed compensatory signal.

## OESOPHAGUS

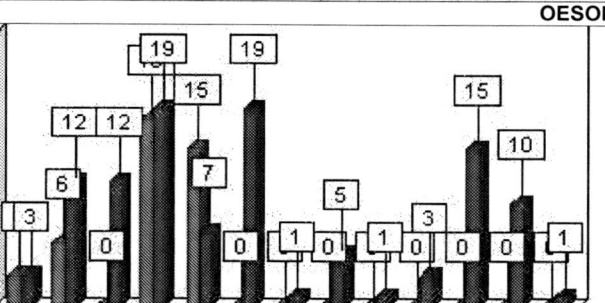

**Chronic Fatigue: Compensatory signal.**
Age-Related Changes: Expressed pathology signal.
Diverticulum: Expressed compensatory signal.
Oesophagitis: Expressed compensatory signal.
Neoplasm: Expressed compensatory signal.
Abnormalities of Development: Compensatory signal.

## STOMACH

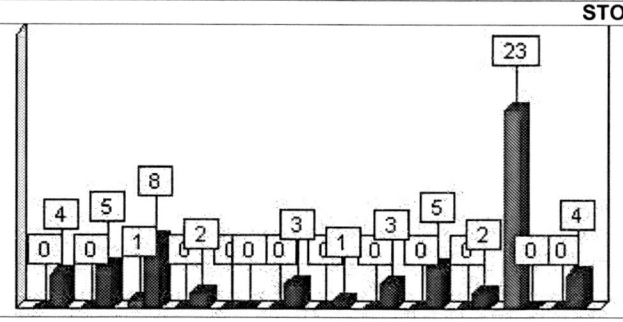

Degenerative Process: Expressed pathology signal.
Functional Changes: Compensatory signal.

250

## DUODENUM

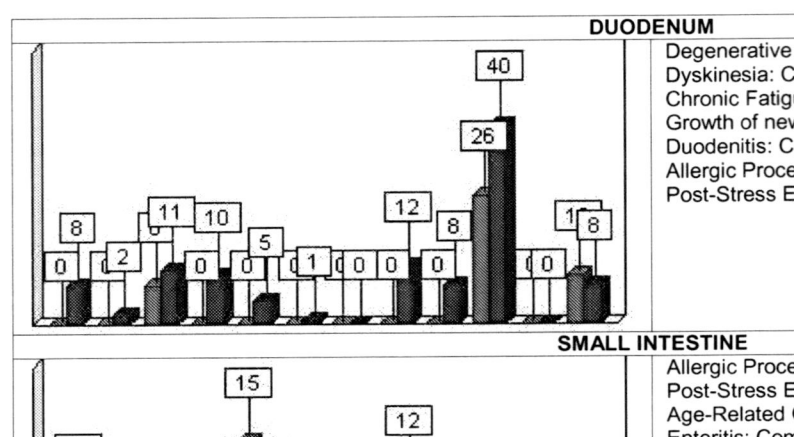

Degenerative Process: Compensatory signal.
Dyskinesia: Compensatory signal.
Chronic Fatigue: Weakening of compensatory abilities.
Growth of new cells: Compensatory signal.
Duodenitis: Compensatory signal.
Allergic Process: Expressed compensatory signal.
Post-Stress Effects: Compensatory signal.

## SMALL INTESTINE

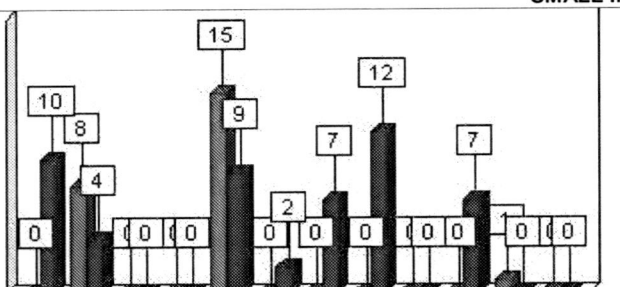

Allergic Process: Pathology signal.
Post-Stress Effects: Weakening of compensatory abilities.
Age-Related Changes: Compensatory signal.
Enteritis: Compensatory signal.
Neoplasm: Expressed compensatory signal.
Diverticulae: Compensatory signal.

## LARGE INTESTINE

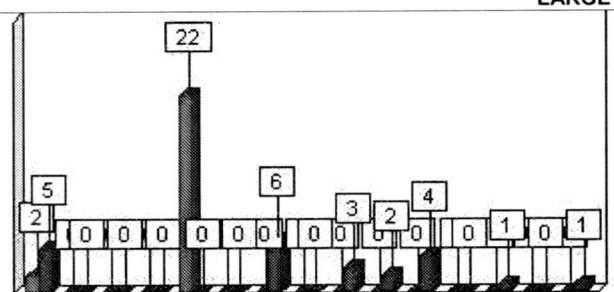

**Chronic Fatigue: Expressed pathology signal.**
Diverticulae: Compensatory signal.
Sigmoiditis: Compensatory signal.

## KIDNEYS

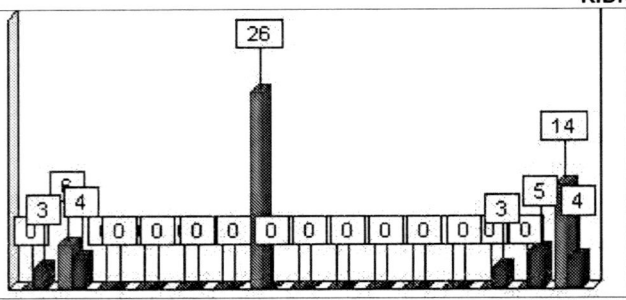

**Chronic Fatigue: Weakening of compensatory abilities.**
Renal Insufficiency: Expressed pathology signal.
Functional Changes: Expressed pathology signal.
Allergic Process: Compensatory signal.

## URINARY BLADDER

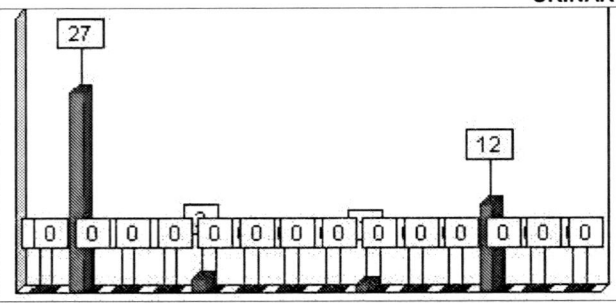

**Chronic Fatigue: Expressed pathology signal.**
Urethral Infections: Expressed pathology signal.

251

## WOMB AND APPENDAGES

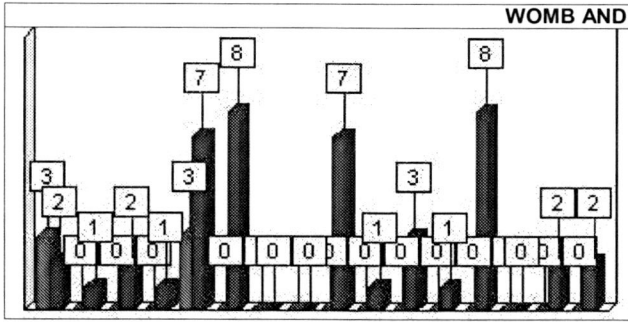

Degenerative Process: Compensatory signal.
Endometritis: Compensatory signal.
Intoxication Effects: Compensatory signal.
Uterine Myoma: Compensatory signal.

## SKELETAL AND MUSCULAR SYSTEM

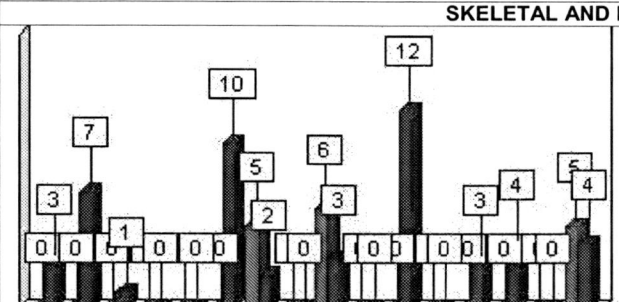

Chronic Fatigue: Pathology signal.
Allergic Process: Pathology signal.
Degenerative Process: Weakening of compensatory abilities.
Arthrosis: Compensatory signal.
Radiculitis: Expressed compensatory signal.
Functional Changes: Expressed compensatory signal.

## 4.13  Assessment of HEART PROBLEMS

### example 14: woman, 53 years, 52 kgs, HEART

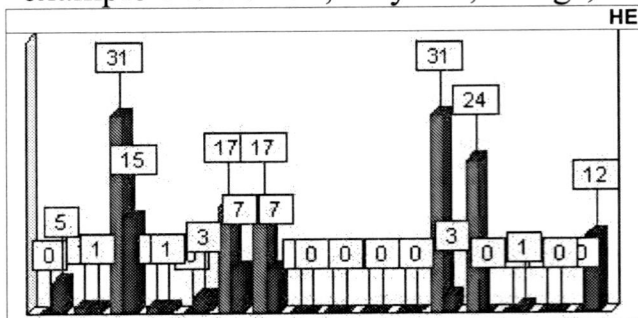

**HEART**

**15/31 Angina Pectoris:  Expressed pathology signal.**
**7/17Cardiosclerosis: Expressed pathology signal.**
7/17 Chronic Fatigue:  Expressed pathology signal.
**3/31 Cardiac Insufficiency:  Expressed pathology signal.**
**0/24 Cardiac Myopathy:  Expressed pathology signal.**
5/0 Ischemic Heart Disease: Compensatory signal.

### example 15: man, 88 years, 77 kgs, HEART

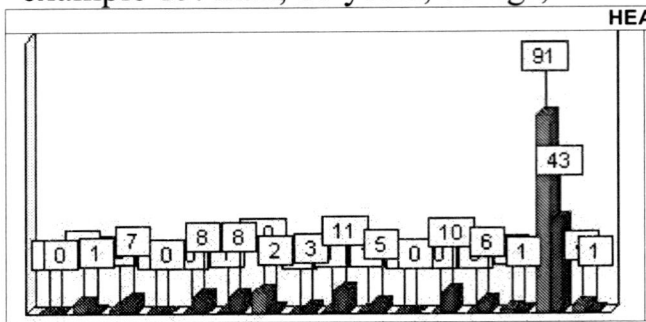

**HEART**

Functional Changes:  Pathology signal.
Chronic Fatigue:  Expressed pathology signal.
**43/91 Impairment of Cardiac Rhythm and Conduction:**
**Expressed pathology signal.**
Tension of compensatory abilities.

### example 16: man, 28 years, 70 kgs, HEART

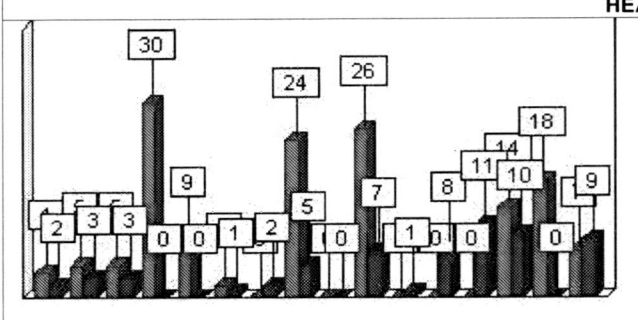

**HEART**

**5/24 Myocardial dystrophy: Expressed pathology signal**
**7/26 Myocarditis: Expressed pathology signal**
10/14 Cardiac Insufficiency: Compensatory signal.
11/0 Cardiac Myopathy: Expressed compensatory signal.
**0/30 growth of new cells: Expressed pathology signal**
**0/18 Impairment of Cardiac Rhythm and Conduction**

### example 17: woman, 32 years, 105 kgs, HEART

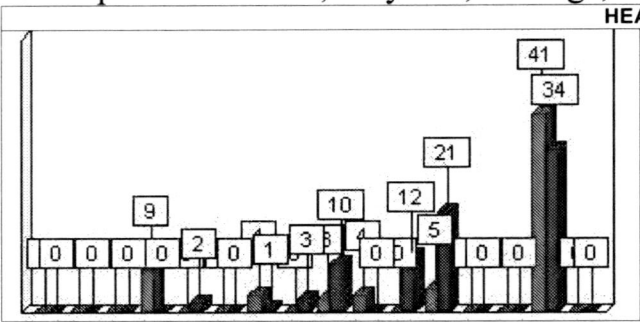

**HEART**

0/9 Growth of new cells:  Expressed pathology signal.
21/5 Cardiac Insufficiency: Expressed compensatory signal.
**34/41 Impairment of Cardiac Rhythm and Conduction:**
**Weakening of compensatory abilities.**

## example 18: man, 64 years, 70 kgs, HEART

| HEART | |
|---|---|
| 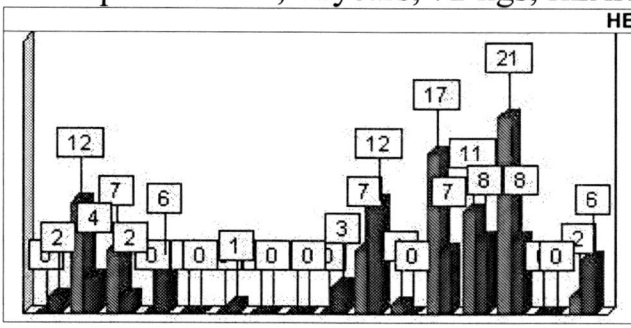 | 3/6 ischaemic heart disease: expressed compensatory signal<br>5/9 cardiosclerosis: expressed compensatory signal<br>14/25 chronic fatigue: expressed compensatory signal<br>**11/19 myocardial dystrophy: expressed compensatory signal**<br>**9/17 myocarditis: expressed compensatory signal**<br>5/6 cardiac insufficiency: expressed compensatory signal<br>3/5 cardiac Myopathy: expressed compensatory signal<br>**13/22 impaired cardiac rhythm & conduction: expressed compensatory signal** |

## example 19: man, 62years, 72 kgs, HEART

| HEART | |
|---|---|
| 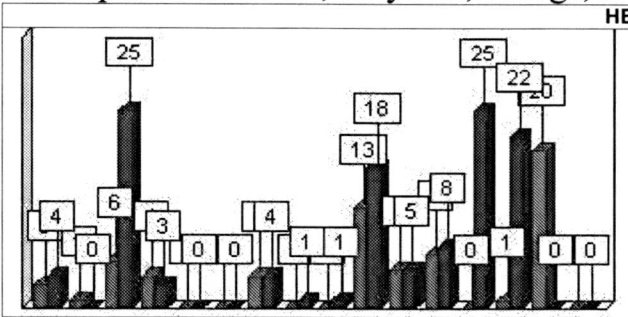 | **12/7 Myocarditis: Compensatory signal.**<br>**7/17 cardiac insufficiency: expressed compensatory signal**<br>**8/11 cardiac Myopathy: expressed compensatory signal** |

## example 20: woman, 59 years, 71 kgs, HEART

| HEART | |
|---|---|
| 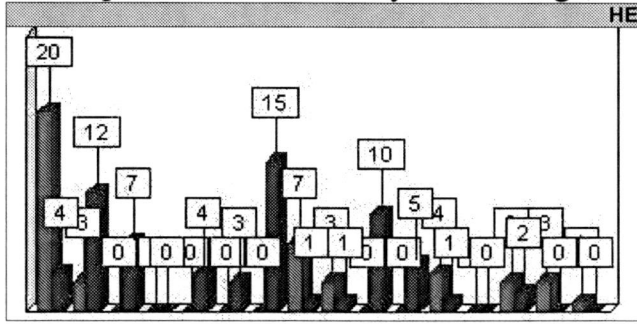 | **25/6 Angina Pectoris: Expressed compensatory signal.**<br>**18/13 Myocarditis: Compensatory signal.**<br>5/5 Cardiac Insufficiency: Compensatory signal.<br>**0/20 Impairment of Cardiac Rhythm and Conduction: Expressed pathology signal.**<br>**25/0 Cardiac Myopathy: Expressed compensatory signal.** |

## example 21: woman, 50 years, 61 kgs, HEART

| HEART | |
|---|---|
| 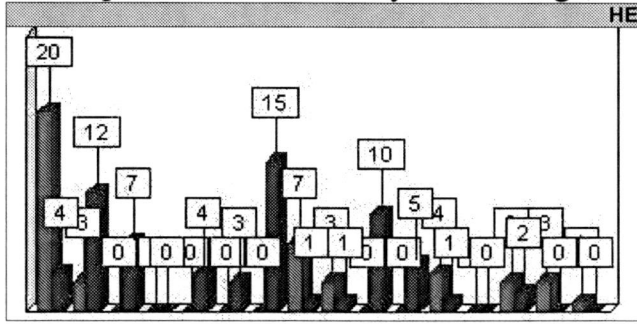 | **0/20 Ischemic Heart Disease: Expressed pathology signal.**<br>1/7 Myocardial Dystrophy: Pathology signal.<br>7/0 Angina Pectoris: Compensatory signal.<br>10/0 Myocarditis: Expressed compensatory signal. |

## 4.14: Assessment of PSORIASIS

example 22: male, 34 years, 55 kgs, PSORIASIS

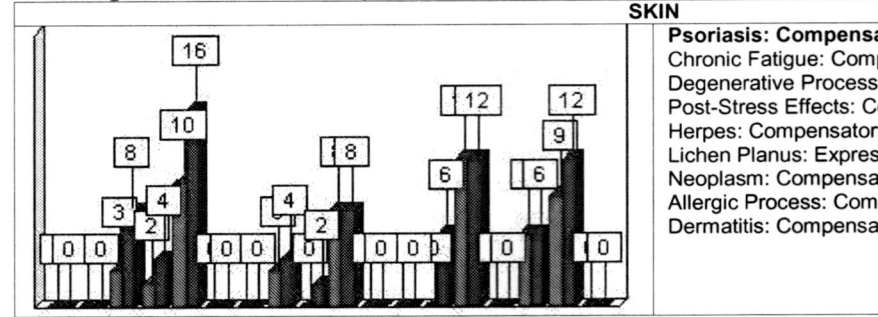

**SKIN**

**Psoriasis: Compensatory signal.**
Chronic Fatigue: Compensated pathology condition.
Degenerative Process: Compensated pathology condition.
Post-Stress Effects: Compensated pathology condition.
Herpes: Compensatory signal.
Lichen Planus: Expressed compensatory signal.
Neoplasm: Compensatory signal.
Allergic Process: Compensatory signal.
Dermatitis: Compensatory signal.

## 4.15 The Effects of Virtual Scanning Therapy

The following case studies have been taken from medical reports on patients treated at various Russian medical institutes.

1. D.M, 16 years old, diagnosis: **Diabetes**, 1 type, heavy form, labile process. Diabetic encephalopathy, polyneuropathy, retinopathy; concentration of sugar in blood was up to 28.4 mmol/l and she was given injections of insulin. After 5 sessions of Virtual Scanning therapy for the cerebrum the level of sugar in the blood was reduced to the 7-9 mmol/l.

2. R.S, 23 years old, diagnosis: **Diabetes**, 1 type, heavy form. Diabetic encephalopathy, polyneuropathy, microangiopathy. Narcotic dependence, concentration of sugar in blood was up to 10-17 mmol/l, he got insulin up to 40 units per day. After 5 sessions of Virtual Scanning therapy the level of sugar in the blood lowed to 5 mmol/l, and was accompanied by hypoglycaemia. It stabilized at 7-8 mmol/l, the insulin dose was reduced and the drug dependency decreased.

3. M.A, 9 years old. Diagnosis: **Enuresis** (involuntary urination 3-4 times per night). The boy received Virtual Scanning therapy for the cerebrum and urinary bladder. After the fourth session the involuntary urination was observed once in 4 days.

4. B.N, 14.5 years old. Complaints for absence of menstruation during 1.5 years against the background of **nervous anorexia**, hypothyroidism. After 2 series of Virtual Scanning therapy for cerebrum menstruation recommenced in 3 weeks.

5. V.Ye.M., 50 years old. diagnosis: **myocardial sclerosis** with rhythm disorders: extrasystolyl sino-tachycardia. Virtual Scanner diagnosis confirmed the diagnosis and revealed an underlying calcium deficit. After Virtual Scanning therapy for cerebrum and heart, supported by mineral supplementation, the patient's condition noticeably improved and the heart rhythm disorders fully disappeared.

6. Patient S., 42 years old. Patient with endogenous **depression**, in the second category of disablement, unable to work or simple house work. Over a period of 8 months he took 2 courses of Virtual Scanning colour therapy for the cerebrum and finally began working not only at home, but also, at the state farm. His suicidal tendencies fully disappeared.

7. Patient Ts., 54 years old. diagnosis: **disseminated sclerosis (MS)**, in the first category of disablement. Complaints: general weakness, shaky walk, moved only with the help of others, irritability, disturbed sleep, bad appetite, weight deficit, depression. After the first course of Virtual Scanning therapy he began walking without any help, put on weight (2kg in 1 month), had good appetite and normal sleep. After the second course of Virtual Scanning therapy for the cerebrum he began doing simple work at home.

8. Patient K., 60 years old. diagnosis: **neuritis** of facial nerve and of the second branch of trifacial nerve (trigeminal neuralgia). Complaints for skin desensitisation of the right face part, speech infringement, and headaches. After the forth session of Virtual Scanning therapy speech improved, by the end of treatment course it was fully restored, and headaches disappeared.

9. Patient J. K, 10 y.o.

Invalided from the age of 5 y.o. with diagnosis **epilepsy**. Suffering c10 attacks every day in spite of taking all necessary medications. Also headaches.

After the first course of treatment with brain module (for 21 days) - all attacks stop. Ceased medications. In 2001 she was given another course of Virtual Scanning therapy. Still no attacks. Clinical investigation showed that the specific local area of the cortex which is responsible for the attacks has disappeared. As a result the categorisation of disability was taken removed/withdrawn.

10. Patient E.A., 43 y.o.

**Slipped/ruptured disc L (lumbar) 3-4 vertebrae and also slipped disc of T (thoracal/chest) 6-7-8 vertebrae resulting in paralysis.** Disorder sensitivity and plegiae left upper limb, left lower limb, disorder of sensitivity and irradiating pain along the sciatic nerve and movement disorder function of left leg.

Following a course of Virtual Scanning therapy for spinal cord and peripheral nervous system the pain in the back had been significantly reduced, sensitivity was recovered in the left part of the body, limp disappeared and irradiating pain on the sciatic nerve disappeared. At the present time she is working as a driver.

11. Patient U., 44 y.o.

Was operated 1987 concerning diffuse toxic nodular goitre third stage (of the thyroid). From 1999 it recurred as **Autoimmune thyroiditis.** She received replacement medication L-Thyroxine and Mercasolil. TTH hormone </= 0.16.

After Virtual Scanning she was given a module for thyroid gland and module for brain. After one month level of TTH is normalised at 4.1

12. Patient C., 44 y.o.

Invalid/disabled for three years with diagnosis **slipped disc of L 3-4 vertebrae, spondylistisis.** Walking with aid of walking stick. Continuous Pain in lumbar region of spine, disorder of sensitivity, disorder of sexual functions, impossible to sit for a long period due to pain.

After Virtual Scanning therapy for spinal cord and peripheral nervous system, sensitivity was restored, low back pain disappeared completely, left the stick after the first course, after second course sexual function improved, and he started to drive his car once again. Disablement was withdrawn, general feeling of well being returned, and well for one year after the treatment.

13. Patient A.S, 14 y.o.

Annually from age of 8yo getting treatment in St Petersburg clinic for **epilepsy**. During clinical investigation clear proven sensitive area of brain responsible for epilepsy. Sedative medication morning and evening,

Virtual Scanning diagnosis of epilepsy. Virtual Scanning therapy for brain and spinal cord. After the first session an intense seizure occurred. Treatment continued with no further seizures/fits. After two months during investigation in St Petersburg clinic the area of the brain associated with the epilepsy no longer showed any anomalies. During a year antiseizures medication terminated, no headaches and no further seizures. Leading an active normal life, fit and without colds or other infections.

14. T.P, 42 y.o.

Was offered an operation for **endometriosis** in Sept 1999.

Virtual Scanning diagnosed endometritis and recommended a course of Virtual Scanning therapy for womb, appendages, and ovaries. Second visit to gynaecologist with diagnostic 'scrape' did not find endometriosis and cancelled the operation Third visit to gynaecologist - full recovery. Presently general condition satisfactory with no complaints.

15. M. S., 42 y.o.

Diagnosis: **slipped disc L 3-5 vertebrae**, offered urgent operation.

After third session of Virtual Scanning therapy for spinal cord, back-pain had disappeared. By the 5th session stopped limping and started to walk normally, and after 8th session full recovery of sensitivity in lower limb. At present, no complaints, active and playing basketball.

16. A.P., 42 y.o.

During 2 years undergoing treatment for diagnosed **plexitis** (right). Movement of right hand restricted, bent/cupped inwards, restricted movement of shoulder joint unable to be moved above horizontal.

After third session of Virtual Scanning therapy for spinal cord he moved his hand out of the cupped position and recovered full range of movements in shoulder joint. After completing this course of treatment full recovery.

17. Svetlana S., 46 y.o.

Operated 1989 with diagnose **diffuse toxic nodular goitre**, in 1999 condition recurred. Taking replacement medications and was offered a second operation.

Two courses of Virtual Scanning therapy for thyroid and brain after which replacement therapy cancelled. After ultrasound it was decided to withhold operation and at the present time her condition is satisfactory without need of replacement therapy.

18. Family couple A. & E., 37 and 43 y.o.

For 8 years their efforts to have a child had failed. She could not conceive. Virtual Scanning diagnosis detected a problem with the man which was **chronic prostatitis** and with the woman, **chronic adnexitis** (inflammation of appendages) and **ovarian cyst**. He was given Virtual Scanning therapy for prostate gland; the woman for womb, appendages and ovaries. She became pregnant within two months and gave birth to a girl of 4.3 kgs.

22. Family couple, S&E.

During 10 years without conception.

He was diagnosed with **oligoazospermi**. She - with **ovarial cyst and abnormal mucous layer of womb.** For the man - Virtual Scanning therapy for prostate gland and for metabolism, and for woman - Virtual Scanning therapy for womb and appendages, ovaries, and brain. It was in need of two courses of therapy with an interval of three months. Pregnancy by caesarean, healthy girl 3.9 kgs

19. Svetlana, 28 y.o.

**Bleeding in the womb** continuously during 8 months she was hospitalised several times in gynaecology dept for scrape of uterus plus conservative treatment plus hormonal treatment without any positive results. Husband put question about divorce. Intense anaemia, erythrocytes 2.8M

After Virtual Scanning therapy for ovaries, womb and appendages, blood discharges started to thicken and suddenly stopped by the end of the fourth session. Finished complete treatment, three months later her menstrual cycle stabilised/normalised. At present moment no complaints, generally good feelings and family stable.

20. V.B., 58 y.o.

Continuous **tinnitus**. Irritability, dizziness, bouts of sickness. Medical treatment over 4 months without positive results. Virtual Scanning diagnosed **Menieres disease**. After 4 sessions of Virtual Scanning therapy for the ear the tinnitus, dizziness and sickness have disappeared. At present moment general feeling is satisfactory. No attacks for 7 months and second course of treatment not required.

21. Valentina, 42 y.o.

Surgeon. **Allergic reaction to latex in surgical gloves.** She was considering a change of career after 20 years surgical experience because her hands were swollen, intense redness, itching which not helping any hormonal or other medication. The condition continued for 18 months.

Virtual Scanning gave diagnosis of **erythema multiforme.** Virtual Scanning therapy for skin and liver relieved the redness and itchiness. At present she is continuing to work without any problem. No reoccurrence in 8 months.

22. Patient S. - woman, 38 y.o., was suffering from severe attacks of **migraine** 2-3 episodes weekly. After first course of informational therapy attacks changes - become easier, she stops take medications/analgetics, 1-2 episodes a month). After second course of treatment – she is free from this condition during 8 months at the moment.

23. Patient K. - woman, 31 y.o., **hypofunction of thyroid gland.** After course of informational therapy patient's conditions significantly improved, which was confirmed by objective paraclinical investigations.

24. Patient M. – man, 40 y.o., is suffering from endogenic **depression**, having 2-nd group of disability. After two courses of informational therapy suicidal tendency is disappeared and he started to work again.

25. Patient P., 14 years, 56 kgs

Complaints: gasping for breath/asthma/asphyxia several times per week, this complaint during 2 years. Investigated by pulmonologist, allergologistigistic, and endocrinologist with diagnosis of **bronchial asthma (hormonal dependent) hypofunction of thyroid gland, and allergy on house dust.** During 1-year different inhalation devices prevented asthma attacks. Virtual Scanning diagnosis detected two destabilised functional systems: system which maintains optimal sleeping pattern and system which maintains optimal breathing level.

Patient received Virtual Scanning therapy for brain and for support of optimal sleeping pattern. After finishing treatment asthma attacks had ceased.

26. Patient S., 38 years, 110 kgs

Complaints: during the last year increasing blood pressure due to stress. His GP and cardiologist diagnosed **hypertension.** Virtual Scanning diagnosis detected pronounced reaction due to stress with disorders in the small intestine, thyroid gland, skin, pituitary gland, adrenal glands, prostate gland, testicles, gall Bladder, spleen, and lungs.

Virtual Scanning therapy for brain and pituitary gland was provided From third till 8th day of treatment patient noticed periodic intensive headache and increased blood pressure during the day, then his condition was stabilized. During the following two months the frequency of these isolated adverse events decreased.

27. Patient G., 55 years, 78 kgs

Was prescribed module for support of **optimal quantity of glucose in blood**. By the 50<sup>th</sup> day of treatment the patient had lost 5 kg without dieting and their general condition was improved.

28. Irena, 12 years

Diagnosis: **Neurosis, night phobias, claustrophobia**, was prescribed a module for supporting optimal sleeping pattern. On first treatment session the girl experienced horror scenes as a result of the flashing colour range on the monitor. After one week of treatment her phobias had disappeared and her night dreams had normalised.

## 4.16  Further Case Studies:

The following case studies conducted over the period 2003-2007 illustrate the broad scope of Virtual Scanning technology:

1. A 10 yo dyslexic child undertook a course of Virtual Scanning therapy. Within 3 weeks there were clear and distinctive improvement in her behaviour.   The first indications of improved writing and reading were indicated by the third consultation. Her end of term report commented upon a leap in her reading ability. Her previous report, as a 10 yo, assessed her reading age to be 2 years behind her calendar age. Within 6 months, as an 11 yo, her reading ability was reassessed as being equivalent to that of a 14yo. Her next set of examination results were 9 grades 1 & 2 (above 70%) and the remaining two examinations as grade 3 (60-70%).

2. A man of 78 years with **type 2 diabetes, circulatory problems and a swollen foot**. Following a course of Virtual Scanning colour therapy over a 6 month period he commented on improved stability of blood sugar levels, improved mobility, improved circulation, improved energy, and dramatically improved quality of life. He now has complete mobility and restored quality of life.

3. A man in his 60's suffering from **severe depression** and who had been treated over many years with many different forms of medication which, he advised, never had any effect on his health: following a course of Virtual Scanner Colour therapy he has been completely free of **depression**.

4. A man in his 60's suffering from **dysarthria** who had been unable to speak, only mumble inaudibly for almost 5 years. His hospital could not identify the problem despite using MRI, checking for Parkinsonism and Alzheimers, and finally was unable to assist him. Virtual Scanner detected encephalopathy, impairment of cerebral circulation, etc. After only 6 days of Virtual Scanning therapy he was able to speak clearly.

5. A lady in her 40's with **migraine** (attacks 2-3 times per week), Tinnitus and other stress symptoms and who reported that medication could not assist her: Following the commencement of Virtual Scanning therapy was free of migraine attacks within 3 weeks, reported to be free of tinnitus within 4 weeks, and reported significantly improved memory which improved her ability to pass examinations, weight loss and general state of health.

6. A man of 50 years with **gastric reflux** which required an endoscopic examination with discussion of possible surgical options undertook a 1-2 week course of Virtual Scanning therapy. The ailment was not detectable at the following medical examination.

7. A lady consulted us about a **duodenal problem**. Virtual Scanning detected a problem with the duodenal ulcer and referred her to her GP who under duress carried out a further consultation and again gave a negative report. Within the week she was admitted to

hospital with blood discharges and spent over one week in hospital being treated for a the misdiagnosed perforated duodenal ulcer.

8. A lady of circa 60 years spent **2-3 years without sleep following a brain operation to remove a cancerous tumour.** She was emotionally unstable. Within 2 weeks of receiving her first therapy she had settled into regular sleeping for 12-14 hours periods. Following 4 months of Virtual Scanning therapy the lady's sleeping patterns became normalized, her demeanor greatly improved.

9. A man of 56 years treated by conventional medicine and by electro-acupuncture for **general poor health, asthma, irregular sleep,** etc; undertook a preliminary course of Virtual Scanning therapy. Following the first module of therapy the patient no longer required their inhaler to treat their breathing insufficiency and had significantly improved sleeping patterns.

10. A man of late 30's, with mobility problems due to severe **inflammation in one knee,** was assessed. The consultation revealed a pattern of 40 cigarettes per day, heavy drinking and marital problems. His report revealed an alarming indication of pathological process development throughout his system. He immediately chose to give up drinking and resolved to reduce his pattern of smoking.

Following the first module of Virtual Scanning therapy, he reported significantly improved mood, less depression, increased relaxation, significantly improved concentration and organisation, reduced cigarette consumption (without increasing weight), and that his general feeling of well-being is greatly improved. Following the second module of treatment the pains in his knee have ceased and he has recovered normal mobility.

11. A lady of 56 years with the after effects of a **head trauma** consulted us after the lack of progress by conventional healthcare. Her initial health was of **migraines and of taking anti-epilepsy medications.** She was fragile, had the appearance of being sedated and was depressed by the effect that her condition was having upon the quality of her life and of the lives of her immediate family. Following several months of Virtual Scanning therapy she no longer required medication, and had recovered happiness, health and wellbeing.

12.     A child of 7 years who found it difficult to sit still, had very **poor reading and writing skills** and found sequencing the alphabet very difficult. He now has a reading and spelling age just above his chronological age, and loves reading – his mother comments: 'getting him to stop is the hardest part!' His fine motor skills (handwriting) are still poor but are believed to have improved.

13. A lady in her mid-40's showed indications of **Chronic Fatigue** starting shortly after her husband had a mental breakdown. Over the previous 4-5 years she had tried many remedies including acupuncture but none had any effect. Her condition was one of

extreme fatigue following short (10 minute) periods of exertion and of aches and pains in her hip. Her cardiovascular system was showing signs of deterioration.

Despite a first month of therapy which brought no improvement (she even considered ceasing treatment), she returned for a reassessment which indicated improvements in some reports. Her Acupuncturist conceded that Acupuncture had achieved nothing in two years of regular treatment, and that she should consider an alternative. As a result she persevered with VS Treatment and, after 3-4 months, showed positive improvement. She was able to jog for short periods while the aches and pains which had plagued her ceased.

14. A lady in her mid-30's suffering facial neuralgia or **Trigeminal Neuralgia**: like many, she had spent many years seeking a cure, travelling widely, and in her own words 'had lost count of the money spent'. In the first week of therapy she advised that her pain had been drastically reduced if not eliminated, and that she was 'delighted with progress'.

15. A man of ca. 60 years, working in security, with **hay fever/pollen allergy**: after one course of therapy lasting 1-2 months he said he could not recall his problem being so insignificant. Each year, he had suffered from the sore throat, streaming eyes, and blocked nose typical of hay fever sufferers. Despite high pollen counts his hay fever was now insignificant.

16. A lady of 57 years: stressed, **frozen shoulder, poor quality and duration of sleep,** emotionally overwrought (breaking down in tears). Her concentration was very poor while taking the test. Her first two consultations were very difficult. After 4 visits her health had dramatically improved, sleep patterns had normalized, the frozen shoulder disappeared, she is now relaxed and content.

## 4.17 Typical Comparative Analyses before and after Treatment

### Male 56 yrs LUNGS AND BRONCHI 1

**Case Study 1:** Virtual Scanning Health Assessment of a 56 year old man before and after Virtual Scanning Treatment for asthma.

Note the strong, indications for the allergic process (2/16) and chronic breathing insufficiency (14/18). In Fig 1b after treatment: the former has been significantly reduced (2/4) and the latter has (4/0) almost disappeared. The assessment of different organs yields an overall picture of the pathology, most aspects of which can be seen to improve with treatment. Note the information about complications to the main pathology yielded by data on the Nose (1c&d)

Initial diagnosis confirms allergic process (2/16) and indications of compensated chronic breathing insufficiency (14/18) are present. Note also (though these are minor signals at below the symptomatic threshold (10 units) the secondary confirmation by the compensatory signal for bronchiectatic disease (5/0 - 4th pair of columns), and the indication of strain caused on the lungs by the signal for chronic breathing insufficiency (1/4 - 3rd pair of columns).

Figure 1a  Male 56 years, Lungs & Bronchi

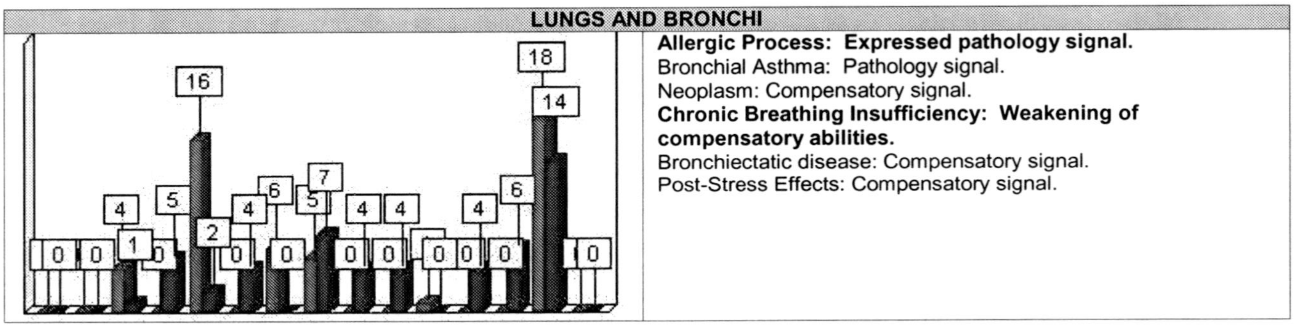

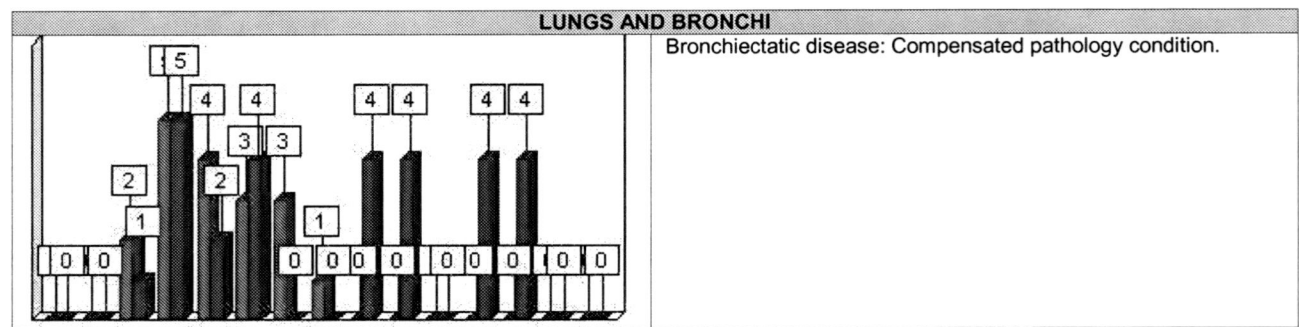

Figure 1b  Male 56 years, Lungs & Bronchi

Post treatment diagnosis shows that the indications of allergic processes and chronic breathing insufficiency have been significantly reduced.

265

Case Study 2: Example of a patient with Chronic Fatigue

A 40 year old male patient with chronic fatigue: initial assessment found indications of uncompensated chronic fatigue signals in six organs, including the brain, liver, pituitary, thyroid, adrenal and blood/peripheral blood vessels. This is illustrated by the prevalence of red signals which are indicative of developing pathology and of the near absence of the blue signals which are indicative the body's natural compensatory abilities.

Figure 2a

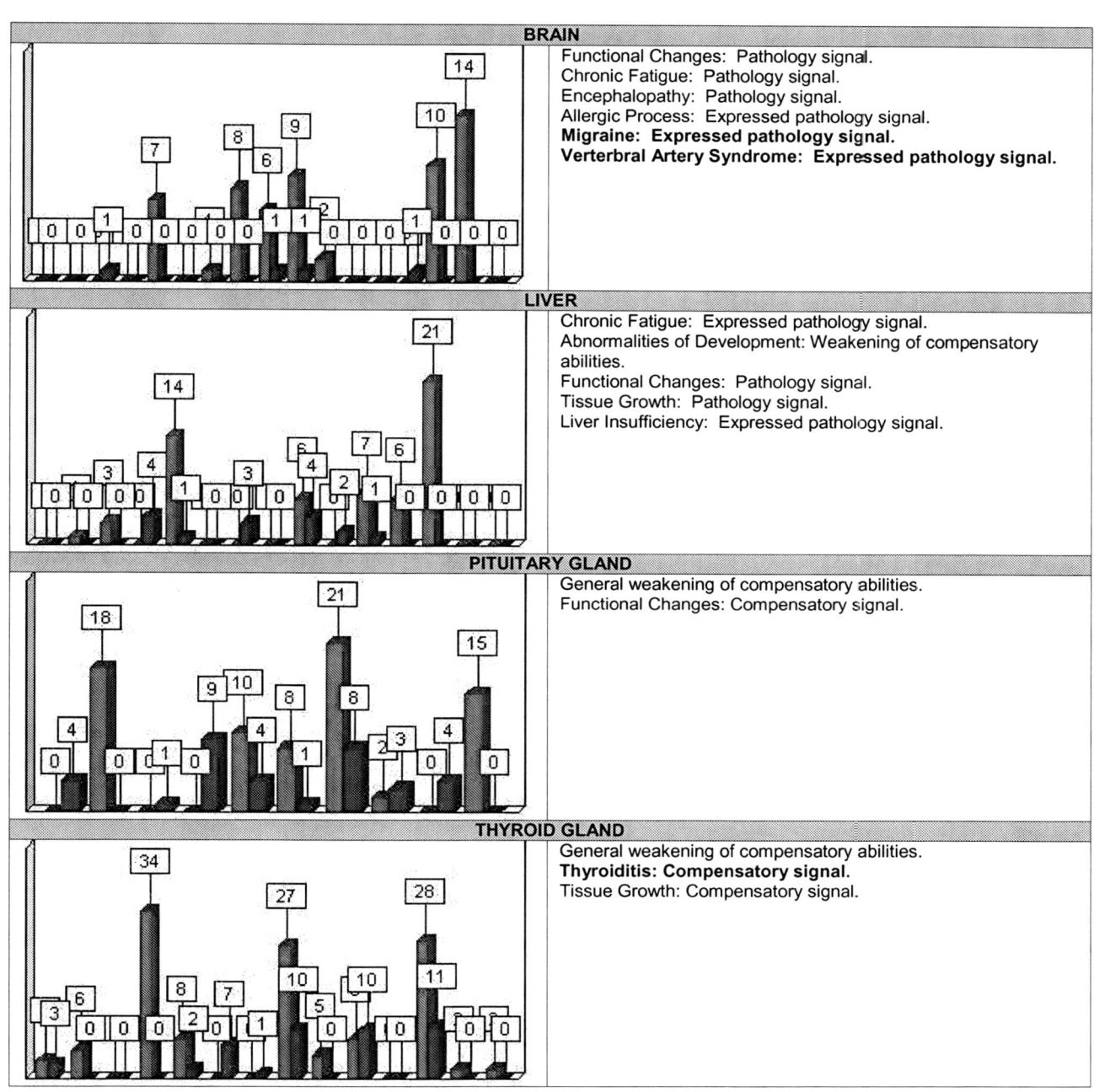

**BRAIN**

Functional Changes: Pathology signal.
Chronic Fatigue: Pathology signal.
Encephalopathy: Pathology signal.
Allergic Process: Expressed pathology signal.
**Migraine: Expressed pathology signal.**
**Verterbral Artery Syndrome: Expressed pathology signal.**

**LIVER**

Chronic Fatigue: Expressed pathology signal.
Abnormalities of Development: Weakening of compensatory abilities.
Functional Changes: Pathology signal.
Tissue Growth: Pathology signal.
Liver Insufficiency: Expressed pathology signal.

**PITUITARY GLAND**

General weakening of compensatory abilities.
Functional Changes: Compensatory signal.

**THYROID GLAND**

General weakening of compensatory abilities.
**Thyroiditis: Compensatory signal.**
Tissue Growth: Compensatory signal.

266

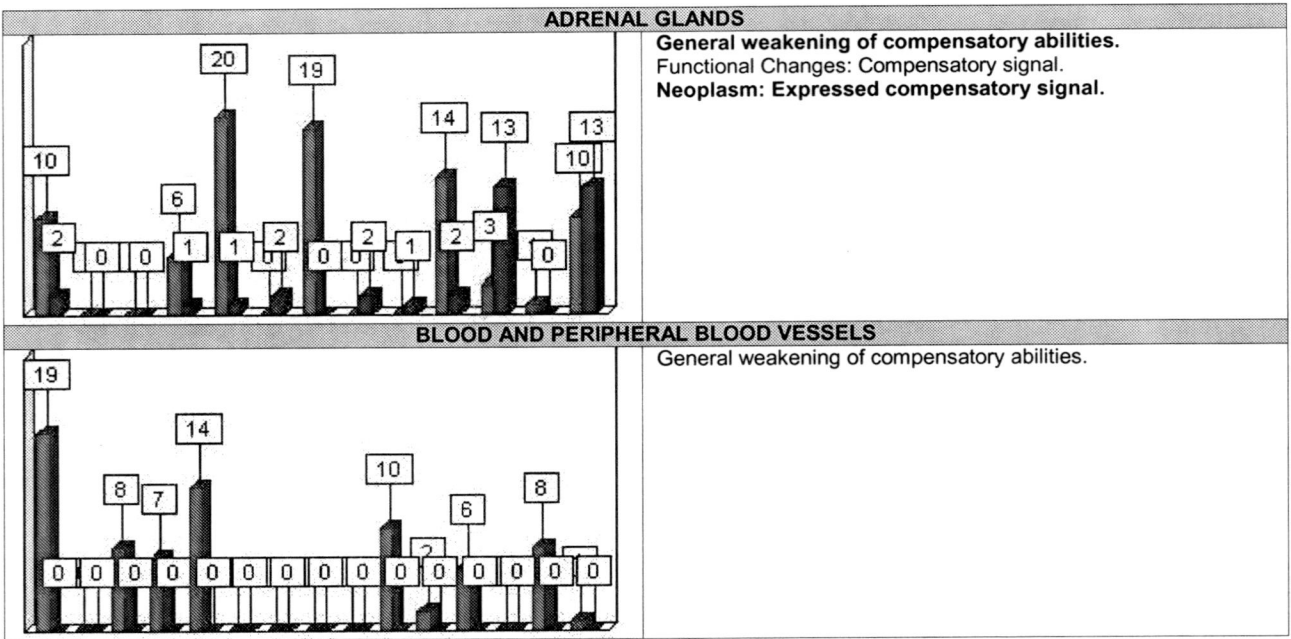

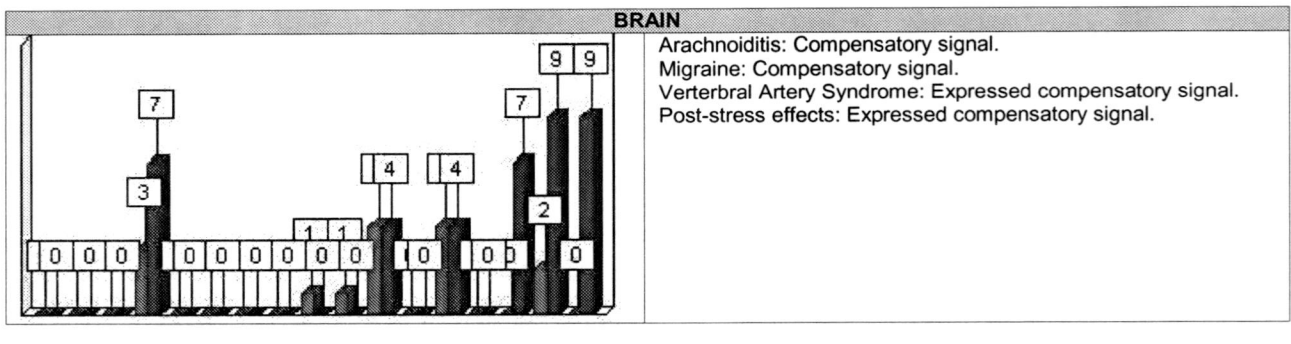

Figure 2b Reassessment after Virtual Scanning Treatment of 40 yrs male from figure 2a.

Note how the organs affected by chronic fatigue or weakened compensatory abilities show improvements from 2a, when they were first measured. The chronic fatigue signals have been reduced or have disappeared, and the ability to compensate for mild pathological conditions has returned in the other organs. The red pathology signals have decreased in magnitude and are no longer uncompensated.

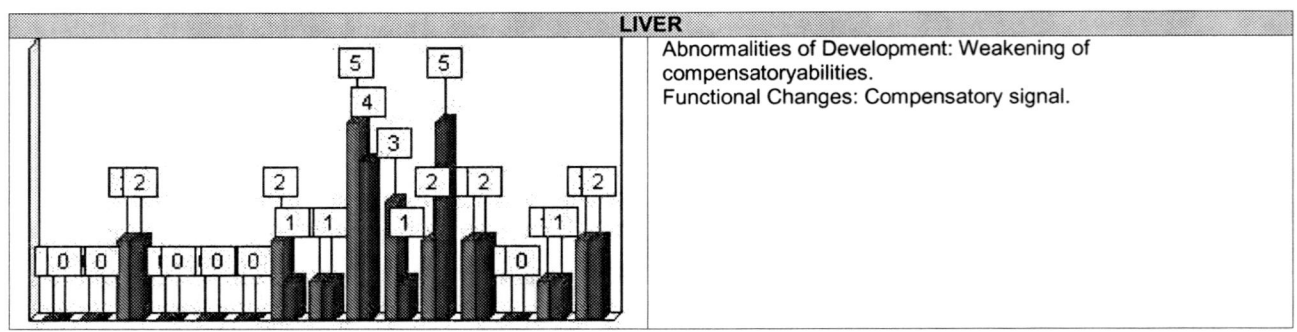

267

## PITUITARY GLAND

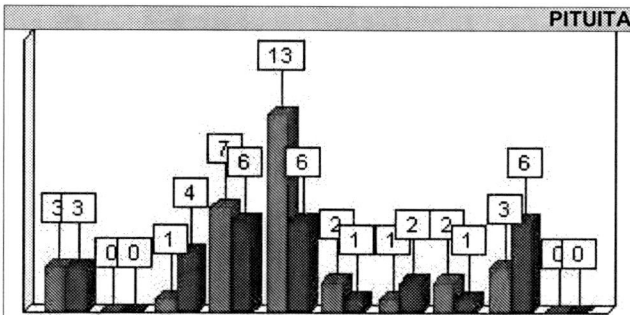

Functional Changes: Weakening of compensatory abilities.
Abnormalities of Development: Expressed pathology signal.

## THYROID GLAND

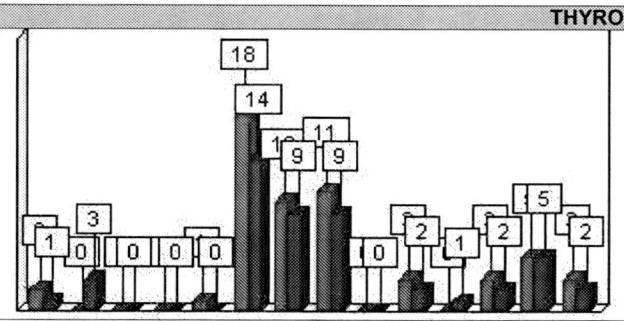

Tissue Growth: Weakening of compensatory abilities.
Hypothyrosis: Weakening of compensatory abilities.
Allergic Process: Weakening of compensatory abilities.
Neoplasm: Compensated pathology condition.

## ADRENAL GLANDS

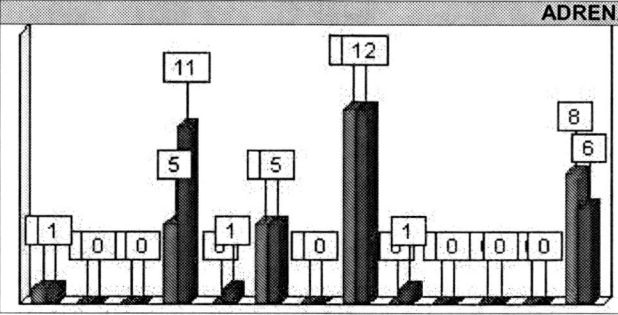

Post-Stress Effects: Compensated pathology condition.
Functional Changes: Weakening of compensatory abilities.
Abnormalities of Development: Expressed compensatory signal.

## BLOOD AND PERIPHERAL BLOOD VESSELS

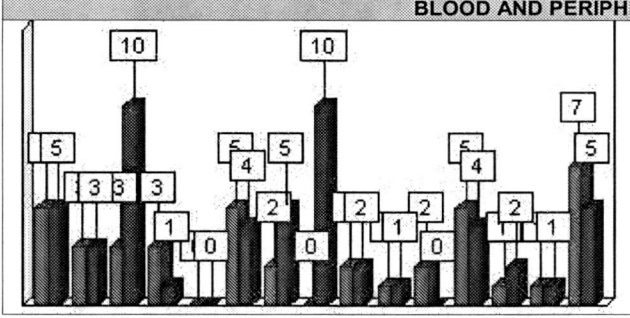

Anaemia: Compensated pathology condition.
Functional Changes: Weakening of compensatory abilities.
Degenerative Process: Weakening of compensatory abilities.
Post-Stress Effects: Weakening of compensatory abilities.
Leukopenia: Expressed compensatory signal.
Haemorrhagic Vasculitis: Compensatory signal.
Neoplasm: Expressed compensatory signal.

268

Case Study 3: Example of Patient with a Range of Unidentified Ailments

**Summary**

Patient seeking treatment for a range of stress-related ailments which could not be identified by conventional medical techniques. Issues identified by Virtual Scanning included calculous prostatitis

**Comparison of Psychological Profiles before and after treatment**

**1.     Before treatment**

| | | | | | |
|---|---|---|---|---|---|
| Imaginary | 1,886 | Anger | 292 | Goodness | 132 |
| Real | 1,346 | Envy | 247 | Patience | 196 |
| | | Injustice | 217 | Labour | 190 |
| | | Sorrow | 204 | Abstinence | 175 |
| | | Guile | 197 | Truth | 166 |
| Mendacity | 25 | Ignorance | 184 | Inventiveness | 199 |

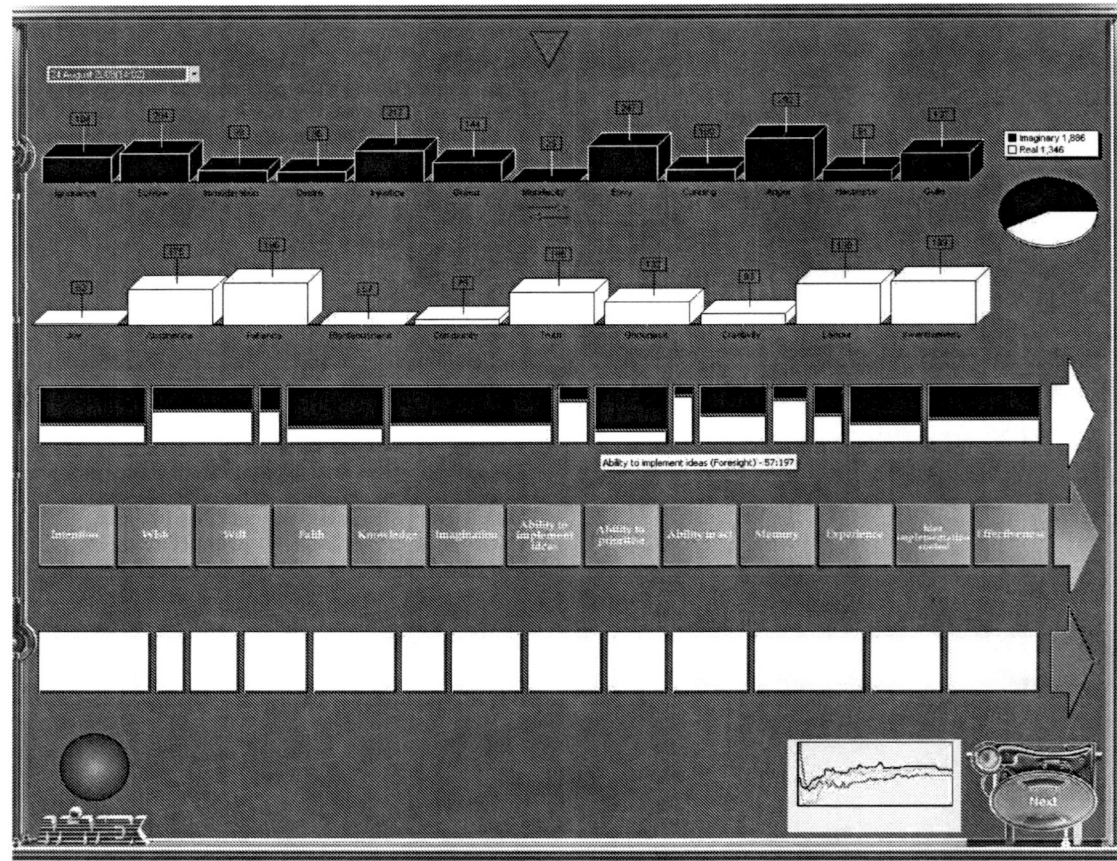

269

## 2.    After treatment

| | | | | | | |
|---|---|---|---|---|---|---|
| Imaginary | 846 | Anger | 107 | Goodness | 98 |
| Real | 686 | Envy | 95 | Patience | 94 |
| | | Injustice | 81 | Labour | 66 |
| | | Sorrow | 77 | Abstinence | 75 |
| | | Guile | 83 | Truth | 89 |
| Mendacity | 53 | Ignorance | 85 | Inventiveness | 73 |

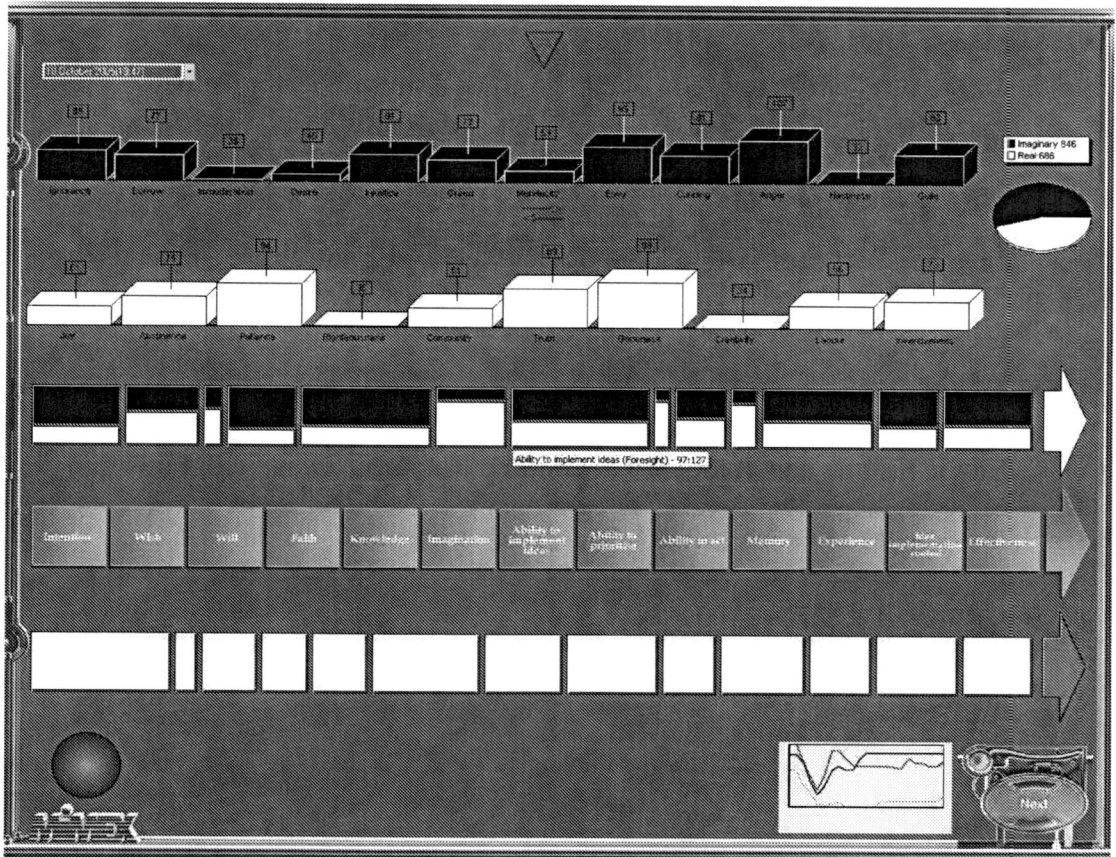

## Summary

The test results improved significantly over a period of three consecutive consultations. Whereas at the first consultation the patient was unable to drive by the third consultation he felt sufficiently improved to drive by himself. There was a marked improvement in his demeanor which was far more relaxed and less confrontational.

The magnitude of positive and negative psychological traits had reduced from over 3,000 units to a more typical level of less than 2,000 units. Moreover the balance of positive (real) and negative (imaginary) traits improved from c 41% to a more typical c 45% illustrating a more balanced and less negative attitude.

## 4.18  Use of Virtual Scanning to monitor various influences on a person's physical and psychological health

For example Virtual Scanning enables us:

1. to monitor the effect of a complementary health therapy

2. to monitor the effect, and hence the safety, of a drug-based therapy

3. to monitor before and after effects of a holiday

4. to monitor the physical and psychological profiles of mental health patients

5.    to monitor the effects of personal interactions between people and groups of people

- the effect of a carer on a patient or vice-versa, of a patient on a carer

- the effect of husband / wife or parent / child relationships

- the interaction of groups at work or in performance oriented environments

6. to monitor the health and psychology of children in an educational environment

7. to monitor changes in health and psychology of delinquents

## 4.19 Weight Loss

Virtual Scanning offers therapy modules specifically for regulation of body weight. Loss of excess weight is often observed as a side-effect of therapy.

Some reported examples of weight loss accompanying Virtual Scanning therapy include:

- Female 82 years, c65kgs, treated for stress-related migraine. 4-5 months therapy reduced both frequency and severity of migraine attacks. She also lost 5 kgs, though her daily routine was unchanged. Her mobility significantly improved.

and from Rusia:

- Hlebnikova A.P., 53 y.o., female, 87 kgs. Excess weight, hypertension. After 20 sessions VS therapy her weight reduced by 11kgs, & waist line 12 cms; blood pressure stabilised; sharply decreased appetite; sense of well-being returned.

- Kozina Z.A., 55 y.o., female, 104 kgs. Excess weight, hypertension. After 40 sessions VS therapy her weight decreased by 21 kgs. Cardiovascular readings stabilised, sleeping patterns stabilised, restored capacity for work.

- Kornauhov U.I., 50 y.o., male, 105 kgs. Excess weight, periodic headaches, erectile dysfunction. After 25 sessions of Virtual Scanning therapy his weight decreased by 17 kgs. Headaches ceased.

## 4.20 DISCUSSION

The information available appears to indicate that Virtual Scanning is able to diagnose a medical condition from the pre-symptomatic level thereby explaining why it could be possible to diagnose a medical condition which could not be diagnosed by conventional medical test procedures. All available data supports the claims by Russian researchers that Virtual Scanning is typically 20-25% more accurate than conventional diagnostic technologies.

It is possible that the data obscures a number of 'false positives' in which medical conditions were falsely diagnosed, or of false negatives in which medical conditions were not diagnosed when in fact they were present. Moreover it would be absurd to claim that the technology is perfect and does not come with imperfections because it is the work of the researcher Dr I.G.Grakov and, as we know, 'people are not perfect and can make mistakes'.

Nevertheless, the available data and examples clearly illustrates the ability of this technology to diagnose conditions (1) before they are subsequently manifest as a measurable symptom (see section 4.2.7) and (2) of the ability to diagnose conditions which were inaccurately diagnosed by the doctor and by the most advanced medical technologies (see section 4.2.6). This illustrates the likelihood that Virtual Scanning is a technology with a significantly greater accuracy than conventional diagnostic test procedures.

Such conclusions are confirmed by the reproducibility of results which are obtained from patients. On each occasion their health results show essential similarities with conventional methods usually accompanied by changes which demonstrate their improving medical condition.

# References

1.  http://www.1stadvantagemarketing.com/advanced-pr/listing/mimex.txt

2.  http://en.wikipedia.org/wiki/Peter_Lesgaft

3.  Patterns of Tremor in Normal and Pathological Conditions: Bishop et al. *J Appl Physiol.*1948; 1: 123-147

4.  Clonus is repetitive, rhythmic contractions of a muscle when attempting to hold it in a stretched state. It is a strong, deep tendon reflex that occurs when the CNS fails to inhibit it.

5.  www.molbiol.princeton.edu/coller/index.php?option=com_content&task=view&id=12&Itemid=26

6.  Hankey.A, Ewing E., New Light on Chromotherapy: Grakov's 'Virtual Scanning' System of Medical Assessment and Treatment, *Evid. Based Complement. Altern. Med.,* Advance Access published on October 5, 2006; doi:10.1093/ecam/nel060

7.  Ewing G., Ewing E., Hankey A, Virtual Scanning: a new system of medical assessment and Treatment Part I: Assessment. *J. Alt. Comp. Med.* Volume 13, (2), 2007

8.  http://www.nym.org/healthinfo/docs/097/doc97drugsremedy.html
    a summary of the specific drugs and remedies for treating a migraine attack

9.  http://www.merckmedicus.com/pp/us/hcp/diseasemodules/migraine/pathophysiology_sub.jsp
    a summary of migraine theories

10. Percutaneous closure of patent foramen ovale reduces the frequency of migraine attacks, *Neurology 2004*; 62: 1399-1401, M. Schwerzmann, S. Wiher, K. Nedeltchev, H. P. Mattle, A. Wahl, C. Seiler, B. Meier, and S. Windecker;

11. Transcatheter closure of patent foramen ovale for migraine prophylaxis: Hope or hype? Tsimikas, *J Am Coll Cardiol* 2005;45:496-498.

12. Blau JN, Thavapalan M. Preventing migraine: a study of precipitating factors. *Headache 1988*;28:481-483.

13. comments attributed to Roses. A, Duke University (Vice-President GSK Pharmacogenetics Division)

14. *American College of Cardiology* March 2005, University of Maryland School of Medicine in Baltimore, Miller M et al

15. *Journal of the American Medical Association* July 2006, Kurth.T et al,

16. Etminan, Mahar; Takkouche, Bahi; Isorna, Francisco Caamaño; Samii, Ali. "Risk of ischaemic stroke in people with migraine: systematic review and meta-analysis of observational studies." *British Medical Journal*, December 13, 2004 doi:10.1136/bmj.38302.504063.8F.

17. DJ Anderson, B.Sc., MB, "The treatment of Migraine with Variable Frequency Photo-Stimulation," in *Headache*, March 1989, pp 154-155:

18. Solomon GD: Slow wave photic stimulation in the treatment of headache - a preliminary study. *Headache* 25: 444-446, 1985.

19. Cohen MJ, McArthur DL, Rickles WH: Comparison of four biofeedback treatments for migraine headache: physiological and headache variables. *Psychosomatic Med* 42:463-480, 1980.

20. Gauthier. J.G., Fournier. A.L., Roberge. C, The differential effects of biofeedback in the treatment of menstrual and nonmenstrual migraine, *Headache 1991*: 31, 2, 82-90

21. Diamond. S, Epstein. M.F, Biofeedback for headache, *Postgraduate Medicine 1982*, 72, 1, 241-9

22. Diamond. S, *Headache*, 41, 2, 183-92, Thermal Biofeedback Treatment; *Clin Cornerstone* 1999, 1, 6, 33-44, Tension-type headache.

23. Van_Hook. E, *Clinical Neuroscience* 1998, 5, 1, 43-9, Non-pharmacological treatment of headaches--why?

24. McGrady. A.V, Bush. E.G, Grubb. B.P, *Applied Psychophysiology and Biofeedback 1997*, 22, 1, 63-72, Outcome of biofeedback-assisted relaxation for neurocardiogenic syncope and headache: a clinical replication series.

25. Burke. E.J, Andrasik. F, *Headache1989*, 29, 7, 434-40, Home- vs. clinic-based biofeedback treatment for pediatric migraine: results of treatment through one-year follow-up.

26. Fentress, D.W., Masek, B.J., Mehegan, J.E., Benson, H, *Developmental Medicine and Child Neurology 1986*, 28, Number: 2, pp. 139-46, Biofeedback and relaxation-response training in the treatment of pediatric migraine.

27. Hoelscher, T.J., Lichstein, K.L, *Biofeedback and Self Regulation 1983*, 8, Number: 4, pp. 533-41, Blood volume pulse biofeedback treatment of chronic cluster headache.

28. Blanchard, E.B., Theobald, D.E., Williamson, D.A., Silver, B.V., Brown, D.A.

29. Temperature biofeedback in the treatment of migraine headaches: a controlled evaluation, *Archives of General Psychiatry 1978*, 35, 5, 581-8

30. Amaral.D.G; Professor of Neurobiology and Psychiatry, University of California, David; *International Meeting Autism Research*, Boston; May 2005; also reported in Van Bothmer. E; *Scientific American Mind*, Vol 17, no5; pages 62-65

31. *New Scientist* November 2006; Ramachandrayan V.S., Oberman. L.M;

32. Autonomic Responses of Autistic Children to People and Objects. Hirstein.W, Iversen.P and Ramachandran. V.S in *Proceedings of the Royal Society of London B*, Vol 268, pages 1883-1888, 2001;

33. EEG Evidence for Mirror Neuron Dysfunction in Autistic Spectrum Disorders; Oberman.L.M, Hubbard. E.M, McCleery.J.P, Altschuler.E.L, Pineda.J.A, Ramachandran. V.S, in *Cognitive Brain Research* Vol 24, pages 190-198, 2005

34. *Journal of Child Psychology and Psychiatry* 2004, Professor Baron-Cohen, University of Cambridge, British Psychological Society annual meeting 2004.

35. Clements J, Wing L, & Dunn G, 1986. Sleep problems in handicapped children: a preliminary study. *Journal of Child Psychology and Psychiatry* 27(3): 399-407.

36. Hering E, Epstein R, Elroy S, Iancu DR, & Zelnik N, 1999. Sleep patterns in autistic children. *Journal of Autism and Developmental Disorders* 29(2): 143-147.

37. Richdale AL & Prior MR, 1995. The sleep/wake rhythm in children with autism. *European Child and Adolescent Psychiatry* 4(3): 175-186.

38. Schreck KA, 2001. Behavioral treatments for sleep problems in autism: Empirically supported or just universally accepted? *Behavioral Interventions* 16: 265-278.

39. Scotson technique; http://www.advancecentre.org.uk/en/index.asp

40. http://www.conradsimon.org/WorkingPaperIntro.shtml

41. *Med Hypoth, 1981*; 7; 673-99  link between adhd, asthma, eczema and other allergic symptoms /consistent with a deficiency of Essential fatty acids

42. *Prostaglan Leukotr Essent Fatty Acids*, 2000; 63; 1-9  difficulty in processing fats

43. *J Pediatr; 1994*; 125; s39-47  deficiency of omega-3-fatty acids

44. *Proc Natl Acad Sci USA*; 1986; 4021-5       deficiency of omega-3-fatty acids

45. *Neuropsychology, 2003*; 17; 458-68 aspartame: neurological effect upon neurological functioning

46. *Sound-and-Light Show as a Stress Reducer*, Howard Millman, www.maaddsg.org

47. *Journal of Proceedings of the National Academy of Sciences*, Professor Ush Goswami, Institute of Child Health at University College London

48. Dr Leon Chaitow: ImmuneSupport.com

49. comments attributed to consultant psychiatrist Dr. Peter White, of London's St. Bartholomews' Hospital

50. Goldstein J. *Chronic Fatigue Syndrome - the Limbic hypothesis,* Haworth Medical Press, 1993.

51. Goldenberg Fibromyalgia, chronic fatigue syndrome and myofascial pain syndrome *Current Opinion in Rheumatology,* 1993;5:199-20810.

52. Bennett R Fibromyalgia and the Facts, *Controversies in Clinical Rheumatism,* 19(1)February 1993 pp45-56.

53. http://www.nil.wustl.edu/labs/hershey/db.htm

54. Dr Shahrad Taheri, *Public Library of Science Medicine December 2004,* The researchers from Bristol University, Stanford University and the University of Wisconsin studied volunteers from the Wisconsin Sleep Cohort Study, a population-based study of sleep disorders.  Impaired sleep

55. Research conducted by Professor Steve Bloom is head of a research team at Imperial College, London's Hammersmith Hospital campus which discovered that pancreatic peptide (PP) is secreted after every meal and signals to the brain to stop eating.

56. http://members.aol.com/profchm/majewski.html   R. H. Logan, Instructor of Chemistry, Dallas County Community College District, North Lake College

57. http://muscle.ucsd.edu/musintro/fattyacid.shtml : University of San Diego, California

58. http://www.endocrineweb.com/pancreas.html

59. *Neuropsychology, 2003;* 17; 458-68 aspartame: neurological effect upon neurological functioning

60. *British Medical Journal,* 2006; 333: 1041-3  children's exercise

61. *Journal of Diabetic Medicine* 2007; 24; 73-80. Hart.C.L, Hole D.J, Lawlor.D.A, Davey Smith G.

62. *Journal of Nutrition,* 2006; 136: 2934-8  exercise

63. report attributed to experts at the US Dept of Energy Brookhaven National Laboratories, Leeds University Dept of Psychobiology, University of Minnesota and Minnesota Obesity Centre  and from the Dept of Neuroscience at Princeton University

64. Buck, L. and Axel, R. (1991) *Cell,* vol. 65, 175-187.  olfaction

65. **http://nobelprize.org/nobel_prizes/medicine/laureates/2004/press.html**

66. *Neuroscience Biobehav Rev.,* 1987, 11 (2) pp. 131-262

67. *Neurosci Biobehav Rev.* 1987 Summer;11(2):131-53, Carbohydrate taste, appetite, and obesity: an overview, **Sclafani A.**

68. *British Medical Journal,* bmjupdates,  4 February 2006

69.    comments attributed to Dr Samuel Klein, Director for the Centre for Human Nutrition, University of Washington School of Medicine, quoted in the Readers Digest 2006.

70.    *New England Journal of Medicine*, 2006; 355: 1991-2002;   low carb diets

71.    *British Medical Journal, bmj* updates, 4 February 2006

72.    www.levinsonmedical.com/uk/info_vitalfacts.php

73.    http://www.hi2u.org/Dyslexic/glue_ear_and_dyslexia.htm

74.    *Archives of Pediatric and Adolescent Medicine*, 6/2000, Wyshak.G

75.    Wyshak.G. et al, "Carbonated beverages, dietary calcium, the dietary Calcium/Phosphorous ratio, and bone fractures in girls and Boys", *Journal of Adolescent Health* 1994, 15, 210
**http://findarticles.com/p/articles/mi_m3225/is_n4_v50/ai_15752799**

76.    *American Journal of Clinical Nutrition* 10/2006, Tucker.K, et al "Colas, but not other carbonated beverages, are associated with low bone mineral density in older women: The Framingham Osteoporosis Study".
**http://www.ajcn.org/cgi/content/abstract/84/4/936**

77.    "Regular cola consumption linked to lower bone density in women" http://www.medscape.com/viewarticle/461898

78.    http://emaxhealth.com/4/7732.html

79.    Reinberg.S, "Cola raises women's osteoporosis risk: caffeine might be the culprit, experts say", *Healthday*, 6th October 2006

80.    *The Lancet* December 2000, 356 (9245): 1911, Birchard.K "Irish concerned about the health effects of stimulant soft drinks".

81.    http://neurology.health-cares.net/dizziness.php

82.    *Photochem. Photobiol. Sci.*, 2004, 3, 102 - 108; The regulatory effect of polychromatic (visible and infrared) light on human humoral immunity; Zhevago.N.A, Samoilova.K.A and Obolenskaya K.D

83.    **http://www.merckmedicus.com/pp/us/hcp/diseasemodules/migraine/pathophysiology_sub.jsp**

84.    Lauritzen M. Cerebral blood flow in migraine and cortical spreading depression. *Acta Neurol Scand Suppl.* 1987;76:1-40.

85.    **http://www.parkinsons.org.uk/shared_asp_files/uploadedfiles/%7B2780F6C3 -891F-497EB838-937B50D44BF1%7D_lowbloodpressure50_01_04.pdf**

86.    **http://www.nym.org/healthinfo/docs/097/doc97drugsremedy.html**

87. Anderson, D. J., Legg, N. J., & Ridout, D. A. (1997). Preliminary trial of photic stimulation for premenstrual syndrome. *Journal of Obstetrics and Gynaecology*, 17(l), 76-79.

88. Bou-Holaigah, I., Rowe, P. C., Kan, J., & Calkins, H. (1995). The relationship between neurally mediated hypotension and the chronic fatigue syndrome. *Journal of the American Medical Association, 2* 74, 961-967.

89. *Fibromyalgia Network Newsletters* : October '90 - January '92 Compendium #2, January 1993, May 1993; Compendium, January 1994, July 1994.

90. Joseph Kalik, Fibromyalgia - diagnosis and treatment, *Journal of Osteopathic Medicine* Feb 1989,10-19.

91. Lindenfeld, K. M., Budzynski, T., & Andrasik, F. (1996). **EEG patterns and chronic fatigue syndrome** *Proceedings of the AAPB 27th Annual Meeting,* Albuquerque, NM.

92. Yunus M. **'Fibromyalgia and other functional syndromes'**, *Journal of Rheumatology* 16(sup 19)69 1989.

93. http://www.cdc.gov/ncidod/diseases/cfs/hot_topics/hot-3.03.htm

94. During February 23-26, 2003, the Centers for Disease Control and Prevention (CDC) and the CFIDS Association of America cosponsored a meeting, *Towards Understanding of Cellular and Molecular Mechanisms of Medically Unexplained Fatigue,* at the Banbury Center, Cold Spring Harbor Laboratory, New York.

95. http://www.cfids.org/about-cfids/research.asp

96. http://chronicfatigue.about.com/cs/fibroresearch/a/fmcfsthyroid.htm

97. http://digestive.niddk.nih.gov/ddiseases/pubs/ibs/

98. Lubar, J. F. (1991). Discourse on the development of EEG diagnostics and biofeedback for attention-deficit/hyperactivity disorders. *Biofeedback and Self-Regulation*, 16(3), 201-225.

99. Russell, H. L., & Carter, J. L.( 1993). A pilot investigation of auditory and visual entrainment of brainwave activity in learning-disabled boys. Texas Researcher, *Journal of the Texas Center for Educational Research*, 4, 65.

100. Sappey-Marinier, D., Calabrese, G. , Fein, G., Hugg, J. W., Biggins, C., & Weiner, M. W, (1992). Effect of photic stimulation on human visual cortex lactate and phosphates using 1H and 31P magnetic resonance spectroscopy. *Journal of Cerebral Blood Flow and Metabolism,* 12, 584-592.

101. Zametkin, A. J., Nordahl, T E., Gross, M., King, A. C., Semple, W E., Rumsey, J., Hamburger, S., & Cohen, R. M. *(1990)*. Cerebral glucose metabolism in adults with hyperactivity of childhood onset. **The New England Journal of Medicine,** 323(20), 1361-1366

**102.** http://www.nhsdirect.nhs.uk/articles/article.aspx?ArticleID=351

103. **http://www.nutrition4health.org/nohanews/NNS02DietMigraineHeadaches.htm**

104. Martin, V.T., Behbehani, M.M., "Headache: Toward a rational understanding of migraine trigger factors," *Medical Clinics of North America* , 85: 1-20, 2001.

105. Gibb, C.M., Davies, P.T., Glover, V., *et al*, *Cephalalgia*, 11:93-5, 1991.

# Chapter 5

# The Value of Virtual Scanning to the Medical Profession

by

**Elena & Graham Ewing**

# Introduction

*The following text uses statistics and data which are available from respected medical journals.*

## 5.1    Defining the Need for improved Medical Technologies

*What do you want to achieve when you visit your doctor? What do you expect of them? Are your expectations realistic?*

Despite the myriad of facts supporting or denigrating the role and effectiveness of drugs; the practitioner has to be believe that he is benefiting the patient otherwise he could not convince the patient to become well. Up to 70% of the therapeutic effect of drugs is attributed to the placebo effect 1 in which the patient attends their doctor in the belief that the doctor will assist them to get well again.

***"The physician's belief in the treatment and the patient's faith in the physician exert a mutually reinforcing effect; the result is a powerful remedy that is almost guaranteed to produce an improvement and sometimes a cure."*** 2-6

The patient:

- attends their health centre and consults their doctor in the expectation that by visiting that they will recover their health;
- listens to their doctor who tells them that they will recover their health if they do as he instructs;
- accepts the doctor's explanation of why they are ill and what will alleviate the symptoms;
- takes the medication/therapy in the belief and expectation that it will alleviate the symptoms;
- makes every effort to recover their health e.g. by isolating themselves, sleeping, keeping warm, reducing stress or removing themselves from the stress influences, exercising and relaxing, etc.

The doctor:

- In most cases the doctor's primary concern is to seek and implement ways to improve the health and wellbeing of their patients.

The process of consulting the doctor – and of treating the patient - involves giving attention, care, comfort, etc. This initiates subtle healing reactions in the body which affect the mood of the subject, and reduce stress; thereby inhibiting the occurrence of further harmful changes and promoting wellbeing.

When a patient consults their GP in most cases it is the patient which tells the GP what is the matter. This contrasts with the high technology approach whereby during the medical consultation we could expect to be tested and advised, by the GP, in precise terms what is the matter with our health.

The GP has 5-10 minutes for a patient consultation, most of which is spent with introductory comments, asking questions, making notes, reading through patient notes, completing forms, etc. They are expected to use their senses, knowledge and experience to discern the symptoms which are of concern to the patient through a brief physical examination and interrogation of typically less than 5 minutes duration. When challenged and unable to resolve the problem they refer the patient to their hospital for further tests where the hospital doctor and consultant are limited by the techniques which are available to them or by the limitations of current knowledge of the medical condition.

In many cases doctors now use the internet [269] to find solutions to the problem. They look up credible medical web sites and scan for reasonable case studies, references, etc, in order to identify and find a solution for the person's ailment.

Based upon our expectations of modern medicine, of the billions of dollars which have been poured into biomedical research, we expect to have a reliable method of medical diagnosis. Yet in many cases the medical profession does not have an accurate and reliable means of diagnosing the health of the patient. As a result there is significant scope for misdiagnosis which can range from 20% in an article reported in the New York Times [7] to 42% as reported by the NPSF [8]. Studies of autopsies illustrate that doctors misdiagnose serious illnesses 20% of the time [9] which implies that the medical statistics have inherent shortcomings. This single reason, of misdiagnosis, is the single most important issue which is responsible for the failure to deliver significantly improved levels of healthcare.

If the GP does not understand what causes an illness, do not understand the nature of the ailment, or are unable to quantify the extent of an ailment, how can they do something about it?

We expect to attend our medical centre and to be advised our health following a rapid test procedure much in the same way that our car is subjected to an auto-diagnosis when in the garage for repair, servicing or MOT. When we meet our doctor we are asked questions and examined in the most rudimentary manner. We rarely receive anything in writing which confirms the diagnosis.

What we receive however is a service which does not measure up to expectations i.e. of what we expect from the most highly funded, allegedly high-tech, industry. Doctors are human and humans make mistakes moreover they are expected to be extremely knowledgeable in so many aspects of medicine. There is a limit to their ability [9], especially so as they age [94]. They are not superhuman.

# What Does the Government Expect
# from the Medical Professions? 37

*The government is legally empowered to look after our health. Look at the issues which have been identified and which need to be improved if the health service is to be improved to meet our needs in the 21$^{st}$ century.*

The NHS plan, which is typical of the healthcare industry, identifies a range of objectives, including, but not limited to, the following:

- to improve quality services and to minimise errors

- to improve efficiency, productivity and performance; to reduce waiting times; and that tests and diagnosis will be carried out on the same day.

- a system of inspection and accountability for all parts of the NHS

- that routine screening will be extended to cover more conditions with emphasis upon prevention

- to tackle the underlying causes of ill-health

- to avoid 'recounting the same details to a succession of staff'

- that GPs are looking for better and more flexible ways of working.

- will be required to empower appropriately qualified, nurses, midwives and therapists to undertake a wider range of clinical tasks

- that information about a patient's care will be copied to the patient

# Medical Diagnosis is Fraught with Errors.

*The single most important issue is that there are very few reliable methods for the diagnosis of a medical condition. Consider the scope for misdiagnosis.*

Every diagnosis is dependent upon the skill of the doctor, the representative nature of the symptoms and samples, limitations of the technology employed, limitations of the test procedure, potential for operator error, and the functionality of the health service [14].

- Each and every set of symptoms varies from person to person [16]. No two people exhibit completely identical sets of symptoms for the same medical condition.

- The biochemical parameters which are used to define health change with age and other factors [17].

- The diagnosis may differ between sexes e.g. a woman's ECG is less likely to be accurate because the woman's arteries are smaller than a man's.

- The patient's symptoms may vary during the day and samples may be affected by external factors such as diet [18,19].

- The cognitive abilities of the GP to diagnose a medical condition varies during the day, with increased work load, with increased age [20, 85, 94]

- Many medical conditions have multiple origins [8] therefore the measurement of one particular biochemical has inherent scope for error e.g. diabetes.

- Medical or diagnostic 'categories' for complex medical conditions lack definition.

- An estimated 30% of medical conditions are of undiagnosable [7] nature.

- Almost all diagnostic procedures are not 100% accurate. Some are significantly inaccurate.

- The ability to determine a medical condition will be dependent upon the sample provided, the test procedure, clinician/operator error, time between sampling and testing, storage conditions for the sample, etc.

- The medical services may not process and report the data correctly [12].

- The accuracy of diagnosis of the best physicians and specialists is not indicative of the diagnostic abilities of the whole medical profession or of every physician.

- The medical statistics may have inherent inaccuracies [20].

On a typical day in the NHS in the UK [13] there are typically 90,000 doctors, 300,000 nurses, 150,000 healthcare assistants, 22,000 midwives, 13,500 radiographers and 15,000 occupational therapists, 7,500 opticians, 10,000 health visitors, 6,500 paramedics, 90,000 porters and ancillary staff, 11,000 pharmacists, 19,000 physiotherapists, 24,000 managers, and 105,000 practice staff in GPs surgeries.

The effect of this expertise is expected to provide a diagnosis which accurately assesses your condition and enables the doctor to provide a course of therapy or medication which will relieve the symptoms of illness and enable you to lead a happy, long and healthy life.

## Diagnosis

There is no gold standard or absolute level against which diagnostic tests can be measured so it is doubtful whether any test is truly accurate.

Most diagnostic tests are based upon the assumption that the level of one chemical, a biomarker, is indicative of the medical condition. In the most simple conditions e.g. of measurement of a bacterial infection, this is a reasonable conclusion; however the body is not a simplistic system but instead is a complex system. Most medical conditions do not observe such simplistic relationships but occur for reasons related to the instability of the physiological systems which regulate the biochemical reactions in the body. Accordingly for tests which are based upon determining the level of a single biomarker in complex medical conditions there is likely to be considerable scope for inaccuracy [23]. As discussed earlier, this can often be confirmed by comparing the results from autopsies and diagnosed cause of death [9].

The accuracy of diagnosis can be influenced by a number of factors e.g.

- some medical technologies have significant limitations yet have not been subject to the same evidence-based requirements which exists for new technologies.

- testing is focussed upon determining the extent of pathology and ignores the mechanisms which maintain the health of the patient.

- there are significant limitations in the detection of a wide range of medical conditions including various cancers e.g. including breast screening [16, 17, 18], cervical cancer, prostate cancer [24, 25], allergies, alzheimer's disease [22], epilepsy [21], migraine [21], multiple sclerosis [15], dyslexia [19], chronic fatigue syndrome [15], diabetes [24], difficulty to differentiate between a bacterial and a viral infection [14], parkinsonism [39,40], myocardial infarction [20], etc.

- using the latest scanning technologies e.g. CAT, PET and MRI scanners, it is often not possible to diagnose a medical condition until the anomaly e.g. a tumour, is large enough to be detected by the scanning technology [24-30]

**There are almost no medical test procedures which are free from misdiagnosis.**

The current generation of biomedical and scanning technologies are only able to identify, qualitatively and quantitatively, the extent of the SYMPTOMS. This is often limited by the extent to which the condition has developed. If the abnormality is not sufficiently large it will not be accurately diagnosed. There is therefore a need for a technology which can detect the pathological processes which are responsible for the development of the condition BEFORE it becomes an abnormality

Based upon the results of the diagnostic tests the patient is prescribed a course of medication i.e. of drugs, therefore each misdiagnosis creates the opportunity for the erroneous prescribing of drugs.

## Therapies/Drugs

The assessment of the efficacy of therapies and drugs is by clinical trials which are comparative procedures. The assessment is therefore subjective, lacking rigour and objectivity.

**'For a study to be truly scientific it must be rigorous, objective, and exact'.**

The objective of a clinical trial is to assess the level of improvement of a new drug or therapy by the process of comparison against other drugs and therapies. These studies are often designed to show the new drug or therapy in the best light [48]. This is achieved by measuring the clinical side-effects and proving the degree of efficacy against a drug which is considered to be less effective for the specific condition. Whilst such practices are the norm in industry – where it is usual to sell the benefits of a product – in the medical context it appears to lack integrity by downplaying the risks associated with the drug or therapy.

It is rare for a drug to be developed which is able to 'cure' the person and to completely remove the medical condition without there being some side-effects. There is therefore no gold standard or absolute level against which the drug can be measured. In fact it may be questionable whether a drug or therapy has been effective in the treatment of a condition for a number of reasons e.g.

(1) the placebo effect in which the patient is considered to benefit from the psychological effect of attending their GP i.e. by the influence of positive psychology [1]

(1) the person's circumstances change and alter the stress-related circumstances which were responsible for the development of their medical condition e.g. the periods of absence from work may compensate for the stress

(2) the person's physiology is naturally able to compensate, adjust and deal with the bacterial or viral causes i.e. their immune system will function effectively and they will recover naturally

The outcome, decided by a regulatory authority, is whether it should be approved and marketed as a drug of choice for a specific medical condition. The final responsibility for the introduction of any new drug or therapy resides with government experts following a process of cost-benefit analysis.

Irrespective, this process leaves significant scope for medical error [10,11]

## Could you imagine.............

Could you imagine attending your medical centre and being asked to undertake a medical test on a computer, following which your GP would invite you into his consultation room and that the GP would advise your complete medical report [32-36]?

Could you imagine that your GP would recommend a course of therapy involving drugs or perhaps the option of other viable non-drug therapies. Such options could include exercise and diet but may also include the new generation of non-drug therapies [32-36].

This is what we envisage to be the future of the medical profession yet the current reality of the medical profession is quite different. The doctor stands accused of being heavily influenced by the drug companies and of being excessively biased towards the use of drugs. For some this accusation is morally repugnant and they prefer to be free of such accusations [49] whilst others just cannot see any alternative to drugs.

# How Can a GP Improve the Services Which They Offer?

*How does a GP, implement the changes to their working practice which bring about the improvements which deliver improved healthcare more efficiently and at lower cost?*

Successive UK governments have variously used the stick and then the carrot to try and achieve the desired levels of improvements but are they able to make the required level of improvements through simple changes to your working practices?

Most GP's are over the age 50 years and have little interest in working harder or introducing radical changes to improve the lives of patients or indeed their own working lives. In the UK in recent years their working hours have declined, not increased. Change is a problem for the over 50's and especially so with radical change. Moreover they do not know what changes can actually make significant improvements. They are human – just the same as the rest of us – and humans make errors! They have ageing eyes and ears and are less able to take in the information from their environment. As they age they become increasingly set in their ways and develop defined and non-negotiable opinions borne out of their life experiences ('been there, seen it, done it!'). They become increasingly prone to make erroneous diagnoses and/or to prescribe the wrong types of medication. They lack the dynamism and idealism which is the hallmark of the younger GP.

The NHS plan identifies the need for better diagnosis, for better working practices and for better therapies but where are the technologies which can make significant change and which can enable the GP to offer a better service?

## The Technology Deficit

The most significant challenge faced by the medical professional is the TECHNOLOGY DEFICIT. In the 5-10 minutes of a consultation the GP does not have the time or capability to make an accurate diagnosis. They are trained as a health professional with the responsibility to manage the health of patients in their practice yet the reality is that they are required to work as a health technician or 'medical clearing house' using techniques and technologies which have distinct limitations.

It is estimated that c30% of medical conditions are of an undiagnosable nature [31] and, that depending upon the journal, a GP's diagnosis can vary from c20% inaccuracy to as much as c80%. There may also be diagnosis of medical conditions which in time will be discredited by future research and technological innovation. It depends upon the terms of reference of the report but nevertheless there is clear indications of the limitations faced by the profession.

Pharmaceutical industry executives [55,] aware of the limitations of conventional biomedicine through their understanding of pharmacogenetics, openly discuss that c90% of drugs are ineffective in c50% of the patients treated. There is therefore, by implication, a significant deficit in the understanding of the origins of many illnesses and the efficacy of many drugs. In addition, researchers have reported that doctors, on occasions, choose drugs in contravention of evidence for their safety and efficacy, and [56] that c21% of drugs are prescribed despite not having been approved for the treatment of the specific ailment.

**If drugs were withdrawn [57]?** When medical professionals withdrew their services in an industrial action this resulted in less deaths. Medical literature records a number of situations where doctors went on strike and that contrary to expectations the death rate had declined during these periods. The investigators attributed the drop in the death rate to fewer drugs and less surgery. The conclusion is therefore that we rely upon drugs to a level which is not in our best interests.

**If antibiotics were not available?** For many of us we would overcome the infection in 7 days and for the rest of us - 1 week! (n.b. antibiotics are essential for those who have a lowered immune system and are vulnerable to such infections.e.g. the elderly).

**If an outbreak of influenza is doing the rounds why does it affects only a small number of us?** This is due to our natural processes of recovery which, simplistically, we refer to as our 'immune system response'.

**Why in near-death incidents do people make remarkable recoveries despite apparently nearing their death as a result of cancers or other very severe illnesses?** There is therefore far more to our health and wellbeing than can be explained by the current biochemical viewpoint.

The GPs faces a challenge which can be regarded as **reactive** and not **preventative** or proactive in its nature. They are focussed upon the treatment of sickness and hence upon alleviating the symptoms of illness and not upon the maintenance of health or upon stimulating the processes which maintain health and stability.

Most drugs merely have the effect of minimizing the symptoms but not of addressing the fundamental causes. The effect is to create a plethora of side-effects and complications which cause yet more need for medical intervention.

Although most GPs recognise the need to deal with the causes of illness their capacity to do something is limited by their limited understanding of the fundamental causes of the illness and of the medical condition. This is so because there is not yet a recognised or accepted theory for the development of illness. Geneticists claim that the role of the genes are the basis of illness but it is also accepted that genetic susceptibility [59] does not lead to illness in most people.

Whereas western researchers consider that stress can worsen an illness, by contrast, Russian researchers [60] have a well accepted theory for the origins of illness which is based upon the homeostatic and allostatic mechanisms, the function of the short and long-term memory to regulate our physiology, the systems-based origins and mechanisms of our mental and physical health, and of the effect of stressors upon these mechanisms i.e. that stress in its various guises is the fundamental cause for most forms of illness.

Complementary health is able to improve to some extent our health and well-being yet it would be folly to consider that complementary health in its current guise can offer significant solutions when compared to the billions of pounds of medical research and subsequently of pharmaceuticals and of medical technologies and therapies. **These complementary therapies are not the solution to the problem due to their inexact nature but they illustrate that there are mechanisms, upon which complementary health approaches are based, which maintain our health.** When these mechanisms are overcome by the stress of our modern-day lives, they result in the development of pathologies, of reduced well-being and of resultant psychological and health effects.

Complementary health has yet to fully address the following issues:

- understanding of the mechanisms associated with specific complementary health therapies
- understanding the side-effects and limitations of a therapy

- having a precise appreciation of the contraindications between therapies

- that no two patients are the same

- the expertise and training which is required for the specific therapy

- the necessity to have a regulatory body to deal with practitioner incompetence and hence for the re-training of practitioners where necessary
- the need to eliminate human error

Complementary therapies are based upon the mechanisms which maintain health, stability and wellbeing which contrasts with the role of the GP and surgeon whose role is to deal with symptoms and pathologies.

With drugs certain side-effects are considered acceptable. It is considered acceptable for patients to experience side-effects e.g. weight-gain, disturbed sleeping patterns, reduced mobility, reduced levels of wellbeing, lowered libido, etc. These are considered to be the acceptable side-effects of medications and of surgical intervention. They are considered to be the price which has to be paid in order to remove the discomforting symptoms associated with the ailment!

Similarly with complementary health there can be side-effects arising from unsuitable therapy e.g.

- of pain arising from poor insertion of acupuncture needles

- of contraindications arising from incompatible therapies e.g. of migraine arising following an aromatherapy massage.
- of digestive discomfort arising from an inappropriate healthfood supplement.

# The Evidence-based Requirement

*What is it actually causes a medical condition? If you are advised that your medical problem is related to the level of a specific biochemical consider why this has occurred. What has caused its overproduction or deficiency?*

To be scientific is to be unsentimental, rational, straight-thinking, correct, rigorous, and exact yet Medicine is a relatively imprecise science. For this reason it is necessary to have a mechanism which proves that new types of diagnostic procedure or therapy are distinct improvements on the existing methods – this is the intended function of clinical trials - yet the application of 'science' [55] lends itself to huge differences of opinion.

Medical decisions are based upon the prevailing level of knowledge and hence of the opinions which medical experts have built over many years. The decisions are not based upon fact but instead upon the subjective processes involved in making decisions.

Some drugs and therapies become the normative treatment of a specific ailment yet advances in knowledge can discredit these drugs and therapies. A literature search quickly reveals how medicine and medical practices have changed through the years [130-132] and how the most horrendous, ill-advised and traumatic medical practices (which poisoned us, separated children from loving families, recommended isolation, removed organs and limbs, made us insane, resulted in the birth of deformed children, accusations of sexual impropriety by parents, etc;) have been discredited and withdrawn.

We are right to question the use of vaccines and drugs and to ask our medical authorities to justify their conclusions and actions.

Until recently (1) atenolol was formerly the recommended standard treatment for high blood pressure until research has resulted in its use being downgraded in 2006; (2) celecoxib has been proven to be unsafe and has been withdrawn despite the clinical data which claimed that the drug was safe for use; (3) cortico-steroid treatment [114] in A&E departments is now being withdrawn because medical statistics have indicated that this form of medication, which suppresses the patient's immune system, causes more harm than good; (4) after over 50 years as the recommended approach in cases of heart attack, mouth-to-mouth resuscitation is no longer recommended. Researchers have recognised that it increases the risk of death. Chest compression [262] is now the recommended approach.

If a system has not yet established standards against which products can be compared it cannot be considered to be scientific [81]. Medicine is comparative, empirical and subjective whereas true science is associated with objectivity and precision. The basis of a clinical trial is to get the drug or product approved or recommended for use and hence to gain revenues for the developing organization – not to prove that it is safe for use which is ultimately the role of government.

293

Claude Bernard [83] describes what makes a theory valid. On cause and effect he states:

**'The scientist tries to determine the relation of cause and effect. This is true for all sciences: the goal is to connect a natural phenomenon with its immediate cause. We formulate hypotheses elucidating, as we see it, the relation of cause and effect for particular phenomena. We test the hypotheses. And when a hypotheses is proved it is a scientific theory. Before that we have only groping and empiricism.'**

Whilst 'to be scientific is to be unsentimental, rational, straight-thinking, correct, rigorous, exact'; medicine, by comparison, can only be considered to be 'as-good-as-is-reasonably-practicable science'[127] which leaves the system of clinical trials wide open to abuse, manipulation, and bias.

In order to be consistent with the principles of a clinical trial, if a study is to be free of allegations of bias it should be free from any pressures and hence can make an unbiased and rigorous scientific report. Moreover the study should, if possible, be compared with a gold standard and not by the subjective comparison of one poorly effective drug or therapy with another. It should also take into account the variability of the patient population [68] and whether the drug has been assessed for this patient grouping [104].

In breast screening, articles support the continued use of breast screening [63] yet up to 10% of women screened could be liable to misdiagnosis - which could lead to an unnecessary mastectomy. Articles focus upon the fact that an estimated 1-3% of women develop breast cancer as a result of the x-ray test procedure. The more concerned researchers comment that 'Breast screening seems driven by belief rather than evidence' [64].

Consider the example of a lady, in her early-mid 50's who went on holiday several weeks following a routine breast x-ray which indicated that she was completely free of cancer. During her holiday a lump formed in her breast with considerable 'discomfort'. Upon her return i.e. within weeks of having her first x-ray, she was re-diagnosed with a virulent form of breast cancer which required her to have one of her breasts removed. It is pertinent to consider how such a condition could have arisen in such a short period of time.

This causes justifiable concern to the extent that some consider that the treatment may be worse than the cure! This is supported by articles in the medical press [69-74] which indicate that "screening leads to more aggressive treatment, increasing the number of mastectomies by about 20% and the number of mastectomies and tumourectomies by about 30%". Such scientific conclusions appear often to be ignored by governments and by the medical industry.

These issues become the subject of further reviews which consider a number of factors including, but not limited to:

- the established views of the medical community,

- the views and reputation of scientific experts,

- the accuracy, impartiality and unbiased reporting of medical results [65-67]

- possible misrepresentation of scientific findings by pharmaceutical, food and beverage companies [48,80].

- representation by those with 'vested interests',

- and political machinations which are designed to evade the issue.

The extent of the problem of misdiagnosis and of the paucity of evidence has not yet been fully explored by the press and the legal profession. Perhaps it needs the legal profession, who represent those who's lives have been affected, to bring pressure on the healthcare profession and government to ensure that change is implemented and to ensure that the industry responds to its legal responsibilities to apply due care and attention when managing the health of the patient.

Whilst it is claimed that breast screening saves 1,400 lives per year at a cost of £3,000 per patient it is also quite conceivable that some of these cases may actually have been caused by the screening procedure.

Take the case of the world-leading pediatrician [75-77, 79] who gave his opinions whilst studiously ignoring the genetic history of families or to take into account the opinion of other experts researching SIDS syndrome (Sudden Infant Death Syndrome) or that future research could lead new insights e.g. that the failure to regulate body temperature may be responsible for SIDS [245].

## People are human – and humans make mistakes.

Clinical Trials are required because of the risk of harm to the patient of the proposed drug or therapy however it takes little account of the fundamental mode of action of the drug or therapy i.e.

**(1) does it focus upon the pathology of the medical condition, or**

**(2) does it focus upon boosting the body's natural processes of compensation?**

This is an issue which has caused great debate between those in complementary health who believe that the clinical trial procedure is not appropriate for the assessment of a complementary type therapy. Drugs are assessed upon their ability to inhibit the progress of pathology whereas complementary health functions by a number of mechanisms ref (1) and (2) above.

The fact that a viewpoint cannot be explained by a currently accepted theory does not mean that it is wrong, in the same way that the conclusions, derived from a clinical trial, are not necessarily right [104].

**'History advises us to be wary of over-relying upon the authoritarian conclusions of our peers when considering judgements on new theories and technologies'.**

# How Likely is a doctor to Make a Mistake?

*We rely upon our doctors to an extraordinary extent. We have implicit trust in their abilities and their advice but is this trust justified?*

Accidental death by the medical profession is considered to be the 3rd (depending upon age) largest cause of death in the US [82]. There are many articles which we can use to illustrate the seriousness of the problem [163-220] e.g.

A survey [68] of 114 American hospital doctors concluded that

- one third had made serious diagnostic errors,

- one third had made mistakes in prescribing,

- one fifth had made mistaken evaluations,

- 11 per cent procedural complications - in 90 per cent of these cases, patients had suffered serious adverse outcomes, of which one third had died.
- 50% of doctors discussed the mistake with their superiors

- 25% of doctors had told the patients themselves or their families.

Attitudes to mistakes and the recognition of the need to make change to working practices appear to depend upon the nature of the institution [85]. Whilst there is recognition of the need to accept responsibility and to discuss mistakes there is also the recognition that this could lead to further repercussions which would have practical and legal implications. The situation is sufficiently serious that second medical opinions [86] have seriously been considered. To illustrate the scale of the problem a 1999 study of cancer patients nationwide by researchers at Johns Hopkins University found that 1.4% of pathology results, 30,000 patients in the US, were misdiagnosed annually and that 20% of the recommended treatments for cancer patients were not appropriate.

Whereas cancer detection was considered to be 98.6% accurate it was also clear that the detection of skin cancer was 97.1% and that the detection of cancers in the reproductive tract was 94.9%. The latest statistics for cervical cancer screening indicates the change from the PAP smear test to the Liquid-based cytology test has increased the rate of detection from 91.0-92.8% which still leaves a significant margin of error.

The accuracy of statistics is also an issue which should be considered and placed in perspective. There are few ways which can be used to assess the accuracy of any diagnostic technology. Perhaps the only 'near gold standard' is to compare the results of death with the results of autopsy [247-251] which illustrates how the prevailing statistics suffer from inherent limitations. Moreover, even the autopsy results have inherent limitations [252].

In recent surveys [54,87] over 40 per cent of people and 35 per cent of doctors said they or their families had been the victim of medical errors.

In the UK it has been estimated that a third of people have experienced some surgical, medication or diagnostic error in the National Health Service over the past five years and that most of the errors involved a misdiagnosis. Of the errors reported it is estimated that c20 % were medication errors and c15 % were errors that occurred during surgery.

Up to 1,490,000- 2,690,000 people are being harmed by medical mishaps every year [88-90] which represents 3-4.5 per cent of the entire population. In the USA, where medicine is considered to be even more aggressive, the problem could be affecting up to 13,450,000 people every year.

More than 30,000 people per year in the UK are killed by doctors, consultants, surgeons, etc; and in the US an estimated 225,000 people die each year due to iatrogenic causes i.e. due to medical cause.

More recently [93] researchers have shown that doctors struggle to calculate drug doses when required to administer adrenaline, lidocaine, atropine, etc. Furthermore a doctors' ability to diagnose is affected by their health which affects their colour vision [94]

There is a massive under-reporting of mistakes [65-67], [88-90] because of fear of litigation. Moreover government officials do not know how many of the reported blunders end in the death of the patient.

"Only 1 in 4 hospitals 'owns up' to the patient when something goes wrong [91]; the rest blame it on the disease itself, while just 1 in 25 drug reactions is ever reported. As it is, 1 in 10 people admitted to a hospital in Britain every year will suffer a mishap or accident that will harm him", said Edward Leigh MP, chairman of the Commons Public Accounts committee.

'If you are in hospital the risk of dying from a medical error is one in 300 [92] whereas by comparison the risk of dying in an air crash is estimated to be one in c10Million'.

This places the doctor at risk of being considered guilty of negligence with considerable legal consequences. By comparison, any driver (commercial or private) who makes a poor decision can be held guilty of driving without due care and attention, causing grievous bodily harm, manslaughter, etc? Consider how a hospital doctor, often working long shifts (when their cognitive abilities including their powers of observation, memory, concentration, visual perception, etc, are undoubtedly affected), is required to make important decisions concerning the treatment of a patient [93,94].

The doctor and/or medical professional is therefore being treated as a special case by virtue of their profession. There is the rule of law for the general public and a special dispensation for the doctor. Medical accidents are not investigated by the Health &

Safety Inspectorate but instead are investigated internally by the hospital [13] and ultimately by the General Medical Council which is run by doctors. One doctor quoted in an article in the New York Times that *"doctors don't go down with their planes."*

A study of people who reportedly had chronic fatigue syndrome concluded that only around 30% of them actually had the condition yet most of them were unemployed and were considered to be depressed. The fact that they failed to meet a defined criteria does not alter the fact that many of them were suffering physiological and not solely psychological ailments [97-99]

If you have prostate cancer or breast cancer, the conventional viewpoint is that cancer is able to be treated the earlier it can be detected, yet your doctor has only a very limited capability to detect these conditions. For the local GP the diagnosis of prostate cancer takes around 148 days to diagnose and breast cancer is diagnosed in around 55 days, yet for those who go to their local hospital it is possible to get a rapid diagnosis because the hospital is able to screen the patient almost immediately [95,96].

Perhaps of greater concern is the access to chemotherapy following surgical removal of a tumour. Surgery is known to enhance the spread of cancer following surgical removal of a cancerous tumour therefore prompt access to chemotherapy and/or radiotherapy is necessary to ensure that the cancer does not re-occur or spread. This is however an issue related to the availability of resources rather than of medical competence nevertheless there is clear need to consider whether surgical removal of a cancer should only be made if there is the prompt availability of the necessary secondary therapies.

The British Medical Association [100] considers that regular medical check-ups including scanning technologies may actually be placing ourselves at an unnecessary level of risk. The x-ray tests which are used to diagnose cancer are considered to increase the risk of developing cancer by one in every 2000 people scanned and also give false positive results.

The standard test for multiple sclerosis is now considered to be the MRI scan which is intended to detect the presence of brain lesions [101] which are associated with this condition yet the presence of brain lesions does not necessarily indicate multiple sclerosis! In fact the test is providing a very large number of false positives thereby illustrating that it is not a very good test.

In the book [102,103]    'A Dose of Sanity' Dr. Sydney Walker provides numerous examples of medical cases that were misdiagnosed as psychiatric problems.

# Do Biomedical Researchers Understand the Influence of Age upon the Effectiveness of a Drug?

*Is the drug safe for use in children or the elderly? Only recently have pharmaceutical companies been obliged to research the effect of drugs upon these patient groups.*

The amount of drug use increases with age. It's been estimated that the average person aged over 70 takes around eight prescription drugs at any one time to treat a variety of conditions associated with ageing yet drug companies rarely test the safety of their drugs on the elderly, and nobody tests for the chemical cocktail from multiple prescribing on anyone.

An estimated 48 million elderly people around the world by 2030, will be affected by diabetes yet the cut-off age for participants in clinical trials of drug treatments is 53 years of age? [104]. In recognition of this fact, drug companies seek to recruit physically fit young adults, often medical students, who are under 25 years of age. This study [104] has discovered that fewer than five per cent of medical studies feature older people.

Some drugs increase the risk of an adverse reaction, and even death, in a vulnerable group and appear in the **'Beers list'** [62], which is a guide to doctors of drugs that are considered to be dangerous when prescribed to an elderly, frail patient.

Furthermore, most drugs are not adequately tested for use in children [246]. A doctor can prescribe the off-label use of a drug to treat a condition for which it was not originally approved. In many cases the adult dose is not adjusted to take into account the child's characteristics.

# Are Drugs Able to Treat the Medical Condition?

*If you are prescribed a drug therapy how likely is it to be able to relieve you of your medical symptoms?*

Leading medical researchers [110,111] are aware that fewer than half of patients prescribed drugs (excluding antibiotics) derive any benefit from them. In medical industry presentations, designed to illustrate the benefit of the pharmacogenetic approach which seeks to design the person-specific drug, researchers have highlighted how '90% of drugs are ineffective in 50% of the population'. This illustrates the efficacy of different classes of drugs work (see below).

## Response rates

Therapeutic area: drug efficacy rate in per cent

|   |   |   |
|---|---|---|
| * | Alzheimer's: | 30 |
| * | Analgesics (Cox-2): | 80 |
| * | Asthma: | 60 |
| * | Cardiac arrythmias: | 60 |
| * | Depression (SSRI): | 62 |
| * | Diabetes: | 57 |
| * | Hepatitis C (HCV): | 47 |
| * | Incontinence: | 40 |
| * | Migraine (acute): | 52 |
| * | Migraine (prophylaxis): | 50 |
| * | Oncology: | 25 |
| * | Rheumatoid arthritis: | 50 |
| * | Schizophrenia: | 60 |

Of around medical 2500 treatments [112] reviewed **15% are rated as beneficial, 22% likely to be beneficial**, 7% as trade off between benefits and harms, 5% unlikely to be beneficial, 4% likely to be ineffective or harmful, and 47%, the largest proportion, as unknown effectiveness.

A study prepared in 2004 [268] revealed that patients who have undertaken chemotherapy in the treatment of cancer increased their 5-year survival rate by less than 2.5 per cent .

## Does the Medical Condition Need to be Treated by a Drug-based Intervention?

*Consider whether a medical condition could be better cured by a regime involving rest and recreation than by drugs or a medical intervention.*

The emphasis upon rest and recreation varies throughout the world. In Germany and Russia, there is a broader acceptance of the value of rest, recovery and rehabilitation which can be provided by health sanatoria and spas. The benefits are recognised by government and costs are supported by government or can be offset against tax. In South East Asia and China there is huge emphasis upon the benefits of massage i.e. feet massage, back massage, etc. **There is a substantial body of evidence that drugs are not necessarily required to improve the health of a patient.**

For those with type 2 **diabetes** a study [106] has illustrated how exercise and good diet is able to make a significant improvement in the quality of life of diabetics, many of whom were obese and hypertensive; and for those with prostate cancer [107, 108] the adoption of a vegetarian diet is also able to bring considerable relief. It is often recognised that **prostate cancer** is the only human cancer that is curable and often does not need to be cured [260,261].

Tennis elbow [109] recovers more quickly alone than with steroid injections. In fact corticosteroid injections appear to be less effective than the resting and recovery approach and appeared to inhibit the rate of recovery.

Around 20% elderly patients in Europe are being prescribed an 'inappropriate' medicinal drug and in the USA c 40% of elderly residents in care homes are being given the wrong drug . The drugs increase the risk of an adverse reaction, and even death, in a vulnerable group. Some of the drugs being prescribed appear on what is known as the 'Beers list' [62], which is a guide to doctors of drugs that are considered dangerous in an elderly, frail patient.

Inappropriate prescribing also adds pressure to a health service, and extra beds have to be found for patients suffering an adverse reaction. Once in hospital, the patient then runs a 20 per cent risk of a further 'inappropriate' drug being prescribed. A research team from Charles University in Prague revealed that inappropriate prescribing varies enormously from country to country in Europe and is typically 12-25%.

In some cases leading researchers [113] are aware that untested therapies, often the standard and approved therapy, may actually be dangerous e.g. the use of corticosteroids for head injury in hospitals was stopped only after a study [114] in 2004 discovered that they significantly increased the risk of death.

## "Don't just do something, stand there!"

Other commonly used but ineffective therapies [120-121] includes e.g. mentoring to address anti-social behaviour in childhood; adenoidectomy versus chemoprophylaxis and placebo for recurrent acute otitis media in children aged under 2 years; the effect of hands-and-knees posturing on the incidence of occiput posterior position at birth; effects of low-dose ramipril on cardiovascular and renal outcomes in patients with type 2 diabetes and elevated excretion of urinary albumin; treating nausea and vomiting during pregnancy.

Ineffectiveness is hard to prove and accept [115]. In each case the type of evidence, its quality, and the potential benefits and harms might convince us that an intervention does more good than harm. If the patient perceives that it has a benefit it seems likely that it will provide comfort, reassurance and will benefit them i.e. it will provide a beneficial placebo effect. If people want to believe there is an effect it can be very hard to persuade them that any effect is too small to be important. An example text extracted from a school textbook illustrates the problem when discussing the dilemma of industries or official organisations trying to convince the public that some thing poses no risk:

**"It is very hard to persuade people that a factor has no effect. This involves *proving a negative.*"**

Others [122] argue that trials done by pharmaceutical companies to obtain drug licences should include sufficient data about the harm and ineffectiveness of the drug rather than focusing upon how it is better than a competitor drug. Some of the most damning evidence concerns the diagnosis and treatment of diabetes [123, 124]. Recent research has concluded that the analysis of available evidence and statistics indicates that improved knowledge about disease does not translate into improved blood sugar control, cholesterol levels, weight management or mortality rates. Despite the available evidence doctors are often left uncertain about the right choice of treatment. To illustrate their dilemma we quote US defense secretary Donald Rumsfeld [125, 126] when dealing with another the highly complex situation (the Iraq insurgency):

*"Reports that say that something hasn't happened are always interesting to me, because as we know, there are known knowns; there are things we know we know. We also know there are known unknowns; that is to say we know there are some things we do not know. But there are also unknown unknowns—the ones we don't know we don't know."*

To make matters worse, this situation is further compounded by the fact that we have a "poverty of medical evidence" in so much of medicine, [127]:

*"only about 15% of medical interventions are supported by solid scientific evidence" – because only 1% of the articles in medical journals are scientifically sound and because many treatments have never been assessed.*

The human organism has an amazing propensity to recover from injury and illness yet there are few if any therapies or drugs which are designed to enhance the body's natural compensatory abilities.

# How safe is the Medical Technology/Therapy?

*We assume that medical technologies must be safe. Are we right to do so?*

The negative effects of electromagnetic radiation [128] upon the human body by electromagnetic radiation is eminently described by Robert Becker. In particular:

## The dangers of medical care: X-rays

X-rays are used to detect physiological disorders such as breakages (of bones) and of physical abnormalities such as cancerous tumours. However, according to reports published in the medical press, an estimated 1-3% of women scanned for breast tumours appear to get cancer as a result of the x-ray procedure [253], or suffer massive damage as a result of operations following misdiagnosis.

X-rays are reported to cause 700 cases of cancer every year in the UK, around 5,700 in the USA, and a total of 18,500 cases overall in 15 developed countries. Cancer risks per cumulative x-ray exposure range from just 0.6 per cent in Poland and the UK, and up to 3.2 per cent in Japan. The findings, made by researchers at Oxford University conclude that radiation is a known carcinogen, and medical x-rays represent 14 per cent of total radiation exposure.

Interestingly, a study [254,255] comments that there is insufficient statistical data to justify the continued use of breast screening.

## The dangers of medical care: CT scans

Patients undergoing a full-body CT (computed tomography) scan are being exposed to a radiation level equivalent to that from the atomic bombs dropped on Hiroshima and Nagasaki. As a result up to one in 400 patients who are scanned will go on to develop a fatal cancer, and those unfortunate enough to have an annual CT scan increase their chances of a fatal cancer by between 4 and 16 times [256-258]. Specific patient groups may be as much as 50% at risk of developing cancer [259].

# How Necessary is the Surgery?

*Consider how necessary is the surgery and what are the outcomes? What are the risks, what could go wrong and what effects could arise following the operation? Will the patient have a better quality of life following the operation.*

There are question marks surrounding the need for a number of surgical procedures. Consider the following examples:

- In removal of the gall bladder [133] the bile duct may be damaged with consequent need for further remedial operations.

- Half of all hysterectomies are due to heavy menstrual bleeding [84, 134]. This may ultimately require the patient to have a hysterectomy yet when researchers sent information about non-surgical options to a number of clinics the number of patients requiring surgery ceased!

- Giving an elderly woman a hip replacement operation may seem a viable option in efforts to improve their quality of life but how many are able to resume a normal life and benefit from the operation? They may not have the bone structure to enable the operation to be a success, the muscle structure to recover the ability to walk, the healing capability to commence the rehabilitation process. They may be so fraught with the stress of the operation that their natural healing abilities are impaired or are damaged by the loss of their normal routines and activities that they lose their mental faculties. They may be left in pain for the rest of their days.

- Operations such as lumbar spinal fusion are considered successful according to the ability to achieve the surgical objective however the patient's viewpoint and consideration of success, hoping for recovery of mobility, is likely to be significantly different.

- Hernia i.e. the inguinal hernia [135], which, in its mild form, can have absolutely no symptoms at all. In a study group only 17% of those who did not have surgery immediately following the diagnosis subsequently required surgery i.e. 83% of patients who would have underwent surgery did not subsequently need surgery!

- Patients who have been advised to have their gall bladder removed to alleviate migraine occurrences. The outcome of their surgery was that they still have their migraine attacks but no longer have their gall bladder.

- Patients who have been identified with borderline cervical smears may be required to have the surgical removal of untypical cells. It is considered a minor surgical procedure yet may condemn women to a lifetime of irregular periods with subsequent effects upon their 'sex life'.

Is it worth giving the drug or carrying out the surgery? What are the long-term implications upon the health, wellbeing and mobility of the patient? Indeed is there a satisfactory mechanism to make such an assessment?

## 5.2      Virtual Scanning - Fullfilling the Need

## What Value does Virtual Scanning Have to the Medical Profession and the General Medical Practitioner (GP)?

Virtual Scanning is based upon the ability to relate cognition to health. Whereas current research refers to this relationship in the most subjective terms [163-220], Virtual Scanning involves the mathematical modeling of the test results to give a completely objective assessment of the health of the patient. It presents a medical practitioner with an astonishing amount of data in a very short period of time.

For those able to complete the short computer-based test, which can be conducted by a medical auxiliary prior to the consultation, it enables the GP to make a rapid and precise assessment of the physical and mental health of the patient and to understand the fundamental origins of their complaint. This reduces the need for further testing, the need for repeat consultations, the scope for misdiagnoses and any erroneous prescribing of drugs.

Armed with this information the GP can decide whether the patient should be referred to the hospital for further investigations or treatment, and/or which is the most appropriate form of therapy. It enables the GP to give a better diagnosis, in less time, at less cost and to be significantly more efficient.

## The ability to prediagnose………

Virtual Scanning enables the doctor to monitor the development of medical conditions from the pre-symptomatic level, **before** they have subsequently been manifest as a symptom and pathology e.g.

1.      a c60 y.o.lady with duodenal complaint. Following several consultations with her GP which failed to diagnose a problem this lady undertook a Virtual Scanning consultation and was advised of the severity of her duodenal condition, being advised that it was almost certainly an ulcerative problem, and that she should request a further consultation with her GP. A further consultation resulted in the GP confirming his previous diagnosis i.e. that there was nothing the matter, and that she should cease wasting his time.

   Within one week of this consultation the lady was admitted to hospital with a perforated duodenal ulcer and of the associated symptoms. The lady spent over 1 week in hospital receiving medication and recovering from the ordeal.

2.      a c40 y.o. lady was diagnosed with **Rhinitis** and commented that she did not have a cold or nasal congestion yet within one week advised that she had subsequently developed a cold with associated symptoms including nasal congestion.

3.      an 84 y.o.man was tested and found to have **type 2 diabetes**. Two years later the diagnosis of diabetes was confirmed by his GP.

4.      a 48 y.o.male. His psychoemotional profile gave extraordinarily high readings of 'Anger' and 'Injustice'. His health profile highlighted a number of medical conditions in various organs including indications consistent with 'degenerative processes' in the prostate gland i.e. indicative of the pre-indications of prostate cancer.

Following two courses of therapy this patient's medical condition was clearly improving. Whereas he had to be driven to the first consultation by his wife – due to his ill health - by the third consultation he was sufficiently well to drive alone to the consultation. After discontinuing the therapy his health declined and 6 –12 months later was diagnosed with prostate cancer .

5.      A 61 y.o.lady was diagnosed with **polyps in her uterus** which was subsequently confirmed two years later and was noticed following an episode of bleeding.

## The ability to diagnose long-standing illnesses………

6.      In response to the request by a financial consultant to justify the claims that Virtual Scanning could diagnose a medical condition we undertook a brief demonstration in a man of c60 years. Within minutes and a brief evaluation of the test results Virtual Scanning indicated that the patient had experienced over many years, and probably since childhood, been predisposed to bouts of pneumonia. The demonstration was brief, concise and successful.

## The ability to track the development and regression of a medical condition…………

Successive tests illustrate the improved health and wellbeing of the patient which are noted as

- Reduced indications in the psychological profile e.g. of anger

- Reduced indications of pathology

- Improved levels of compensation

## Where does Virtual Scanning fit into the Medical Spectrum?

The medical spectrum comprises a spectrum of technologies and medical expertise which can be summarized as follows:

**Figure 1**

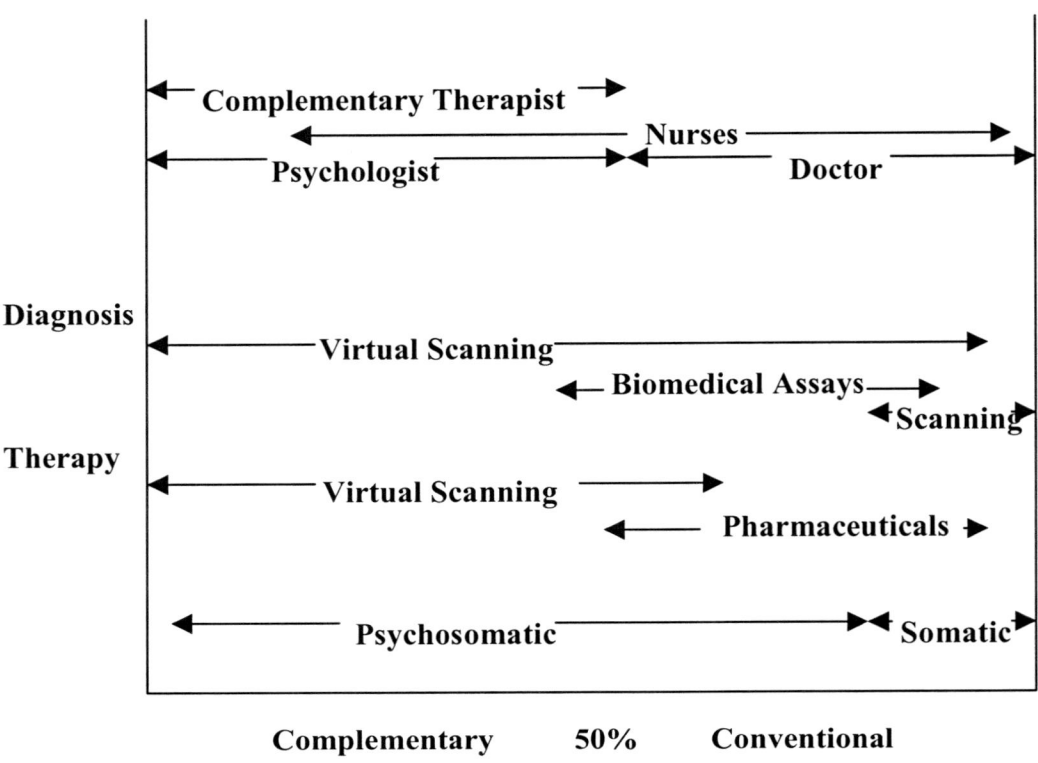

**Healthcare Spectrum**

The above diagram is not intended to make conclusions about efficacy but instead illustrates how the expertise is spread. The conventional healthcare model is served by the doctor and psychologist who are ably supported by nurses. It is the nurse who is required to provide regular contact and comfort to the patient. Unsurprisingly many nurses are trained in complementary medical techniques. As complementary medicine is based upon enhancing wellbeing it has conceivably greater applicability to the health of a patient by contrast to the role of the doctor who is involved in the diagnosis and treatment of pathology. The role of the nurse in the healing process should not be under-estimated.

Diagnosis of a medical condition is provided mainly by the patient and doctor. The technologies employed to diagnose pathology are provided by histology and radiography i.e. assays of fluids, tissues and scanning technologies which can locate a physiological anomaly such as a tumour. Virtual Scanning is able to provide a broad-spectrum diagnosis which would simplify the process of diagnosis. It would make the diagnosis quicker, and more precise – requiring sophisticated medical technologies to confirm the diagnosis and perhaps to locate the precise sight of the anomaly – and it would dramatically reduce the cost of testing. Expensive diagnostic techniques would be required to verify results instead of screening – for positives **and negatives**.

As a therapy Virtual Scanning offers a non-drug alternative for the treatment of disorders which have psychosomatic origins. It is not able to treat conditions which are genetic or which are due to physical injury and where the condition is clearly of an irreversible nature.

# The Scope of the Technology

Virtual Scanning is a cognitive technology therefore it can only be used by those who are able to complete the test which restricts the test to those of typically 7 years and above, and those who have not yet progressed to an age or stage of life where their cognitive abilities have been lost..

It provides a huge amount of information about the health of the patient and enables us to have information about health from the pre-symptomatic level. It facilitates the identification of factors which have caused the condition rather than the pathologies which are the symptomatic consequences. Accordingly it is of value as an inexpensive screening technology (similar to the auto-diagnosis of a vehicle) which augments the wide range of sophisticated and expensive medical diagnostic technologies which are used to determine the extent of pathological development e.g. histological, biochemical, and scanning technologies.

**Virtual Scanning should be of interest to those who wish to improve the ability to diagnose and treat illness.**

**This would include:**

- the **medical practitioner** who wishes to have more information available in order to make a more thorough and accurate medical diagnosis

- **insurance companies** who wish to reduce the costs associated with misdiagnosis, the damaging side-effects of therapies which increasingly lead to compensation claims by patients, and the costs due to illness and absenteeism.

- the **patient** who wants to be diagnosed and treated with much less risk and greater effectiveness

- **governments** who wish to reduce the cost of providing healthcare and who wish to provide a better service.

- **health and safety** organizations who wish to improve their ability to monitor the health of patients and hence to minimize the risk of industrial incidents, and accidents in our everyday lives, which cause so much misery

- the **patient** who seeks to have a precise report of their medical condition which is of course their 'human rights'.

- the Medicines and Healthcare Products Regulatory Agency in the UK and other legal bodies which are charged with the responsibility for **patient safety**

- **recruitment** companies which can use the information to make better selection of employees

- **employers** which can also use the information to improve the productivity of working teams and to reduce industrial incidents

- **education**al organisations which are involved in the assessment and treating of learning disorders

- organizations which deal with **delinquency** where an estimated 80-90% of offenders have learning disabilities

- and in the **family** where it can be possible to determine and treat the reasons for dischord between family members.

Virtual Scanning Therapy is not a replacement for drugs nor is it ever likely to be. Drugs are clearly and indisputably associated with the treatment of medical conditions and in particular the treatment of the symptoms of pathology/illness and hence are clearly associated with the ability to prolong life. It is inconceivable that modern life could be conducted without the support of the various categories of drugs which are necessary in life and death situations.

The value of Virtual Scanning therapy is in quality of life situations where subtle and often not-so-subtle psychosomatic influences destabilise the function of our physiological systems and hence are responsible for the symptoms of illness which are so damaging for our quality of life and for our feelings of wellbeing.

Based upon the data which is available from Russian researchers, Virtual Scanning appears to be able to:

- improve quantity and precision of data which is available to diagnose a medical condition
- monitor the progress of any medical therapy

- re-establish the stability and/or function of the body's physiological systems and organs
- augment the function of drugs which have the effect of severely destabilizing the body's physiological systems e.g. in chemotherapy
- reduce the amounts of drugs required e.g. of insulin required by type 1 diabetics

- improve and accelerate the body's ability to recover from illness or injury

- re-establish mental health, cognition, stability and wellbeing

Although Virtual Scanning has a significant effect in the treatment of many medical conditions the use of drugs is the established way. The market is structured around the status quo provided by the healthcare industry which is oriented around the need for pharmaceutical medications which satisfies society's demands the quick fix which only drugs appear able to provide.

## Virtual Scanning is the ideal option for those:

- who, through strongly held convictions, no longer wish to use drugs,

- for whom drugs are less effective (i.e. for those who are typically over 50 yo),

- with a medical condition which cannot be accurately diagnosed or treated using conventional means,
- who do not wish to be affected by drug side-effects.

# Example

1.      A lady of mid 40's with **trigeminal neuralgia** advised that she had travelled widely seeking a solution for her ailment. She had spent thousands of pounds seeking a cure and advised that she often consumed a bottle of wine in the evening in efforts to relieve the pain.

   Whilst Virtual Scanning did not completely remove the ailment it did however reduce the extent of the discomfiture to the extent that the lady considered it manageable. She wrote to her local pain clinic describing the improvement to her health

2.      A lady of c 60 years sought a remedy for the **stress** of dealing with her ailing, elderly husband.

   After one month of Virtual Scanning therapy she commented that her feelings of wellbeing could only be described by the word 'sparkling' and that she had not felt so well for many years. Her GP commented that he was surprised that she was in such good health despite the stress of her personal circumstances

3.      A lady of c62 years (Chapter 4, case studies from UK, no2) was relieved of **migraine**s by Virtual Scanning therapy. She comments in a letter:

   "Of course the people closest to me, my family, have seen the most dramatic change in my health. They have commented on the fact that I am far more relaxed and calmer. I am less likely to let situations upset me. I have become far more confident and have a more positive attitude to life in general".

3.      a lady, mid-50's had decided to avoid surgery because she did not want to risk becoming injured, damaged or invalided as a result of the surgery to treat the **sarcoma** affecting the lymph nodes on her neck; and was looking for a non-drug alternative. She was extremely emotional. Her husband, whom she had asked for divorce, was struggling to cope with the stress.

   Virtual Scanning was used to treat them both. She was at that time trying some other therapies and had a very bad experience with some people who treated her with some form of oxygen therapy. Her face was in lumps, bumps, discoloured – she looked terrible and felt very ill. Virtual Scanning Therapy over a six month period steadily improved her health. Her medical report, obtained from her oncologist, reveals that she is now completely free from any detected biomedical indications of cancer. The CAT scans do not detect the presence of any tumours although she continues to have swollen lymph glands. Nevertheless he insists that there is the possibility that she has cancer and he wants her to have surgery.

Her relationship with her husband is greatly improved. Their psychological 'ratio of success' has recovered from a dismal 40% to 100% which is a normal or slightly above average figure for a well adjusted couple. Whereas before disaster was looming now there is no more discussion of divorce and they are much happier, stable, and planning for the future.

Virtual Scanning has not been the only therapy used. She considers that Virtual Scanning has been responsible for her greatly improved mental/psychological/emotional stability and for much of her improvement. She has been augmenting the therapy with various herbal remedies.

## 5.3    The Placebo Effect

*As discussed in the earlier part of this chapter and in Chapter 3:*

The placebo effect is the sum total of positive psychological effects which stimulate the body's compensatory response to illness. It is therefore able to reduce or eliminate the development of pathology. It is the flow of sensory data or energy.

**Figure 2**

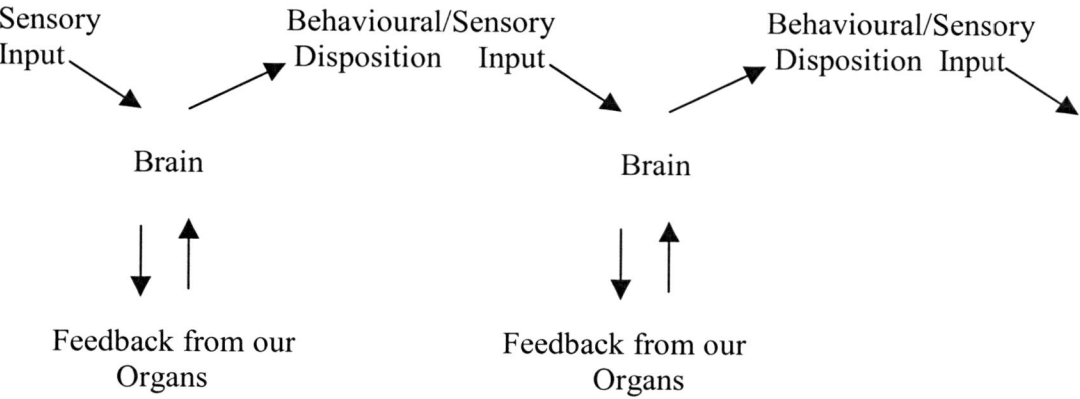

As data is cumulative we can assess the interaction between people or effects. This is a specific capability of Virtual Scanning and is described in detail in Chapter 2.

The technology's ability to assess the interaction between two or more people illustrates how two people could have a positive re-enforcing effect or whereby one could have a demotivating and de-energising effect on the other.

As we have discussed previously the patient

- attends their health centre and consults their doctor in the expectation that by visiting that they will recover their health;
- listens to their doctor who tells them that they will recover their health if they do as he instructs;
- accepts the doctor's explanation of why they are ill and what will alleviate the symptoms;
- takes the medication/therapy in the belief and expectation that it will alleviate the symptoms;
- makes every effort to recover their health e.g. by isolating themselves, sleeping, keeping warm, reducing stress or removing themselves from the stress influences, exercising and relaxing, etc.

With few exceptions, the medical process is engineered by accident or design to optimise the flow of data which is a part of the healing process. Even the process of attracting patients to take part in clinical trials of new drugs takes advantage of the opportunity to emphasise the benefits of the new drug, of technological innovation, and of raising the patient's expectations.

This is recognised by health psychologists and specialists in other related disciplines such as Neuro-Oncology and PsychoNeuroImmunology who recognise the power of the thought processes to influence the levels of biochemistry and hence of our mental and physical health.

The Positive thought processes which stimulate our immune system improve our health whilst the negative thought processes and stress effects lower the level of immunochemicals thereby damaging our ability to fight infection. This is subsequently manifest through the development of pathologies.

The placebo effect is therefore a reflection of the levels of the positive thought processes and of their ability to influence the levels of our immune system. Placebo is associated with positive psychological effect and of raising the levels of the immune system whilst nocebo is associated with the negative effect associated with stress which would lower the levels of the immune system.

As outlined in earlier chapters Virtual Scanning is based upon recognition of the fact that the human is a complex biofeedback system (figure 2 above) which is regulated by the brain and which involves the exchange of sensory information with our environment. The brain regulates the body's physiological systems and hence the function of the organs; whilst stress affects the autonomic nervous system and the body's stability. There is therefore a mechanism associated with the regulation of the body's stability i.e. homeostasis, and a mechanism associated with the body's instability. The latter is recognised as allostasis which is potentially manifest as pathology. Accordingly consideration of the placebo effect must consider that drugs and placebo operate by two entirely different mechanisms and that each is mutually dependent.

The homeostatic system regulates the body's physiological systems and the function of the organs. This maintains our health. If destabilised pathology develops and affects brain function which in turn affects the stability of the body's physiological systems and organs.

The body is therefore a dynamic system in which the body's stability, and hence our function and behaviour, is continuously increasing and decreasing in response to the wide range of experiences, encounters and stresses which affect all aspects of our function. Any medical condition is therefore in a dynamic process or equilibrium in which it is stable, worsening or improving [264-266].

Such is the nature of medical debate that each discipline puts their own unique slant on the explanation. As a result the flow of what is essentially data becomes lost in scientific gobbledegook and the inevitable academic need for categorisation and sub-categorisation of symptoms involving terms such as 'pseudoplacebo', 'superplacebo', 'placebo' and 'nacebo' [263, 267].

Placebo is a highly complex issue involving elements which we would ascribe to 'nature' and to 'nurture' e.g.

- genetic profile of the person perhaps including blood type, personality type, etc

- the person's current health and mental condition

- environmental effects and psychosocial effects including exposure to stress effects.

These issues can be addressed at different levels of brain function e.g.

- At the conscious level –    by overtly conscious thought processes (beta wave) involving discussion and association with need.

- At a subconscious level –    by influencing the covert and subconscious thought processes (alpha & theta wave)

- At a health level –    by stimulating the processes which regulate our health (delta wave)

Medical conditions can therefore be influenced at different levels of 'consciousness'. They act synergistically (see Chapter 1, figure 1a) and have an effect upon the other levels of consciousness.

- The flow of data at the conscious level (beta wave) affects sub-conscious thought which subsequently affects our health i.e. the approach of psychology, cognitive behavioural therapy, etc.

- The flow of data at the sub-conscious level (alpha and theta wave) affects behaviour but also affects our health e.g. using the power of association of thoughts, hypnotherapy and meditation.

- The flow of data at the basic level (delta wave) affects the underlying levels of sub-conscious and conscious thought.  This could perhaps explain how music can be used to stimulate health by its association with a past event. The memory of the past event would be associated within the brain with the person's health at that time.

There is therefore the basic level of biochemical function upon which consciousness is projected or is manifest ie that the basic biochemical function, regulated by the delta and theta brain waves, are necessary for the more active functions involved in data processing, thought and behaviour. These are implicitly linked to the placebo effect.

There is nothing sinister about the placebo effect. It is merely a reflection of the natural mechanisms which the body uses to maintain stability, health and wellbeing.

The important issue is to recognise the fundamental importance of positive thinking and of how to motivate the person to have a life involving positive thinking, an active lifestyle, good diet, etc; and the avoidance of issues which induce poor mental and physical health.

Virtual Scanning illustrates how the advent of new technology can bring a greater level of understanding to issues such as the placebo effect.

# References:

1. Petr Skrabanek and James McCormick, *Follies and Fallacies in Medicine, p. 13.,* *pub:* Prometheus

2. *Journal of the American Medical Association* 1955, 159, 1602-6

3. *Clin Psychology Rev,* 1993: 375-391

4. *Journal of the American Dental Association* 1976, 92: 755-8

5. http://skepdic.com/placebo.html

6. **http://www.fda.gov/fdac/features/2000/100_heal.html**

7. February 26, 2006, *New York Times*

8. **http://www.wrongdiagnosis.com/intro/common.htm**
   *National Patient Safety Foundation,* phone survey in 1997.

9. http://www.dailymail.co.uk/pages/live/articles/news/news.html?in_article_id=415562&in_page_id=1770#StartComments

10. *British Medical Journal,* March 18,2000

11. http://www.quic.gov/Report/

12. www.pathologyconsult.com

13. Brennan.T.A. Hospital peer review and clinical priveleges actions: to report or not to report. *Journal of the American Medical Association* 1999, 282, 381-2

14. http://apiii.upmc.edu/live2001/Gupta/Anatomic%20Pathology%20Errors%20APIII_Gupta.ppt

15. http://www.acceleratedcure.org:8080/article.pl?sid=06/08/03/1045218&mode=nested

16. Zackrisson et al, *British Medical Journal* 332, pp 499-500, 538-41

17. *British Medical Journal* 2001;323:956, Gotzsche et al

18. Thornton.H, Breast screening seems driven by belief rather than evidence, *British Medical Journal* March 16, 2002; 324(7338): 677 – 677

19. **http://news.bbc.co.uk/1/hi/education/4205932.stm**; comments attributed to Professor Julian Elliot, Durham University; reported in **the Times Educational Supplement** 2nd September 2005

20. **www.quic.gov/report/** In 24% myocardial infarction was not diagnosed clinically, 60% confirmed on autopsy. In 33% heart failure was not diagnosed clinically but only on autopsy, 66% confirmed on autopsy.

21. *Cephalalgia,* Online Early, doi:10.1111/j.1468-2982.2006.01245.x
    The impact of education on the diagnostic accuracy of tension-type headache and migraine: a prospective study, N Karli , M Zarifoglu , S Erer, K Pala & N Akis

22. http://www.wrongdiagnosis.com/news/pet_scans_have_a_91_accuracy_for_alzheimer_s_diagnosis.htm

23. *Journal of the National Cancer Institute*, February 8, 2007, Reports Of Prognostic Tumor Markers Often Inadequate, Kyzas.P.A. et al

24. *Radiology, 1991; 178; 447-451*

25. *British Medical Journal, 1991; 303; 205*

26. *The Lancet 2002; 359; 1643-7*

27. *Am J Roentgen, 1994; 162; 189-194*

28. *Am J Roentgen, 1990; 154; 1229-1232*

29. *J. Magn Res Imaging, 1992; 2; 721-8*

30. *Am J Roentgen, 1990; 154; 1229-1232*

31. comments attributed to Dr David Green, *Civitas*

32. Medical Assessment and Treatment
*Evid. Based Complement. Altern. Med.*, Advance Access published on October 5, 2006; doi: doi:10.1093/ecam/nel060

33. Virtual Scanning, *Journal of Alternative & Complementary Medicine*, Volume 13 no2; Ewing G., Ewing E., Hankey A.

34. Kalpana Joshi, Alex Hankey, and Bhushan Patwardhan
Traditional Phytochemistry: Identification of Drug by 'Taste'
*Evid. Based Complement. Altern. Med.*, Advance Access published on October 5, 2006; doi: doi:10.1093/ecam/nel064

35. Alex Hankey,  Studies of Advanced Stages of Meditation in the Tibetan Buddhist and Vedic Traditions. I: A Comparison of General Changes
*Evid. Based Complement. Altern. Med.*, Advance Access published on July 31, 2006; doi: doi:10.1093/ecam/nel040

36. Alex Hankey, CAM and Post-Traumatic Stress Disorder
*Evid. Based Complement. Altern. Med.*, Advance Access published on July 6, 2006; doi: doi:10.1093/ecam/nel041

37. NHS plan

38. *Pediatrics*, 2006; 118: 34-40;

39. Hughes AJ, Daniel SE, Ben-Shlomo Y , Lees AJ. The accuracy of diagnosis of parkinsonian syndromes in a specialist movement disorder service. *Brain* 2002;125:861-870.

40. Hobson P, Holden A, Meara, *Age and Ageing* 1999, 28, 341-6

41.   *British Journal of General Practitioners*, 2003; 53: 441-5

42.   *http://en.wikipedia.org/wiki/Pharmacogenomics*

43.   http://www.msnbc.msn.com/id/3079362/

44.   *Journal of General Internal Medicine,* Volume 16 Issue 5 Page 325,May 2001

45.   *British Medical Journal*, 2004; 329: 966-8

46.   Hobson P, Holden A, Meara *Age and Ageing* 1999, 28, 341-6

47.   *Seizure,* 2006; 29 September;  NICE states that misdiagnosis rates for epilepsy in the UK are between 20-31 per cent

48.   *Medical Journal of Australia*, 2005, http://www.theage.com.au/news/investigations/drug-companies-manipulating-trials/2006/08/06/1154802756201.html?page=2

49.   http://www.nofreelunch.org/

50.   http://www.wrongdiagnosis.com/d/diabetes/tests.htm

51.   *New England Journal of Medicine*, 2003; 349: 335-42.

52.   *Journal of the American Medical Association*, 2005; 294: 66-70

53.   *The New York Times*, February 26, 2006

54.   *New England Journal of Medicine*, 2002; 347: 1933-40

55.   report attributed to Dr Allen Roses, Duke University, published in the Daily Telegraph.

56.   *Journal of the American Medical Association*, 2005; 293: 1348-58

57.   *British Medical Journal*, 2006; 333: 1041-3; http://www.chebucto.ns.ca/~waterbuf/Profile.html

58.   *Journal of Nutrition*, 2006; 136: 2934-8

59.   comments attributed to Lander.E, MIT

60.   Bekhtereva et al

61.   comments attributable to Dr Chris Parker at the Royal Marsden Hospital

62.   Fick DM, Cooper JW, Wade WE, Waller JL, Maclean JR, Beers MH. Updating the Beers criteria for potentially inappropriate medication use in older adults: results of a US consensus panel of experts. *Arch Intern Med*. 2003;163:2716-2724

63.   *British Medical Journal*, 332, 538-41; *British Medical Journal*, 332, 499-500

64. Thornton.H., Breast screening seems driven by belief rather than evidence *British Medical Journal*, March 16, 2002; 324, (7338): 677 – 677

65. 'Pharmacy-coordinated program...' Gilroy GW et al, *Am J Hops Pharm* 1990 Jun;47(6):1327-33

66. *Am J Hosp Pharm* 1988 May;45(5):1086-9 Kimelblatt BJ et al,

67. 'Under-reporting of AD reactions...' *Br J Clin Pharm* 1997 Feb; 43(2):177-81, Moride Y et al...

68. Harris L. Coulter PhD, author of 'The Controlled Clinical Trial: an Analysis'

69. 'The treatment may be the problem'; M E Godfrey *British Medical Journal*, 27 Oct 2001;

70. *The Lancet* 2001;358:1340-2

71. *British Medical Journal* 2001;323 ( 10 November ) The agonies of evidence

72. *British Medical Journal* 2001;323:1131 ( 10 November ) Office of NHS cancer screening programme misrepresents Nordic work in breast screening row

73. *British Medical Journal* 303, 5 October 1991 "The poverty of medical evidence"

74. Dr Robert Good in :*The Immunoglobin A System*" 1973, pages 514 - 515

75. Emery J. L. Sudden Infant Death: *Modern Medicine* October 1984 pgs 9 - 11 *"Are we asking the right questions?"*

76. Emery J. L. *British Medical Journal* 18 November 1989 volume 299 pg 1240 "Is sudden infant death syndrome a diagnosis? Or is it just a diagnostic dustbin?"

77. Rognum, T., *Acta Paediatr* 85: 401 - 3, 1996. "SIDS or not SIDS? Classification problems of sudden infant death syndrome"

78. comments attributed to Dr Anne Fausto-Sterling: http://www.bcholmes.org/tg/brainsex.html

79. http://www.meactionuk.org.uk/Professor_Sir_Roy_Meadows.htm

80. *Journal of Public Library of Science*, January 9 2007; Ludwig.D, MD, PhD, Lesser.L, MD, Ebbeling.C, PhD, Goozner.M and Wypij.D, PhD.

81. *British Medical Journal*, 2004; 329: 966-8;

82. *Journal of the American Medical Association* July 26,2000, 284, 4, 483-5; *National Vital Statistics Report* (US), Vol. 50, No. 15, September 16, 2002

83. *An Introduction to the Study of Experimental Medicine* (1865), Claude Bernard

84. *British Medical Journal*, 2003; 327: 1243-4

85. *Journal of the American Medical Association*, 24 April 1991

86. Tarkan L  Value of second opinions is underscored in study of biopsies. *New York Times* April 4,2000  D7

87. YouGov.com; *Daily Telegraph*, 11 January 2006

88. Leigh, *British Medical Journal* 2006, 333:59; Parliamentary Public Accounts Committee Report: *A Safer Place for Patients: Learning to Improve Patient Safety*

89. *Journal of the American Medical Association* 2000, 284, 4

90. *N Engl J Med*, 2002; 347: 1933-40, Views of Practicing Physicians and the Public on Medical Errors  *Robert J. Blendon, Sc.D., Catherine M. DesRoches, Dr.P.H., Mollyann Brodie, Ph.D., John M. Benson, M.A., Allison B. Rosen, M.D., M.P.H., Eric Schneider, M.D., M.Sc., Drew E. Altman, Ph.D., Kinga Zapert, Ph.D., Melissa J. Herrmann, M.A., and Annie E. Steffenson, M.P.H.*

91. *Journal of the American Medical Association* 2005;293: 1348-58. Hospital leaders don't like mandatory reporting of medical errors.

92. www.guardian.co.uk/uk_news/story/0,,1941120,00.html

93. *Journal of Clinical Practice* 2007; 61; 189-194

94. *British Journal of General Practitioners*. 1999 June; 49(443): 469–475. Colour vision deficiency in the medical profession, Spalding.J.A, International Colour Vision Society

95. *British Journal of Cancer*, online release at: www.bjcancer.com,doi:10.1038/sj.bjc.6602587;

96. McPherson K, Hemminki E. Synthesising licensing data to assess drug safety. *British Medical Journal* 2004;328: 518-20.

97. Yunus M. 'Fibromyalgia and other functional syndromes', *Journal of Rheumatology* 16(sup 19)69 1989;

98. *New England Journal of Medicine*, 2003, 349: 335-42;

99. *Journal of the American Medical Association*, 2005; 294: 66-70

100. *British Medical Journal*, 2005; 332: 475

101. *British Medical Journal*, 2006; 332: 875-8

102. Walker, Sydney M.D., *"A Dose of Sanity"*, (pub: John Wiley & Sons Inc., 1996.

103. Moir, Anne & David Jessel, *"A Mind to Crime"*, pub: Signet Books, 1995

104. *British Medical Journal*, 2005; 331: 1036-7

105. *New England Journal of Medicine*, 2006; 355: 1991-2002;

106. *British Medical Journal, bmj* updates, 4 February 2006

107. *J.Urol*, 2005; 174:1065-1070; Adoption of a Plant-Based Diet by Patients with Recurrent Prostate Cancer, Nguyen et al;

108. *Integr Cancer Ther.*2006; 5: 214-223

109. *British Medical Journal*, 2006; 333: 939-41

110. comments attributed to Professor Allen Roses, worldwide vice-president of pharmacogenetics, GlaxoSmithKline; Duke University

111. Why do doctors use treatments that do not work? Jenny Doust and Chris Del Mar, *British Medical Journal* 2004 328: 474-475.

112. http://www.clinicalevidence.com/ceweb/about/knowledge.jsp *British Medical Journal of Clinical Evidence*

113. *British Medical Journal* 1999;319: 652-3  Haynes B Can it work? Does it work? Is it worth it? *; The Times*, 7 September 2006

114. comments attributed to Prof Roberts of the London School of Tropical Medicine: presented to the *British Association for the Advancement of Science* in September 2006.

115. comments attributed to Archie Cochrane, *British Medical Journal* 328, 7438, 473

116. Why do doctors use treatments that do not work? Jenny Doust and Chris Del Mar, *British Medical Journal* 2004 328: 474-475.

117. Roberts H, Liabo K, Lucas P, DuBois DL, Sheldon TA. Mentoring to address anti-social behaviour in childhood. *British Medical Journal* 2004;328: 512-4.

118. Koivunen P, Uhari M, Luotonen J, Kristo A, Raski R, Pokka T, Alho OP. Adenoidectomy versus chemoprophylaxis and placebo for recurrent acute otitis media in children aged under 2 years: randomised controlled trial *British Medical Journal* 2004;328: 487-90.

119. Kariminia A, Chamberlain ME, Keogh JM, Shea A. Randomised controlled trial of the effect of hands-and-knees posturing on the incidence of occiput posterior position at birth. *British Medical Journal* 2004;328: 490-3.

120. Marre M, Lievre M, Chatellier G, Mann JFE, Passa P, Menard J. Effects of low-dose ramipril on cardiovascular and renal outcomes in patients with type 2 diabetes and elevated excretion of urinary albumin: a randomised, double-blind, placebo, controlled trial (the DIABHYCAR study). *British Medical Journal* 2004;328: 495-9.

121. Harker N, Montgomery AA, Fahey T. Treating nausea and vomiting during pregnancy: case outcome. *British Medical Journal* 2004;328: 503-6.

122. Pound P, Ebrahim S, Sandercock P, Bracken M, Roberts I. 'Where is the evidence that animal research benefits humans?'*British Medical Journal* 2004; 328: 514-7.

123. *American Journal of Cardiology*, Volume 95, Issue 11 , 1 June 2005, Pages 1290-1294, 'Diabetes-Related Knowledge, Atherosclerotic Risk Factor Control, and Outcomes in Acute Coronary Syndromes', Sánchez .C.D, Newby.L.K, McGuire D.K, Hasselblad .V, Feinglos M.N, Ohman E.M.

124. Duke University Medical Centre, June 2, 2005

125. *Disarmament documentation. Back to disarmament documentation, June 2002. Defense secretary Rumsfeld press conference, June 6. "Secretary of Defense Donald H. Rumsfeld, press conference at NATO headquarters, Brussels, Belgium, June 6, 2002," US Department of Defense transcript.*

126. www.acronym.org.uk/docs/0206/doc04.htm (accessed 20 Feb 2004).

127. David Eddy, Professor of Health Policy and Management 73 at Duke University, North Carolina, *British Medical Journal*

128. Becker.R, Cross Currents, The Perils of Electropollution, http://www.energyfields.org/science/becker.html

129. comments attributed to David Eddy, Professor of Health Policy and Management at Duke University, North Carolina,

130. Dr Robert Good, *The Immunoglobin A System"* 1973, pages 514 - 515

131. Breast screening seems driven by belief rather than evidence *British Medical Journal*, March 16, 2002; 324(7338): 677 – 677

132. *British Medical Journal* 303, 5 October 1991

133. *Journal of the American Medical Association*, 2003; 290: 2168-73

134. *British Medical Journal*, 2003; 327: 1243-4

135. *Journal of the American Medical Association*, 2006; 295: 285-92

136. Craik FIM, Salthouse TA. *Handbook of Aging and Cognition*. Hillsdale, NJ: Erlbaum, 1992.

137. Smith GE, Petersen RC, Parisi JE, et al. Definition, course, and outcome of mild cognitive impairment. *Aging Neuropsychol Cogn* 1996;3:141–7.

138. Brayne C, Gill C, Paykel ES, et al. Cognitive decline in an elderly population—a two wave study of change. *Psychological Study of Medicine* 1995;25:673–83.

139. Youngjohn JR, Larrabee GJ, Crook TH. Discriminating age-associated memory impairment and Alzheimer's disease. *Psychol Assess* 1992;4:54–9.

140. Hänninen T. Age-associated memory impairment: A neuropsychological and epidemiological study. *Neurologian klinikan julkaisusarja* 1996;39

141. *Diagnostic and Statistical Manual of Mental Disorders*, 4th ed: *American Psychiatric Association*, 1994, 684.

142. Levy R. Aging-associated cognitive decline. *Int Psychogeriatr* 1994;6:63–8

143. Rubin EH, Storandt M, Miller JP, et al. A prospective study of cognitive function and onset of dementia in cognitively healthy elders. *Arch Neurol* 1998;55(3):395–401.

144. Bolla KI, Lindgren KN, Bonaccorsy C, Bleecker ML. Memory complaints in older adults: Fact or fiction? *Arch Neurol* 1991;48:61–4.

145. Lezak M. *Neuropsychological Assessment*, 3rd ed. New York: Oxford, 1995.

146. Spreen O, Strauss E. *A Compendium of Neuropsychological Tests: Administration, Norms, and Commentary*. New York: Oxford, 1991.

147. La Rue A. *Aging and Neuropsychological Assessment*. New York: Plenum, 1992.

148. Nussbaum, PD, ed. *Handbook of Neuropsychology and Aging*. New York: Plenum, 1997.

149. Ferris SH, Kluger A. Commentary on age-associated memory impairment, age-related cognitive decline and mild cognitive impairment. *Aging Neuropsychol Cogn* 1996;3:148–53.

150. Rediess S, Caine ED. Aging, cognition, and DSM-IV. *Aging Neuropsychol Cogn* 1996;3:105–17.

151. Solfrizzi V, Panza F, Torres F, et al. High monounsaturated fatty acids intake protects against age-related cognitive decline. *Neurology* 1999;52(8):1563–9.

152. Jarvis MJ. Does caffeine enhance absolute levels of cognitive performance? *Psychopharmacology (Berl)* 1993;110(1–2):45–52.

153. Perrig WJ, Perrig P, Stahelin HB. The relation between antioxidants and memory performance in the old and very old. *J Am Geriatr Soc* 1997;45(6):718–24.

154. Di Carlo A, Baldereschi M, Maggi S, et al. Prevalence and risk factors of age-related cognitive decline: The Italian longitudinal study on aging (ILSA). American Academy of Neurology, 50th Annual Meeting [abstract] P04.103.

155. Kilander L, Nyman H, Boberg M, et al. Hypertension is related to cognitive impairment: a 20-year follow-up of 999 men. *Hypertension* 1998;31(3):780–6.

156. Williams P, Lord SR. Effects of group exercise on cognitive functioning and mood in older women. *Aust N Z J Public Health* 1997;21(1):45–52.

157. Emery CF, Huppert FA, Schein RL. Relationships among age, exercise, health, and cognitive function in a British sample. *Gerontologist* 1995;35(3):378–85.

158. West RL, Crook TH. Video training of imagery for mature adults. *Appl Cogn Psychol* 1991;6: 307–20.

159. Caprio-Prevette MD, Fry PS. Memory enhancement program for community-based older adults: development and evaluation. *Exp Aging Res* 1996;22(3):281–303

160. Abraham IL, Neundorfer MM, Currie LJ. Effects of group interventions on cognition and depression in nursing home residents. *Nurs Res* 1992;41(4):196–202.

161. Myers BL, Badia P. Changes in circadian rhythms and sleep quality with aging: mechanisms and interventions. *Neurosci Biobehav Rev* 1995;19(4):553–71. Published erratum appears in *Neurosci Biobehav Rev* 1996;20(2):I–IV.

162. Dori D, Casale G, Solerte SB, et al. Chrono-neuroendocrinological aspects of physiological aging and senile dementia. *Chronobiologia* 1994;21(1–2):121–6.

163. Bismark, M., Dauer, E., Paterson, R., Studdert, D. (2006). Accountability sought by patients following adverse events from medical care: the New Zealand experience. *CMAJ* 175: 889-894

164. Guckin, M., Waterman, R., Shubin, A. (2006). Consumer attitudes about health care-acquired infections and hand hygiene.. *American Journal of Medical Quality* 21: 342-346

165. Yeon, H. B., Lovett, D. A., Zurakowski, D., Herndon, J. H. (2006). Physician Discipline. *J. Bone Joint Surg. Am.* 88: 2091-2096

166. Crone, K. G., Muraski, M. B., Skeel, J. D., Love-Gregory, L., Ladenson, J. H., Gronowski, A. M. (2006). Between a Rock and a Hard Place: Disclosing Medical Errors. *Clin. Chem.* 52: 1809-1814

167. Gallagher, T. H., Garbutt, J. M., Waterman, A. D., Flum, D. R., Larson, E. B., Waterman, B. M., Dunagan, W. C., Fraser, V. J., Levinson, W. (2006). Choosing Your Words Carefully: How Physicians Would Disclose Harmful Medical Errors to Patients.. *Arch Intern Med* 166: 1585-1593

168. Gallagher, T. H., Waterman, A. D., Garbutt, J. M., Kapp, J. M., Chan, D. K., Dunagan, W. C., Fraser, V. J., Levinson, W. (2006). US and Canadian Physicians' Attitudes and Experiences Regarding Disclosing Errors to Patients.. *Arch Intern Med* 166: 1605-1611

169. Berlin, L. (2006). Will Saying "I'm Sorry" Prevent a Malpractice Lawsuit?. *Am. J. Roentgenol.* 187: 10-15

170. Stelfox, H T, Palmisani, S, Scurlock, C, Orav, E J, Bates, D W (2006). The "To Err is Human" report and the patient safety literature.. *Qual Saf Health Care* 15: 174-178

171. Wolf, M. S., Davis, T. C., Tilson, H. H., Bass, P. F. III, Parker, R. M. (2006). Misunderstanding of prescription drug warning labels among patients with low literacy. *Am J Health Syst Pharm* 63: 1048-1055

172. Stebbing, C., Kaushal, R., Bates, D. W. (2006). Pediatric medication safety and the media: what does the public see?. *Pediatrics* 117: 1907-1914

173. Berney, B., Needleman, J. (2006). Impact of nursing overtime on nurse-sensitive patient outcomes in new york hospitals, 1995-2000.. *Policy Politics Nursing Practice* 7: 87-100

174. Cleopas, A, Villaveces, A, Charvet, A, Bovier, P A, Kolly, V, Perneger, T V (2006). Patient assessments of a hypothetical medical error: effects of health outcome, disclosure, and staff responsiveness.. *Qual Saf Health Care* 15: 136-141

175. Bria, W. F. II (2006). Applied Medical Informatics for the Chest Physician: Information You Can USE!--Part 2.. *Chest* 129: 777-782

176. Tamblyn, R., Huang, A., Kawasumi, Y., Bartlett, G., Grad, R., Jacques, A., Dawes, M., Abrahamowicz, M., Perreault, R., Taylor, L., Winslade, N., Poissant, L., Pinsonneault, A. (2006). The Development and Evaluation of an Integrated Electronic Prescribing and Drug Management System for Primary Care. *J. Am. Med. Inform. Assoc.* 13: 148-159

177. Murff, H J, France, D J, Blackford, J, Grogan, E L, Yu, C, Speroff, T, Pichert, J, Hickson, G B (2006). Relationship between patient complaints and surgical complications. *Qual Saf Health Care* 15: 13-16

178. Dunn, K L, Reddy, P, Moulden, A, Bowes, G (2006). Medical record review of deaths, unexpected intensive care unit admissions, and clinician referrals: detection of adverse events and insight into the system. *Arch. Dis. Child.* 91: 169-172

179. Needleman, J., Buerhaus, P. I., Stewart, M., Zelevinsky, K., Mattke, S. (2006). Nurse Staffing In Hospitals: Is There A Business Case For Quality?. *Health Aff (Millwood)* 25: 204-211

180. Jagsi, R., Kitch, B. T., Weinstein, D. F., Campbell, E. G., Hutter, M., Weissman, J. S. (2005). Residents Report on Adverse Events and Their Causes. *Arch Intern Med* 165: 2607-2613

181. Duclos, C. W., Eichler, M., Taylor, L., Quintela, J., Main, D. S., Pace, W., Staton, E. W. (2005). Patient perspectives of patient-provider communication after adverse events. *Int J Qual Health Care* 17: 479-486

182. Elder, N. C., Jacobson, C. J., Zink, T., Hasse, L. (2005). How Experiencing Preventable Medical Problems Changed Patients' Interactions With Primary Health Care. *Ann Fam Med* 3: 537-544

183. Boudville, N. (2005). The predictable effect that renal failure has on H2 receptor antagonists--increasing the half-life along with increasing prescribing errors. *Nephrol Dial Transplant* 20: 2315-2317

184. Hibbard, J. H., Peters, E., Slovic, P., Tusler, M. (2005). Can Patients Be Part of the Solution? Views on Their Role in Preventing Medical Errors. *Med Care Res Rev* 62: 601-616

185. Gallagher, T. H., Levinson, W. (2005). Disclosing Harmful Medical Errors to Patients: A Time for Professional Action. *Arch Intern Med* 165: 1819-1824

186. Sachs, B. P. (2005). A 38-Year-Old Woman With Fetal Loss and Hysterectomy. *Journal of the American Medical Association* 294: 833-840

187. Shaw, R, Drever, F, Hughes, H, Osborn, S, Williams, S (2005). Adverse events and near miss reporting in the NHS. *Qual Saf Health Care* 14: 279-283

188. Walsh, K E, Kaushal, R, Chessare, J B (2005). How to avoid paediatric medication errors: a user's guide to the literature. *Arch. Dis. Child.* 90: 698-702

189. Beer, Z., Guttman, N., Brezis, M. (2005). Discordant public and professional perceptions on transparency in healthcare. *QJM* 98: 462-463

190. Leape, L. L., Berwick, D. M. (2005). Five Years After To Err Is Human: What Have We Learned?. *Journal of the American Medical Association* 293: 2384-2390

191. Stryer, D., Clancy, C. (2005). Patients' safety. *British Medical Journal* 330: 553-554

192. Werner, R. M., Asch, D. A. (2005). The Unintended Consequences of Publicly Reporting Quality Information. *Journal of the American Medical Association* 293: 1239-1244

193.   Sorokin, R., Riggio, J. M., Hwang, C. (2005). Attitudes About Patient Safety: A Survey of Physicians-in-Training. *American Journal of Medical Quality* 20: 70-77

194.   Burroughs, T. E., Waterman, A. D., Gallagher, T. H., Waterman, B., Adams, D., Jeffe, D. B., Dunagan, W. C., Garbutt, J., Cohen, M. M., Cira, J., Inguanzo, J., Fraser, V. J. (2005). Patient Concerns about Medical Errors in Emergency Departments. *Acad. Emerg. Med.* 12: 57-64

195.   Holder, A. R. (2005). Medical Errors. *ASH Education Book* 2005: 503-506

196.   Altman, D. E., Clancy, C., Blendon, R. J. (2004). Improving Patient Safety -- Five Years after the IOM Report. *New England Journal of Medicine* 351: 2041-2043

197.   Crigger, N. J (2004). Always Having to Say You're Sorry: an ethical response to making mistakes in professional practice. *Nurs Ethics* 11: 568-576

198.   Kachalia, A., Studdert, D. M. (2004). Professional Liability Issues in Graduate Medical Education. *Journal of the American Medical Association* 292: 1051-1056

199.   Berlin, L. (2004). Outcome Bias. *Am. J. Roentgenol.* 183: 557-560

200.   Mazor, K. M., Simon, S. R., Gurwitz, J. H. (2004). Communicating With Patients About Medical Errors: A Review of the Literature. *Arch Intern Med* 164: 1690-1697

201.   Tuttle, D, Holloway, R, Baird, T, Sheehan, B, Skelton, W K (2004). Electronic reporting to improve patient safety. *Qual Saf Health Care* 13: 281-286

202.   Schwappach, D. L. B., Koeck, C. M. (2004). What makes an error unacceptable? A factorial survey on the disclosure of medical errors. *Int J Qual Health Care* 16: 317-326

203.   Woolf, S. H., Kuzel, A. J., Dovey, S. M., Phillips, R. L. Jr (2004). A String of Mistakes: The Importance of Cascade Analysis in Describing, Counting, and Preventing Medical Errors. *Ann Fam Med* 2: 317-326

204.   Kuzel, A. J., Woolf, S. H., Gilchrist, V. J., Engel, J. D., LaVeist, T. A., Vincent, C., Frankel, R. M. (2004). Patient Reports of Preventable Problems and Harms in Primary Health Care. *Ann Fam Med* 2: 333-340

205.   Aarts, J., Doorewaard, H., Berg, M. (2004). Understanding Implementation: The Case of a Computerized Physician Order Entry System in a Large Dutch University Medical Center. *J. Am. Med. Inform. Assoc.* 11: 207-216

206. Mazor, K. M., Simon, S. R., Yood, R. A., Martinson, B. C., Gunter, M. J., Reed, G. W., Gurwitz, J. H. (2004). Health Plan Members' Views about Disclosure of Medical Errors. *Ann Intern Med* 140: 409-418

207. Devers, K. J., Pham, H. H., Liu, G. (2004). What Is Driving Hospitals' Patient-Safety Efforts?. *Health Aff (Millwood)* 23: 103-115

208. Studdert, D. M., Mello, M. M., Brennan, T. A. (2004). Medical Malpractice. *New England Journal of Medicine* 350: 283-292

209. Berlin, L. (2003). Radiologic Malpractice Litigation: A View of the Past, a Gaze at the Present, a Glimpse of the Future. *Am. J. Roentgenol.* 181: 1481-1486

210. Herndon, J. H. (2003). One More Turn of the Wrench. *J. Bone Joint Surg. Am.* 85: 2036-2048

211. Aiken, L. H., Clarke, S. P., Cheung, R. B., Sloane, D. M., Silber, J. H. (2003). Educational Levels of Hospital Nurses and Surgical Patient Mortality. *Journal of the American Medical Association* 290: 1617-1623

212. Sage, W. M. (2003). Medical Liability And Patient Safety. *Health Aff (Millwood)* 22: 26-36

213. Shanafelt, T., Adjei, A., Meyskens, F. L. (2003). When Your Favorite Patient Relapses: Physician Grief and Well-Being in the Practice of Oncology. *J. Clin. Oncol.* 21: 2616-2619

214. Berwick, D. M. (2003). Errors Today and Errors Tomorrow. *New England Journal of Medicine* 348: 2570-2572

215. Wade, J. G. (2003). Patient safety in anesthesia - continuing challenges and opportunities/La securite du patient en anesthesie - possibilites et defis permanents. *Canadian J. Anesthesia* 50: 319-322

216. Robblee, J. A., Nicklin, W. L. (2003). Views of Practicing Physicians and the Public on Medical Errors. *New England Journal of Medicine* 348: 1184-1185

217. Milstein, A., Adler, N. E. (2003). Out Of Sight, Out Of Mind: Why Doesn't Widespread Clinical Quality Failure Command Our Attention?. *Health Aff (Millwood)* 22: 119-127

218. Gallagher, T. H., Waterman, A. D., Ebers, A. G., Fraser, V. J., Levinson, W. (2003). Patients' and Physicians' Attitudes Regarding the Disclosure of Medical Errors. *Journal of the American Medical Association* 289: 1001-1007

219. Hsia, D. C. (2003). Medicare Quality Improvement: Bad Apples or Bad Systems?. *Journal of the American Medical Association* 289: 354-356

220. Lee, T. H. (2002). A Broader Concept of Medical Errors. *New England Journal of Medicine* 347: 1965-1967

221. Anderson G, Poullier J-P. Health Spending, Access, and Outcomes: Trends in Industrialized Countries. New York, NY: The Commonwealth Fund; 1999.

222. Schuster M, McGlynn E, Brook R. How good is the quality of health care in the United States? *Milbank Q.* 1998;76:517-563.

223. Kohn L, ed, Corrigan J, ed, Donaldson M, ed. To Err Is Human: Building a Safer Health System. Washington, DC: National Academy Press; 1999.

224. Starfield B. Primary Care: Balancing Health Needs, Services, and Technology. New York, NY: Oxford University Press; 1998.

225. *World Health Report* 2000. Accessed June 28, 2000.

226. Kunst A. Cross-national Comparisons of Socioeconomic Differences in Mortality. Rotterdam, the Netherlands: Erasmus University; 1997.

227. Law M, Wald N. Why heart disease mortality is low in France: the time lag explanation. *British Medical Journal* 1999;313:1471-1480.

228. Starfield B. Evaluating the State Children's Health Insurance Program: critical considerations. *Annu Rev Public Health*. 2000;21:569-585.

229. Leape L.Unnecessary surgery. *Annu Rev Public Health*. 1992;13:363-383.

230. Phillips D, Christenfeld N, Glynn L. Increase in US medication-error deaths between 1983 and 1993. *Lancet.* 1998;351:643-644.

231. Lazarou J, Pomeranz B, Corey P. Incidence of adverse drug reactions in hospitalized patients. *Journal of the American Medical Association* 1998; 279:1200-1205.

232. Weingart SN, Wilson RM, Gibberd RW, Harrison B. Epidemiology and medical error. *British Medical Journal* 2000;320:774-777

233. Wilkinson R. Unhealthy Societies: The Afflictions of Inequality. London, England: Routledge; 1996.

234. Evans R, Roos N. What is right about the Canadian health system? *Milbank Q.* 1999;77:393-399.

235. Guyer B, Hoyert D, Martin J, Ventura S, MacDorman M, Strobino D. Annual summary of vital statistics1998. *Pediatrics.* 1999;104:1229-1246.

236. Harrold LR, Field TS, Gurwitz JH. Knowledge, patterns of care, and outcomes of care for generalists and specialists. *J Gen Intern Med*. 1999;14:499-511.

237. Donahoe MT. Comparing generalist and specialty care: discrepancies, deficiencies, and excesses. *Arch Intern Med*. 1998;158:1596-1607.

238. Shi L, Starfield B. Income inequality, primary care, and health indicators. *J Fam Pract*.1999;48:275-284.

239. If it doesn't work, stop it: Medicine is a science of prediction and intervention , *British Medical Journal* 2004;328:1015

240. Ludovic Reveiz, *British Medical Journal* 2004 328: 1015.

241. If it doesn't work, stop it: I don't know, Simon M Loader, *British Medical Journal* 2004 328: 1016.

242. If it doesn't work, stop it: Summary of rapid responses, Caroline White, *British Medical Journal* 2004 328: 1016.

243. Nothingness: the role of journals, Richard Smith, *British Medical Journal* 2004 328: 0.

244. *British Medical Journal* 1996; 313:13-16 (6 July) **Misdiagnosis** of the vegetative state: retrospective study in a rehabilitation unit.

245. Krous.H, UCLA, San Diego

246. *Archives of Pediatrics and Adolescent Medicine*, published online March 5, 2007

247. A Comparison of the Antemortem Clinical Diagnosis and Autopsy Findings for Patients. O'Connor et al. *Acad Emerg Med*.2002; 9: 957-959

248. *Surg Gynecol Obstet*. 1992 Sep;175(3):227-32, The results of autopsy of patients with surgical diseases of the digestive tract. **Barendregt WB, de Boer HH,** Kubat.K.

249. *Hunan Yi Ke Da Xue Xue Bao*. 1999;24(3):275-6. A comparative analysis of clinical and pathologic diagnoses in 79 pediatric autopsy cases Zhao L, Yian Y, Chen R.

250. *Forensic Science International*, Volume 71, Issue 1, Pages 75-76 E. Ambach, The inadequacy of death certificates claiming myocardial infarction without autopsy verification.

251. Sweeney.P.J, 'Parkinsons Disease -an Overview' http://www.clevelandclinicmeded.com/diseasemanagement/neurology/parkinsons/parkinsons.htm

252. Choe.J, Misdiagnosis occuring in a course of autopsy. *Korean J Leg Med*. 1991 Oct;15(2):56-57.

253. *The Lancet*, 2004; 363: 345-51

254. *British Medical Journal* 2001;323:956, Gotzsche, P. C;

255. *British Medical Journal* 2002 324: 677 Thornton.H

256. *Radiology*, 2004; 232: 735-8;

257. *Journal of the American Medical Association*, 2004; 292: 1669

258. *British Medical Journal*, 2004; 329: 849-51, Picano E.

259. Journal of Clinical Oncology, June26, 2006

260. *J.Urol*, 2005; 174:1065-1070; prostate/lifestyle

261. Adoption of a Plant-Based Diet by Patients with Recurrent Prostate Cancer Nguyen et al. *Integr Cancer Ther.*2006; 5: 214-223

262. *The Lancet*, 2007; 369: 882-4

263. MeyerU.A, Kindli R, *Ther Umsch.* 1989 Aug;46(8):544-54, Placebos and Nocebos.

264. Sapirstein.G 1995, *'Listening to Prozac but Hearing Placebo'* ;

265. Are drug and placebo effects in depression additive? *Biological Psychiatry*, Vol 47, Issue 8, pp 733-735 Kirsch.I

266. *Prevention & Treatment.* 1(1), Jun 1998, Kirsch.I; Sapirstein, G

267. Understanding the Placebo Effect in Complementary Medicine, pub Churchill Livingstone, Section 2. Ernst.E pp 17-29.

268. *Clinical Oncology* (2004) 16: 549e560, The Contribution of Cytotoxic Chemotherapy to 5-year Survival in Adult Malignancies, Morgan.G, Wardy.R, Barton.M.

269. 26th November 2006, The Daily Mail

# Chapter 6

# The Implications of this New Generation of Medical Technologies

### by

**Graham Ewing**

It is not that technologies of this nature are considered to be impossible. In the Scientific American journal a highly respected academic and ethicist ₁ openly discusses the future implications of this new generation of technologies which would have the capability to download the contents of the brain and have the ability to diagnose and treat disease.

Uri Geller, amongst others, has written about the technology and articles have been featured in national newspapers in Russia, UK and occasionally in articles in the scientific and popular press in UK, EU, etc.

In this chapter we outline the implications arising from the introduction of a technology of this nature. This is the future. Virtual Scanning is the first of this new generation of technologies. Others will inevitably follow.

## 6.1    Biomedicine

*Is it possible that the biomedical approach overlooks issues which are fundamentally important to our health?*

That drugs perform a valuable function in the treatment of illness is not in dispute, but their effectiveness is often limited because researchers lack an adequate level of understanding of the precise cause(s) of the medical condition. They focus upon the treatment of a generic population whilst overlooking the differing physiology of the different age groups; fail to recognise that each of us is completely unique; and that the symptoms of an illness are rarely identical for each of us. Such issues are recognised by pharmacogeneticists who are developing a drug-based approach which, it is hoped, will be able to develop drugs which are more appropriate for the individuals genetic type.

Most medical research is devoted to the development of new technologies and new drugs which it is claimed will reduce the incidence of illness. The evidence, available in the medical industry's own journals, is that this is not the case. In fact the incidence of illness is rising alarmingly in the major industrialized nations of the world yet no-one appears able to question conventional wisdom. For every new drug that is developed there is a corresponding range of side-effects which develop. This is the logical outcome of the drug-based approach and if the body is regulated by physiological systems as described. Most pharmacologically active substances adversely affect the ability of the brain waves to regulate our physiology. There is significant amounts of evidence that drugs may actually be contributing to illness and that they adversely affect our physiological stability. The medical journals are full of reports which catalogue the side-effects of drugs and of the drugs which are used to treat side-effects.

There are no drugs which do not have side-effects. Even drug supplements such as insulin have side-effects because they are administered in far greater quantities than is required by the body. Whereas in the past when drugs were developed with the most rudimentary knowledge of the body's biochemistry the side-effects were relatively slight, the latest knowledge of the biochemical processes enables drugs to be developed which have greater efficacy but which also have very much greater side-effects. It appears unlikely therefore that there will ever be a drug which is free from side-effects.

The conventional wisdom is that it is our genes which are responsible for our character and health yet new evidence is emerging that this is no longer an accurate conclusion. It indicates only that we are predisposed to have a medical condition under the right set of conditions, that the function of the genes can be affected by stress, and moreover that there are differing morphological types of the genes which are involved in our function. Recent research into the new subject of epigenetics i.e. reversible, heritable changes in gene function that occur without a change in DNA sequence and how our lives are shaped in part by your ancestors life experiences; questions the long-held assumptions regarding the functions of the genes.

Stress acts to depress our immune system therefore if we stimulate our immune system we will to some extent reduce our vulnerability to stress and infection. By contrast over-stimulation of the immune system will be accompanied by a range of conditions e.g. allergies, etc.

Each of our physiological systems involves the complex interaction of a number of factors. For example our digestive system is dependent upon the control of pH; the quality (cell content), pressure and volume of blood; temperature; removal of toxins and by-products; osmotic pressure; etc. Each of our physiological systems works in a logical, sophisticated and complex manner as outlined in this and most medical textbooks.

If we can maintain our health and wellbeing our susceptibility to stress will be reduced and our vulnerability to infection will be reduced thereby reducing our need for antibiotics. If we lead less stressful lives we will remain more healthy and hence will have less need for medical intervention therefore by understanding that our physiological systems are regulated by the brain waves we can start to understand that the function of specific categories of drugs can be improved. The success of anticancer therapies is widely recognised and the statistics clearly illustrate how anticancer medications have reduced the number of people who die from cancer but this is not the end of the story. The survival rates of those who have been treated is abysmally low. Many people who contract cancer and are treated by chemotherapy appear to suffer from the inability of their system to function normally thereafter [2]. If anticancer drugs have a destabilising effect upon the brain waves it is reasonable to assume that therapies which can improve brain wave function, and immune system function, will complement the role of chemotherapy and improve survival rates.

Indeed why people contract cancer still remains a mystery in many cases. It is widely accepted that cancers form and are destroyed by killer t-cells however in many people the production of killer t-cells becomes inadequate and cancerous tumours form. **Is it possible, as so many believe, that the effect of stress and the associated production of stressor substances, and of impaired immune system function; depresses the function of our systems and cells to the extent that our natural ability to deal with illness is reduced to a disastrous level?**

This viewpoint is reinforced by noting that under stress the most benign of substances can become biologically active to the extent that they can affect our physiology and also that stress affects our cognitive processes [3].

**The principles behind Virtual Scanning, as outlined in earlier chapters, provides a fundamental philosophy which does not contradict any established biomedical research. It does however illustrate the regulatory nature of the physiological processes which control all aspects of our function and biochemistry.**

## 6.2    Vaccines

One of the most most sensitive areas of medical debate centres around the use of vaccines which are considered to be the most important vehicles which the medical profession can use to eradicate illness.

This approach overlooks the vulnerability of the immature central nervous systems of young children to 'toxic insults' arising from the vaccination. There are also significant concerns surrounding the mass vaccination of children and adults using multiple vaccines [4] which are controversial and alleged by some observers and researchers to be responsible for autistic spectrum disorders in children and perhaps also for Gulf War Syndrome in soldiers.

**Evidence-based fact analysis:**

The evidence-based factual analysis, the approach often used by epidemiologists, allows us to evaluate the effect of specific factors on demographic groups **e.g. in 'Amish' communities** [5,6] **the children do not have autism.** These families live a religious lifestyle in large groups which reject modern culture and scientific progress in favour of a simplistic lifestyle. As they live without pharmaceuticals, vaccines and artificially enhanced foods they are an ideal study group. The occurrence of Autism is almost non-existent in an Amish community and is far below the rates of occurrence which are seen in those who have been vaccinated.  No matter how eloquent the argument one fact remains: those who do not have vaccinations of any sort do not get autism.

Epidemiologists [6] should be encouraged to research why auto-immune diseases have become increasingly common but were relatively rare in recent years. Diabetes been rising steadily in the west yet is not a significant health issue in the under-developed countries of the world.

For children who at risk of developing autistic spectrum disorders there is a logical safety-first argument that the use of vaccines should be delayed until (1) the child's immune system becomes more mature i.e. giving the injection when the child is older; (2) ensuring the child's immune system is at a satisfactory level; or (3) giving single vaccines instead of multiple vaccines.

For some vaccines, dissent has been focussed upon the use of mercury-containing 'thimerosal' as a preservative however, whilst mercury poisoning is considered by many to be associated with impaired brain function, the removal of thimerosal from vaccines [7-10] has not been linked to a reduction in autism.

If we consider the brain as a data processing or computing entity consider what would happen if you pressed several keys on your keyboard simultaneously – the computer would crash. Is it possible that by giving multiple vaccine to a vulnerable child we risk the same phenomena – and cause the brain's software to crash?

Similarly for an adult combatant who is under stress following news of their imminent posting to a war zone and of the hectic period prior to their departure should they be given their vaccinations when they are not under stress and/or that the vaccinations should be given singly over a prolonged period of time. Under stressful situations it is recognised that the activity of substances, hitherto considered to be 'benign', can become 'malignant' and therefore cancerous.

Consider the body as a complex data-processing entity i.e. a 'soft-ware'; which processes our receipt of data from our environment. By doing so we can understand that it is this receipt of data which affects the body's biochemistry. Now consider that multiple vaccines could dramatically confuse the ability of the body to process data 13 and hence could affect the body's physiological systems and the body's physiological and psychological stability. As you can see from the accumulated body of data in the first chapters this is an interesting viewpoint with merits and few, if any, limitations.

In vaccines for the treatment of flu in the elderly and against bird flu, the claimed benefits appear not to match the facts. Flu vaccine is almost completely ineffective 11. Moreover the US drug regulator, the Food and Drug Administration (FDA), has asked Roche to reveal that Tamiflu 12 can cause the patient to become delirious and declare that self-injury, confusion and delirium are not uncommon. It can also cause anaphylactic shock, serious skin reactions, nausea, vomiting, bronchitis, insomnia, vertigo, suicidal tendencies, etc.

The risks from being immunised with the flu vaccine may outweigh the benefits and place you at risk of developing the neurological disorder Guillain-Barre syndrome 12. This attacks the nervous system thereby causing weakness, tingling and might eventually lead to paralysis.

Further indications of the risk from vaccines indicate that the meningitis vaccine can cause Guillain-Barre Syndrome 13. In the US, 15 teenagers and two adults developed Guillain-Barre Syndrome after being given a version of this vaccine and in October 2005 a further five cases were reported. The 14 FDA now estimates that the vaccine is causing 1.25 cases of Guillain-Barre Syndrome for every million vaccinations whereas an estimated one in 100,000 adolescents between 11 and 19 years of age contracts meningitis each year of which about 10% suffer severe consequences of the infection i.e. death or disability. There appears to be little difference in risk between having the vaccine or not.

Further indications of the safety risks associated with vaccines are illustrated by the 15 DtaP (diphtheria, tetanus and whooping cough) vaccine. It has been discovered that two-thirds of the children in a study suffered a reaction around the vaccinated area observed as a reddening of the skin which could be considered to be indicative of a more serious condition. Many of the children said their arms and legs were aching and sore following the vaccination.

The introduction of the HPV (human papilloma virus) vaccine for the treatment of cervical cancer is circumstantial and the conclusions upon which it has been developed appear liable to be misinterpreted [19]. The National Cancer Institute[16, 21, 22] in the US is not yet convinced that the link between HPV and cervical cancer is proven (quote: "It is important to note, however, that the majority of high-risk HPV infections go away on their own and do not cause cancer") The rate of occurrence is typically 3-4 per 100,000 and the occurrence of cervical cancer happens typically 20-50 years after infection [17]. Perhaps, as with so many other conditions, stress exascerbates the situation - and that a particular stress-event could, when exposed to one or more of the HPV strains, lead to lowered immunity which is subsequently manifest as cervical cancer.

Most of the research [18] appears to be based upon assumptions and conjecture - since proliferating cells i.e. growing cancer cells, would be more susceptible to infection than resting cells, the viruses would be indicators, rather than causes, of abnormal proliferation. It does not yet prove the link. Moreover the HPV vaccine is associated with a range of side-effects including headache, gastroenteritis, appendicitis, pelvic inflammatory disease, asthma and bronchial spasms, and arthritis [23]. Perhaps, as seems likely, the risks outweigh the benefits [24]. Quote:

**"Nobody at Merck, the CDC or FDA know if the injection of Gardasil (HPV vaccine) into all pre-teen girls -- especially simultaneously with hepatitis B vaccine -- will make some of them more likely to develop arthritis or other inflammatory autoimmune and brain disorders as teenagers and adults".**

Perhaps of greater concern is the PCV vaccine [25] which has been developed to treat pneumococcal meningitis, septicaemia and pneumonia yet in the US in the first two years of the vaccine's introduction there have been 4,154 reports of side-effects (15%) and 117 deaths - from pneumococcal meningitis, pneumonia, and septicaemia. It is likely that this vaccine is offering little protection against these conditions.

All vaccines depress our immune system. The lymphatic system carries lymphocytes throughout our body and maintains control over our cellular function. If the lymphatic system becomes congested, arising from the injection of large molecular sized proteins (foreign tissues in the vaccines), this could be expected to create problems for the lymphatic system, allergic reactions, etc. This may explain the apparent similarity of vaccine side-effects and lymphatic diseases [26]. It is possible therefore that vaccination does not confer immunity against a pathogen but instead leads to its manifestation in other ways and that attempts to eradicate the naturally occurring pathogen (e.g. polio, measles, whooping cough, etc) are now displaced by other 'newer' medical conditions eg. multiple sclerosis, autism, allergies/asthma, auto-immune diseases, diabetes, cancer, and neurological problems. This is a very real concern.

For instance could non-vaccinated HPV strains become more dominant in the future. There are precedents e.g. some of the seven strains of pneumococcus contained in 'prevnar' vaccine have been displaced by some of the > 80 other strains which are not present in the vaccine.

Some leading epidemiologists and immunologists are now extremely concerned [50, 51] that vaccines based upon the use of live-virusses could actually be creating a new generation of diseases, genetic mutations, or worse.

Whereas the introduction of vaccines was expected to eradicate specific illnesses there is proof of the reverse [52].

Consider some of the facts

- [53] half the victims of whooping cough in 1987 and 1991 in Ohio state had been vaccinated against it according to their medical records.

- [54] Between 1981 and 1987 the occurrence of hepatitis B increased from 550 per million to 630 per million

- [55] Of 867 infants who received BCG vaccine and had tuberculin tests, 36% per cent developed allergies, including asthma.

- Withdrawing smallpox vaccination led to a reduction in the incidence of TB. It is considered that smallpox vaccine reinforced Koch bacilli - which explains the widespread occurrence of TB in the 19th century.

- the epidemic of polio followed the introduction of the diphtheria vaccine. Diphtheria vaccination when coupled with whooping-cough vaccination was considered to increase the virulence of the polio virus.

- [56] Polio vaccination, coupled with other, routine vaccinations, is alleged to have contributed to the overload of the immune system and evolution of acquired immunodeficiency syndrome.

- The eradication of scarlet fever was replaced by measles and diphtheria.

- [57, 58]. Some research has revealed similarities between vaccines and the protein structure of myelin. Accordingly any loss of myelin could affect the structure and function of the nervous system. Any vaccination could therefore trigger encephalitis and if accompanied by demyelination could hinder normal development of the brain and lead to behavioural problems. An estimated 20% of children in the US have at some time suffered from these type of effects.

- Vaccines produce antibodies thereby affecting the stability of the brain waves and hence of the body's physiological systems. If so, this will affect the extent of physiological and neurological development. There appears to be evidence to support such a conclusion e.g. the clinical observation that many autistic children with raised body temperature appear to lose their autistic symptoms.

**The principles behind Virtual Scanning provides a fundamental philosophy which does not contradict any established biomedical research. It illustrates the regulatory significance of the physiological processes which regulate all aspects of our biochemistry and our function.**

There is much to be gained by understanding how our immune system can be stimulated to act against illness.

## 6.3    The Future Provision of Healthcare

*How is the government going to achieve the objectives laid out in the NHS plan? How is the GP going to make the improvements which are required? Which technologies are going to assist them to achieve their objectives? Which technologies are able to reduce the cost of providing healthcare?*

**Governments** are faced with the dilemma of how to improve the level of services provided whilst balancing the budgets of the government departments. Healthcare expenditure is a massive proportion of the tax spend. The challenge is how to recognise, encourage and approve the new innovative technologies which improve the level of services whilst reducing the cost of healthcare, education, etc.

Virtual Scanning is the first new medical technology which can enable a government to improve the provision of general medical services and also to reduce the cost of providing medical diagnosis and treatment.  The introduction of this technology enables the **GP** to have all necessary data about the health of the person and hence to be more informed. This moves the emphasis for improved medical diagnosis from secondary care (i.e. the hospital) to primary care (i.e. local health centres)

For the **elderly** it conceivably provides a means of addressing the malaise which is often associated with increased age i.e. the problems associated with increased weight, reduced blood circulation, reduced energy levels, reduced mobility and generally reduced levels of wellbeing.

For the **young**, of typically >7 years, it conceivably provides a means of ensuring optimal mental and physiological development and hence improves their ability to concentrate, memorise, function; which affects their performance in education, sport, etc.

For those in **patient-carer/therapist relationships** it provides a means of stimulating the brain's compensatory mechanisms which, as outlined in chapter 4, may be inhibited due to illness, injury or stress.  It can be of value in overcoming the status quo which often exists between carer/therapist and patient and which could be preventing the patient becoming well i.e. that the carer's job is to look after a patient and the patient's task is to sit and be looked after whereas ideally we should instead be seeking a situation where the carer or therapist's job is to make the patient well and the patient should understand that they are being looked after in a manner which is intended to optimise their chances of recovery.

Every new diagnostic technology, every new drug ADDS cost, and makes the process of diagnosis more and more complicated, with the consequent requirement for more and more people at greater and greater cost.  The use of MRI scanners and other highly expensive medical scanners, upon which the government and medical profession places great reliance, can only diagnose a medical condition when it has developed into a physical abnormality which is sufficiently large to be diagnosed e.g. a tumour. It does little to reduce the burden of diagnosis and misdiagnosis or to reduce the cost of remedial operations.

Moreover the cost of each test – circa £750 per scan – is an astonishing increase in cost, especially so, bearing in mind that the majority of these tests are screening tests which yield a negative or provide information which has little value.

What is required is a technology which can provide a quick and cheap broad-spectrum diagnosis which can subsequently, and if required, be confirmed by a specialist diagnostic technology e.g. an MRI scanner, x-ray, ultrasound, etc; and hence can significantly reduce the cost of medical diagnosis.

**The implications of these findings** for all aspects of medicine are intriguing e.g.

- Whereas the measurement of blood pressure in the arm is related to our health Virtual Scanning can identify the physiological systems, organs and medical conditions, which are responsible for the condition.

- Whereas a sphygmomanometer is used to determine blood pressure in the arm of a patient it has limited relevance to the blood pressure in the spinal chord or brain which is conceivably responsible for migraine, stroke, etc.

- Whereas a patient would comment upon having poor sleeping patterns it can now be possible using Virtual Scanning to determine the precise causes (stress-related, systems-based and/or somatic) for the poor quality sleep.

- Various forms of 'invasive' and hazardous medical technologies which are currently used for screening i.e. to detect the presence or absence of a medical condition, can now be augmented by the broad-spectrum screening technology, Virtual Scanning, which enables the 'invasive' medical technologies to be used to confirm the medical diagnosis in the most serious cases.

- Whereas nutrition is important when considering a person's health it is now possible using Virtual Scanning to identify the destabilized systems which affect blood flow to the digestive system (quality of the blood, blood pressure, blood volume, body temperature, pH), hence regulating the stability of our digestive system and hence which affect our ability to absorb minerals, vitamins, etc.

The huge amounts of data which are available from a Virtual Scanning assessment enables the medical services, for the first time, to seriously contemplate the possibility that medicine could move from a symptoms-based approach to a preventative or cause-based approach and that this could serve as a truly comprehensive screening programme for the population.

# Virtual Scanning is the only technology which can conceivably enable the NHS to fulfill the objectives laid out in the NHS plan.

There would be potentially massive political implications and significant cost-savings, if a technology of this type was proven and adopted by the NHS, based upon

- introducing new methods of working,

- reducing the incidence of illness,

- introducing preventative screening and hence to identify the progression of illness before it requires the most expensive drugs or surgical procedures,
- reducing the requirement for medical diagnoses,

- being able to provide a comprehensive patient health report during the patient consultation i.e. 'at the press of a button'.
- reducing the requirement for some categories of drugs,

- reducing the need for expensive medical technologies,

- reducing the need for unnecessary surgical procedures,

- reducing the legal liability of the medical profession arising from misdiagnosis and misprescribing of drugs,
- reducing the scope for hospital-transmitted infections

- reducing the cost of healthcare

## 6.4 Could Diabetes and Obesity be due to the Destabilization of the Body's Physiological Systems?

*Instead of looking for a biochemical approach which is related to organ dysfunction should we be looking one step further up the hierarchical ladder? Is it a problem with the regulatory systems?*

There are multi-biochemical origins of type 1 and type 2 diabetes. Over 14 diagnostic test procedures are unable to reliably diagnose the precise biochemical origins of the medical condition:

- diabetes is reaching epidemic scale proportions in western society. It is a condition of affluence and is not prevalent to any significant extent in societies which have a traditional low fat diet and where the expenditure of energy and hence of physical exercise is a significant part of their working day.

- exercise can dramatically reduce and/or eradicate type 2 diabetes

- excess weight and the 'fast-food diet' is heavily implicated and is considered to be an important factor [45,46]

- vegetable oils and/or animal fats are heavily implicated and considered to be an important factor yet an eskimo's diet comprises large amounts of fat yet they do not have heart disease

- cholesterol is processed and regulated by the liver, duodenum and gall bladder [38]

- stress is known to exascerbate the condition

- chronic diabetes affects the various systems of the body and hence can be considered to be largely responsible for the development of multiple side-effects of varying degrees of severity

- diabetes is related to poor memory, concentration, etc

- light therapy is known to have a positive therapeutic effect upon the condition

- diabetes is an age-related condition

- mineral depletion is often detected in the diabetic [37]

The biochemical or reductionist approach fails to differentiate between the symptoms of illness and the causative factors. The glib answer 'that the absence of a single biochemical is responsible' does not fit the prevailing facts nor does it explain how the level of the various biochemicals became destabilized.

Researchers are seeking the holy grail or the magic bullet which can magically treat the condition yet the reality is that diabetes - either as type 1 or as type 2 – has multiple origins and that the biochemical approach fails to explain the complex nature of the condition.

Some of the latest drugs being developed for the treatment of obesity target the endocannabinoid receptors in the brain thereby reducing cravings and increasing energy expenditure but are also responsible for a number of side-effects which for example affect the reproductive system. Moreover the precise mechanisms for these drugs are often unknown and the gains at, in some cases, typically 5-10 kgs pa, are hardly worth the trouble by comparison to other alternatives such as 'weightwatchers'.

Interestingly researchers have concluded that if you lose weight and then stop the treatment that the person's weight will often return to the previous high level.

Virtual Scanning offers an approach which can explain a number of the issues e.g.

- the effect of the metabolic rate and hence of the increased prevalence of diabetes with age and with increased weight

- that stress exascerbates the condition

- that light and colour have a positive therapeutic effect which can reduce the body's need for insulin in the type 1 diabetic and which can eradicate the symptoms of diabetes in the type 2 diabetic

**These issues illustrate that diabetes and obesity have origins which are related to the stability of the body's physiological systems.** If so we would expect to see conditions which were associated with the stability of the body's physiological systems e.g.

- indications of impaired function of the heart

- variable blood cell content

- variable blood pressure

- problems with the blood vessels

- digestive problems

- variable body temperature

- destabilized pH

- sleeping problems

- appetite problems

349

These result in mineral depletion, skin problems, poor excretion, loss of energy, increased weight, fungal infections, erectile dysfunction, thirst, etc. Other reported side-effects include stroke, kidney disease, diabetic retinopathy, sciatica, heart disease, numbness and tingling feet, cramps in the legs, swollen skin tissues, blurred vision, chest pain, shortness of breath, slowed reaction times, and long-term memory problems [42].

**The body's physiological function is managed by short-term memory and long-term memory.**

As the body has a mechanism of homeostasis which is responsible for the body's stability this manages the function of the various physiological systems of the body. This is the long-term memory. In the pancreas this effectively/directly or indirectly manages the production of insulin which is responsible, in situations of excess food, for the conversion of glucose into triglycerides which is the mechanism for storage of glucose as fat. If the levels of proteins which regulate the production of insulin are destabilized and the levels of insulin are at too high or too low a level this will affect appetite, food consumption and weight.

**Diets** which are known to be effective include the vegetarian diet which excludes most fats and the Atkins diet which includes fats and excludes vegetarian produce. How do we resolve these apparently contradicatory diets? What is the explanation? Does blood type play a role?

Increasingly it is becoming a concern that it is not just the use of trans fats which are the problem but that excess use of vegetable origin oils may in fact be the problem. Whilst the use of trans fats are associated with heart problems their replacement by unsaturated vegetable oils merely reduces the problem [101]. It does not eliminate the problem.

In addition vegetables deliver minerals and vitamins which catalyse the processes of digestion whereas meats are more difficult to process and reside longer in the digestive tract.

Vegetables (including bread, pasta and rice) and meats are processed by the digestive system at different rates. If we eat vegetables they are processed by the digestive system into nutrients and blood glucose (relatively rapidly) whereas if we eat meats they are processed by the digestive system into protein, nutrients and blood glucose (over a much longer period). In each case the digestive system produces pancreatic enzymes which are appropriate to digest vegetables or meat.

If we eat vegetables and meat simultaneously the digestive system produces enzymes which is appropriate to digest vegetables AND meat. The glucose which is derived from the digestion of vegetables satisfies the immediate need for blood glucose and the glucose which we derive from the digestion of meat follows later. Is it possible that the meat is digested more quickly, or perhaps more slowly, if we eat meat and vegetables simultaneously? Irrespective, the result is that we accumulate glucose which is surplus to requirements and which is subsequently stored as fat.

Researchers have now established that obesity causes the breakdown of a brain system that regulates appetite and that the function of the 'arcuate nucleus' in the hypothalamus is affected by an excess of leptin [34].

Our appetite and feelings of satedness are regulated by a mechanism which involves the levels of proteins [35] and in particular of the proteins leptin, ghrelin, and pancreatic peptide. If for example our **sleep** is disturbed this has an effect upon the levels of these proteins and consequently we eat to excess. When being fed too much food the body produces excess insulin beyond normal requirements.

Under normal circumstances the body uses the natural reservoir of **blood glucose** which is stored in the liver and organs of the body to produce energy and the associated level of insulin is therefore, for the normal levels of energy requirements, maintained at a low level; however at high level of energy requirements e.g. running, etc, in which the metabolic rate is raised and the body's energy requirements exceed the available blood glucose reserves the body starts to increase the production of insulin in order to convert the available fat reserves into blood glucose and hence into energy.

Chromium is known to catalyse and/or regulate the processes which use insulin. If chromium (or any other minerals or substances which are essential minor components of the process of converting glucose into energy) is not present in the diet or the processes which absorb chromium from the diet are dysfunctional e.g. due to destabilized levels of intestinal flora, gut pH, impaired blood flow to the intestines, etc; this will result in higher levels of insulin as the body attempts to compensate.

The means that your ability to burn fat is mostly dependent upon on the processes which use oxygen. Consequently if energy is required more rapidly than oxygen can be delivered to the muscles the body switches to the less efficient anaerobic pathways. So your ability to burn energy is based upon the size and condition of the muscles, their ability to store oxygen and subsequently their ability to change to the slower anaerobic pathways which convert the available fat reserves into glucose.

Increased muscle mass increases the ability to burn calories by up to 10 calories per kg muscle.

Exercise designed to burn calories at a greater rate than can be replenished by the body (frequency, magnitude and longevity).

- rapid spurts of exercise burn energy

- sustained programmes which deplenish the body's glucose reserves therafter requiring the body to produce energy from fat reserves.

As the rate of production of insulin is slow the cessation of exercise is not accompanied by an immediate cessation in the production of insulin but by a steady slow-down of insulin production. During this period the body continues to burns energy and to convert available food into blood glucose, but also burns fat as necessary in order to replenish the body's blood glucose and hence re-establish the homeostatic stability of the blood glucose system.

50% of our energy requirements fuel the activity of the brain. Cholesterol is the main raw material for production of acetyl-choline which is an essential neurotransmitter for brain activity without which we could not function. Too much cholesterol is clearly associated with thickening of the blood and too little with impaired neural function. The consequences of too much blood cholesterol are of stroke or heart attack, and in the case of too little blood cholesterol, of dementia, parkinsonism, etc.

With soft drinks the body produces an excess insulin. In the situation of excess sugar the body produces sufficient insulin to convert the sugar although the rate of increase of blood glucose is rapid and the subsequent end of supply of blood glucose is also very rapid. Accordingly the body has difficulty managing the supply of insulin.

When artificial sweeteners are used in soft drink manufacture the body is tricked to believe that it is about to receive a supply of sugar. Consider the following possibility: that it commences the production of insulin – which results in an excess of insulin which rapidly absorbs the available blood glucose. The surplus is subsequently converted into fat reserves. The result is that the child has a rapid high or 'buzz' followed by a 'low' and hence of hunger, cravings, anger, misbehaviour, etc. In such cases the excess of insulin consumes the available blood glucose leading to an effect which is conceivably the precise opposite of the intended effect. Furthermore as insulin is a hugely reactive protein this conceivably results in the reaction of insulin with susceptible components of its environment. This could be manifest as damage to the cells of the islets of langerhans, to the blood cell walls and walls of the heart, etc; i.e. as the side-effects of diabetes.

The child's behaviour of cravings, anger and misbehaviour is just the body's way of drawing attention to the fact that his biochemistry is destabilised, that he is hungry and that he wants to rectify the matter by obtaining food.

In the event that the body's physiological systems are desynchronized the body's metabolism will be affected, that the levels of proteins (insulin, glucagons, etc) which are required will be affected, and that the mechanisms which convert glucose into fat will be adversely increased or decreased, that the mechanisms which convert fat into glucose will also be adversely increased or decreased. As **blood pressure** and **blood glucose** are affected this will have a consequent effect upon the digestive system, condition of skin, memory and concentration. As the **digestive system** is affected this will affect the **pH** of the digestive system and hence the absorption of minerals. As the digestive system is affected then so too will be the **excretory system.**

This is supported by studies which illustrates that it is the quality of a person's food intake which is important rather than the quantity. They compared in a separate study of the Mediterranean diet, which is rich in fruits, vegetables, cereals and olive oil, and which avoids processed foods i.e. with adequate levels of protein, vitamins, minerals, natural oils with an omega-3 type component, and slow-release carbohydrates. The researchers found that overweight people who stuck to the diet were very unlikely to become obese, while people of standard weight didn't become overweight.

Supporting this line of thought other researchers have postulated 'that heavy intakes of large amounts of fat can override the body's controlling mechanism and that this would lead to lower levels of neurotransmitters which may explain their need for binge quantities'. This would to some extent be consistent with the conclusion that a diet which is low in protein would be consistent with the production of low amounts of neurotransmitters and hence of difficulties in regulating sleeping and eating; and of difficulties with sleep patterns, memory, concentration, etc. In other words the body would seek to compensate for low amounts of protein, and hence of neurotransmitters, by increasing its intake of food which would be accompanied by large increases in the levels of insulin.

Moreover it is highly likely that the use of fats and oils to deliver flavours in foodstuffs has the effect of reducing the ability of the body to metabolise vitamins and minerals which are essential for catalysing all biochemical processes in the body and hence for good bodily function.

Have you ever consider why we have an ability to detect substances through smell and taste? What is the function of these senses? Researchers have proven how these senses function yet overlook the fundamental use of these senses. Whereas they conclude that odour and taste are essential for sensory stimulation relating to our ability to sense our environment they ignore the far more significant possibility that taste is a function related to the regulation of our diet.

Indeed if pheromones are molecules which, through the nose and tongue, can influence different social behaviours in animals (and if these affect the function of GPCRs), it is entirely logical to make the connection that the taste buds of the tongue have yet another function, which is associated with the sense of taste and which is involved in the processes which regulate our diet.

Knowledge of the function of flavours, odours produce the most appetizing components. A consequence of their function may be that this can over-ride the natural mechanisms which regulate diet.

Finally, in order to illustrate that diabetes (type 2) is a failure of our physiology a study [37] of 72 patients were subjected to a programme involving diet and exercise, monitored by a GP. This illustrated that diabetes can be controlled without drugs.

Examples of how Virtual Scanning can be used to regulate the physiological systems and hence regulate appetite and weight are listed in 4.19.

## 6.5 Medical Insurance

*Consider what would happen if all patients who suffered at the hands of the medical profession were to sue for compensation.*

If all patients who were misdiagnosed; given the wrong drugs; suffered a drug side-effect, medical negligence or incompetence; or who were otherwise mistreated; were to take legal action for compensation that the full effect would bankrupt the NHS.

This would certainly focus the minds of those who administer the NHS to adopt the best and safest measures to diagnose and treat a patient.

The lack of a satisfactory medical technology/alternative has prevented the insurance industry implementing changes which could affect how we look after our lives. Consider what would happen if our health insurance were to be provided by private companies and that our premiums were linked to our age, weight, and lifestyle (smoking, diet, drink/alcohol, recreational drugs).

If improved health is to be achieved by government it is necessary to introduce an incentive for people to take responsibility for matters which are under their control.

This would mean e.g.

- the cost of misdiagnosis, and resulting claims for compensation, would be paid by the GP's insurance policy – therefore the insurance company would have a vested interest in ensuring that the GP used the best available technologies

- the cost of medical negligence arising from misdiagnosis would be paid by the doctor or hospital's insurance company

- that sports injuries would be paid by sportsmen who hold valid private insurance policies which would cover the cost of their treatment.

- those in car accidents would have the cost of their medical care covered by the insurance policy of the person who caused the accident

- those who smoke would pay greater insurance premiums

- those who are overweight would pay greater insurance premiums

- those who cause injury to others would be held responsible and would compensate for damage to person or property.

Virtual Scanning provides the means to implement a system of this nature.

## 6.6    Education

*The process of REPETITION, REPETITION, REPETITION is not just the basis for learning in the educational environment but shapes our health and our thought processes through our exposure to all aspects of our lives.*

Repetition, the process of **adaptation**, influences all aspects of our lives e.g. where we live, the type of house in which we choose to live, types of beer which we drink, types of car which we drive, types of soft drinks which we consume, types of clothes we wear, our political viewpoints, etc, etc.

Everything in our lives is shaped by our exposure to sensory experiences and to those influences which particularly resonate with our genetic profile, now studied as *PsychoSocial Genomics* 55, which predisposes you to become an athlete, artist, academic, scientist, mechanic, cook, etc. This process is known as 'learning' which, at different stages of our lives, becomes dominated by our neural functions i.e. of perception, imagination, memory and associative thinking and of decision-making.

This process, although adopting subtle variations, is fundamentally based on the ability to place ideas in our brain and influence our thoughts and behaviour.  The process is known as education or learning, advertising, branding, influencing and in the most-extreme case of brain-washing.  It is used to fashion our knowledge and beliefs; influence our purchases, political views; and to propagate our way of life. This process defines what are our wants, desires and dreams; and defines our ability to achieve these objectives.

We adapt to our environment to an extraordinary extent. For some this will be a challenge, to align their abilities with achievable objectives, to shape their destiny and achieve. For others this may create stress from a life of perceived under-achievement. If they under-achieve and are continually reminded, by overt or covert means, that they are 'a failure' they will grow to accept that they are less intelligent, less able, 'a failure' and therefore their attitudes and expectations will be 'of failure'. No matter what they achieve in their lives they will have to confront the opinions which have been planted in their brain – when at an impressionable stage of their lives - that they are less worthy, less capable and 'a failure'.

If a belief is established from the earliest age it is likely that the person will grow into adulthood holding this belief irrespective of the prevailing facts and evidence.  It is for this reason that the advertising industry attempts to influence the youngest, and most vulnerable, in society with the happy experiences which are associated with the advertised product.

For a child rejected by the educational system, perhaps through underachievement, they adapt to their environment and seek sensory stimulus, to communicate, and to exist outside of the conventional and traditional mode of development i.e. the educational system. This would result in them becoming, for example, a racing driver, entrepreneur, etc; to prove that they can achieve.

For others the rejection by the educational system and their upbringing in lesser surroundings perhaps with a familial tradition of dishonesty, theft, etc; could result in their adapting to the same stereotypes and pursuit of non-conventional ways of survival which could ultimately lead into delinquency and prison. The importance of education, to teach a child the basic philosophies of life, cannot be under-estimated.

A child brought up in a stable environment with sufficient sensory stimulation and the right type of sensory stimulation will learn from these experiences to be a well-balanced individual, assuming that the negative experiences of their non-family lives do not have a significantly adverse effect; whereas a child raised in an unstable environment may be less aware of the accepted behavioural limits and behave in an apparently hectic, chaotic, and irregular manner.

Sensory deprivation is the most widely used form of punishment in society and ranges from (1) standing a child at the punishment step or standing in the corner wearing the dunces cap, (2) of being excluded, dismissed or 'getting the sack', (3) of 'solitary confinement' or 'being sent to Coventry'. Such techniques of exclusion and deprivation are based upon our fundamental need for sensory stimulus and of the stress created by their effect.

The act of putting prisoners together in a highly stressed, testosterone-charged environment is probably the exact opposite of what is actually required by the process of punishment, remediation and rehabilitation. Sending people to prison risks that they become better criminals through their association with others who have similar problems, and from the tuition of other more experienced prisoners. It is imperative to educate through repetition, repetition, repetition the justification to become law-abiding people and to show the benefits of such a course of action. Being law-abiding must be proven to be a better option than being delinquent. Moreover the punishment must be appropriate to the age and circumstances of the delinquent. For instance the punishment for an 18y.o who is born in poverty should not be similar to that meted out to a man of 55 y.o. who lives in relative wealth.

Consider the effect of advertisers and broadcasters to influence our spending patterns but also their ability to influence our patterns of behaviour. These organisations have a responsibility to represent our society in a balanced manner and not to over-sensationalise issues or to make inaccurate depictions of modern life which could influence the opinions of the most vulnerable and impressionable. They have a responsibility to make a positive effort to represent civilised behaviour and hence to raise the standards of society and counteract regressive or primitive behaviour.

The education system is designed to treat children irrespective of their social background and abilities. This was not always the case when we look back at the history of schools and the changes from the grammar school system to the comprehensive school system.

In any education system it is necessary to consider a number of issues including:

- The ability of the teachers to teach

- The teaching methods

- The learning methods

- The ability of the children to learn.

The **ability of teachers to teach** has undergone dramatic changes and ensures that these people have the time and resources to teach in a quality manner however there remains question marks over the **teaching methods** in the most basic and important issue i.e. of reading. The method used has been in debate for many years – analytic or synthetic phonics however if you consider the following paragraph you will understand that the issue is not yet resolved.

*'I cdnuolt blveiee taht I cluod aulaclty uesdnatnrd waht I was rdgnieg. The phaonmneal pweor of the hmuan mnid. Aoccdrnig to a rscheearch at Cmabrigde Uinervtisy, it deosn't mttaer in waht oredr the ltteers in a wrod are, the olny iprmoatnt tihng is taht the frist and lsat ltteer be in the rghit pclae. The rset can be a taotl mses and you can still raed it wouthit a porbelm. Tihs is bcuseae the huamn mnid deos not raed ervey lteter by istlef, but the wrod as a wlohe. Amzanig huh? yaeh and I awlyas thuohgt spleling was ipmorantt !'*

This proves that neither method is a truly accurate reflection of how we read although it would be ridiculous to argue that we should discard either method. It does indicate that the issue should be open to further discussions.

Despite all of the changes which have taken place since the introduction of the comprehensive school system, and despite the contribution by educational psychologists, there has been little consideration of the latter two factors: the **'learning methods'** and the **'ability of the children to learn'**.

It can be argued that one of the most significant contribution appears to have been the recognition of the value of nutrition and of its relationship to the mental abilities of children throughout their time at school yet as outlined earlier in this book these findings are not new but are in fact a symptom of the failure of government and academia to recognise the importance of the factors which affect the health and hence the learning abilities of our children. Many of these 'new' research findings are not 'new' but are, it appears, the updating of research which was conducted in the 30's, 50's, etc. New developments indicate that this approach is not yet the solution to the problem.

**Poor diet, arising from a fast-food diet, undoubtedly affects the physiological development of the mind and body's of our children**. This developmental disorder is manifest in ways which affect memory, concentration, and cognition. We recognise it, to some extent, through tests which assess the ability of a child to hear, read and write.

The issue is considered by many to be a reflection of a person's personality and their genes yet many who have been educational underachievers have gone on to be achievers in their adult lives. Some, identified as dyslexic, have gone on to be world-leading sportsmen and businessmen so the issue cannot be considered to be the simplistic reflection of who and what you are. It must also take into account that these people were not able to express themselves in the learning environment due to a combination of factors which affected their ability to memorise, concentrate, read, write, etc.

Most research has focussed on the assessment of the presenting symptoms in order to categorise these people however there has been relatively little research into the origins of the condition. **It takes the emergence of a new technology, Virtual Scanning, to cast light upon the fundamental origins of learning difficulties which affect children.**

Flashing Light therapies have existed since the 1930's, originally as 'photic stimulation' and more recently as biofeedback, and the flashing light therapies of empirical nature, which are marketed for the treatment of dyslexia.

Clinical trials of the flashing light therapies have shown promise since their first use in the 1930's. A great deal of research into this type of therapeutic approach was shelved following the discovery of sulpha drugs which were used for their antibacterial properties and which are widely considered to have been the precursor of penicillin. These have failed to make progress due to the empirical nature of the research 47 which, as can be seen from this publication, could only be overcome with the use of the most advanced mathematics and the power of the computer. Despite this set back flashing light therapies have continued to attract interest and are widely associated with a number of observations including the power to improve intellect.

In the dyslexic condition, hitherto considered as the sole domain of psychologists, Virtual Scanning has identified a range of medical issues which have an effect upon the child's ability to concentrate and hence to learn. Virtual Scanning appears to be the only technology in the world which is able to give such a comprehensive and detailed report and hence make such conclusions.

Further research illustrates that the flashing light therapies are associated with improved IQ. and that children who suffer from ADD and ADHD are often shown to have brain-wave patterns which have a high theta component and a low beta component, and hence which are associated with their ability to concentrate. (Further reading of brain wave research 59-93)

Consider the effect of the above factors in relation to the modern mineral and vitamin deficient diet often involving 'drinking acidic, carbonated drinks, often with high levels of Sodium, Phosphates, Sugar, and additives (e.g. Tartrazine, Caffeine, Aspartame, etc), often packed in Aluminium cans'.

By virtue of their chemical constituent soft drinks are designed to induce changes to the functional systems of a child and hence to induce changes to

- Acidity thereby affecting the mineral balance;

- the child's ability to concentrate - associated with the effect of caffeine;

- the pancreatic system involving large release of insulin;

and the effect of

- artificial colourants, nucleosides and salt in artificial flavourings, and artificial sweeteners.

These have been which have been implicated in child hyperactivity and educational underachievement for many years.

## 6.7 Delinquency & Criminality

Often associated with educational insufficiency a very high percentage of delinquents (estimated to be over 90%) are known to have learning inhibition e.g. as dyslexia, attention deficit disorder, and various associated learning disorders however to conclude that delinquency is the direct product of educational insufficiency which has a biological basis [27] should be considered a gross oversimplification of a highly complex issue.

The statistics available differ from country to country and of course the remit of each study differs. In the US [28,29] there is an estimated 2million people in prison of which c70% are functionally illiterate; and c40% of youth delinquents in detention centres have learning disabilities including dyslexia. By comparison [30] of the c90-100,000 people in prison in the UK the extent of learning problems varies: 80% of prisoners have poor writing skills, 50% have reading difficulties and 65% have trouble with numeracy although the level of those with dyslexia is not considered to be significant from the normal population (4-10%) but is instead considered to be related to their social background.

Nevertheless there must be influences which, directly or indirectly, have an effect upon a person's predisposition to delinquency e.g.

- Social/family background – if raised within a stable family environment

- Any **medical conditions** which have an effect upon a person's ability to learn and concentrate

- Alcoholism, drug-taking, etc which feeds crime – alcohol, nicotine and caffeine are now recognised to be highly addictive and damaging to our health. They significantly affect our behaviour and mental stability.

The study of brainwaves and in particular the alpha and theta waves has been widely studied [31] although much of the research has an empirical basis. Nevertheless researchers have understood how they can generate sufficient alpha waves and hence induce a deeply relaxed state - a state as deep as that reached by people who'd meditated for years – and that this can be used to reduce stress and anxiety and to help manage pain.

More recently [32] it has been demonstrated that by boosting the alpha and theta waves of chronic alcoholics it has been possible to achieve an unprecedented 80 percent abstinence rate, compared to 20 percent in the comparison group which received conventional medications including antidepressants. Moreover, when the participants in the study were followed up five years later, their recovery rate remained at 70 percent.

The same principle applies to all aspects of behaviour which, as outlined earlier in this book (chapters 1&3), illustrates how our mental decision-making is directly influenced by our biochemistry, which is regulated by the brain waves, and which is in turn affected by the two primary influences or data inputs i.e. of stress and diet.

**Virtual Scanning enables us to identify and treat those psychosocial issues** which, as outlined in earlier chapters.........

- involve dietary factors,

- affect stress levels,

- are manifest as health issues,

- are conceivably manifest as alcoholism and drug-dependency,

- affect a person's ability to learn, memorise and concentrate,

and ultimately affects their progress through the educational system and which could ultimately affect their employability, self-esteem, and ability to succeed in life.

## 6.8    Sporting Achievement

Virtual Scanning is considered by the Director of the Lesgaft Institute (Vysochin Yu), to be the single most effective means of improving an athlete's performance. It is now used by various Russian sports institutes to improve the performance of their athletes. As Professor Vysochin was in charge of the medical preparation of athletes for competition at the 1980 Olympiads his comments should be seriously considered.  Bearing in mind that Russia remains one of the top two the leading sporting nations it seems reasonable to conclude that Russian sports physiologists understanding of physiological function remains more advanced than the experts of most other nations.

Virtual Scanning has been used to prepare Russian athlete's for the 2000 and 2004 Olympiads. Russian athletes consistently perform at the highest levels of sporting achievement throughout their careers.

The understanding of the physiological functional systems which regulate our health facilitates an unparalleled understanding of the processes which inhibit and relax the organism against the extreme influences of the various stress factors which subsequently result in homeostatic infringements and in a distortion of the oxygen and carbon dioxide ratio in the organism.

Considering the background of stress effects and of the associated homeostatic infringements which affect performance, Virtual Scanning therapy activates the relaxation processes and decreases excitability; regulates the nervous processes; improves regulatory function of the central nervous system and coordinates the physiological systems. This significantly improves the function of the skeletal muscles.

Further aspects of the effectiveness of the therapy includes: significant improvement of movement regulation and coordination; increased effectiveness of the central nervous system, neuromuscular, cardiovascular, respiratory, neuro-endocrine and other systems; improvement of muscular blood supply and muscular activity energy supply; acceleration of the reduction processes and resynthesis of energy resources; and finally leads to homeostasis and increase physical efficiency or the "second wind" effect" .

Accordingly by understanding the principles [33] it can be possible to improve the performance of athletes who have to run faster over short distances, lift more weights, run faster for longer distances, or which involve a combination of performance, balance and skills e.g. as in football.

Take the example of a professional footballer (see chapter 4: page 74)

Age 21 years with a history of broken bones which had occurred on several occasions in this young footballers career and which were affecting his ability to appear for the club each week.  We note from the test report indications of chronic fatigue in the endocrine system and osteoporosis which supports

This can be explained by a history of drinking and overtraining; perhaps with poor diet an overindulgent social life and poor sleeping patterns. This would result in an underperforming endocrine system, and in particular the pituitary and adrenal glands, which results in progressive decalcification of the bone structure and hence a susceptibility to breakages.

Further indications of anaemia, leukaemia and phlebitis may also be indicative of poor energy levels and of conditions which could ultimately result in the premature termination of this footballers career.

The ability to diagnose these conditions earlier in the footballer's career could have resulted in remedial action which could have prolonged his career and improved his ability to perform or to have been used to guide him into another career. This information would also have been invaluable to the club to judge whether to continue to invest in this footballer.

Over-exercising can be as damaging to health as under-exercising and in women can result in menstrual dysfunction and problems with bone metabolism [35]. Low bone mass can result in poor muscle and ligament development – there is simply not enough good quality bone upon which ligament and muscle are bound – which subsequently is manifest as susceptibility to muscle and ligament injuries. If there is not sufficient bone mass this will affect muscle development but also the quantity and quality of the white blood cells in the immune system and the ability to convert blood glucose into energy. As all systems are to some extent inter-connected it can reasonably be expected to affect the stability of all other physiological systems including the quantity and quality of red blood cells which affect the ability to absorb oxygen.

*** 

The psychology of an athlete is considered to be an essential requirement for good performance and psychological training and conditioning is considered essential for good athletic performance, especially by sporting coaches in the US.

In general a young athlete's performance is affected by stress. It is almost legendary that a sportsman performs so much better in practice than under competitive conditions. The ability to deal with anxiety can dramatically reduce an athlete's ability to perform at the peak of their abilities. Most athlete's ability to perform increases steadily throughout their years of adult maturity which is coincident with improved mental function and hence of improved brainwave function. (Further reading [94-100])

Virtual Scanning is the first technology which is precisely able to determine and to alleviate the limiting psychological and physiological factors which affect an athlete's performance.

## 6.9    Military & Performance-related Professions

*Would the military actually wish to know whether their staff is fit for deployment or not [48].*

The military recognises that the soldier is the most vulnerable link in the completion of military tasks. Their ability to perform under the most extreme stress undoubtedly affects their ability to think and perform as planned and to achieve military objectives.

From recognition of 'shell-shock' as perhaps the most extreme response to pressure there is a muted recognition that the combat arena provides the most far-seeking examination of the character of a combatant and moreover that the magnitude and extent of exposure to stress will result in the steady development of stress-related disorders which will affect

- the level of their performance in the combat arena

- their ability to recover during rest periods

- the levels of health services which are required to support combatants

- the levels of compensation which may be awarded to former combatants

- and finally, the future ability to recruit soldiers

Stress undoubtedly affects the ability of the combatant to think clearly and lucidly. It affects their ability to sleep and consequently it steadily and insidiously affects all aspects of their physiology. It affects the level of energy which they can function and it affects their ability to act promptly as instructed and as required to complete a manoeuvre with least risk.

It is for this reason that entertainment, and R&R, of the troops is considered to be essential to maintain good morale and functionality. On the other hand, at the most extreme levels of stress, it can be responsible for acts of apparently complete disregard for personal safety.

Virtual Scanning has the ability to diagnose the psychological, psycho-emotional and health profiles of a combatant which can be invaluable in determining the suitability of personnel for combat operations and of establishing when combatants should be considered for less onerous non-combat duties. Moreover, through therapy, it potentially (in the right circumstances) provides a temporary solution during deployment where therapy can be used to reduce the stress of the combat situation [48,49]

What would happen if the pressures of war were considered to be unreasonable and beyond that to which any combatant should be exposed? Could this lead to a dramatic reduction in the use of troops as a means of delivering a military initiative?

## 6.10 Recruitment

*Consider how technology could affect the ability to recruit an employee and to monitor and optimise their performance in the work environment.*

As a result of personal problems in their social/home lives, or of failing health, increasing age or increasing weight, the patient could for example become predisposed to emotional, psychological and health changes which would affect their ability to function in the work environment. Virtual Scanning would have massive benefit for the recruitment industry which would be better able to select and place good employees and, moreover, for the employer who could routinely check the health of their employees. This information could be used to enable the employer

- to adhere to their legal obligations to look after the health of their employees (and if necessary employees families).

- to minimise lost time due to illness and hence to reduce the need for additional staff or overtime payments.

- to minimise accidents in the workplace which are due to stress and consequently of lesser levels of concentration which result in adverse, careless and potentially dangerous occurrences.

- to examine how a worker is coping with unusual work systems and projects e.g. including long hours, shift working, etc.

- to examine less productive work groups i.e. to locate the reasons for the lowered productivity and failings of the group.

- to examine options to change work patterns, group structures, members of the team, etc

- to recruit employees which can fit into an established team

- to examine an employee's suitability for promotion

- to maintain a harmonious and positive working environment.

- to examine the orientation of employees towards alcoholism and the use of recreational drugs

- to examine the failure of interpersonal relationships which may for example explode as outburst of anger, frustration and negative outbursts which would result in lost time, lost productivity, etc.

For the recruitment company this could lead to a massively improved service to the client which will lead to better placements, better performance by these new employees, and ultimately to a recognition by the employer of the improved calibre of employee from the employment agency.

The ability to work with the client and to monitor the psychology and health of employees will lead to better performance, less turnover of staff, a more harmonious work environment, and ultimately a more cost-effective service with less time spent on resolving staff problems and ultimately less expenditure on staffing. This will result in an improved reputation, greater loyalty from existing clients, and an increased portfolio of satisfied clients.

The employer will benefit by being able to work with an organisation which can provide a comprehensive and competitive programme which is able to provide and monitor the ability of staff to perform as required.

The employee will benefit by having the support of an organisation which can assist them to resolve stress-related issues which would ultimately reduce their effectiveness, their prospects for promotion, their job satisfaction, and ultimately that they would leave seeking other opportunities.

## 6.11 Detection and Treatment of Mental Health Issues

*If a person becomes mentally unwell due to the effects of stress could this process be reversed by understanding how stress has affected their ability to function and by using appropriate therapies to reverse this process?*

An estimated 90% of mental health patients have a physiological ailment. In fact some psychologists [31] have considered that various conditions considered to be psychological may in fact be the result of a physiological disorder e.g. bowel blockage, lupus, brain tumors, hyperthyroidism, Lyme disease, Tourette's and Klinefelter's syndromes.

Current research [39] illustrates that men and women with schizophrenia are significantly more likely to have one or more of 46 common chronic health conditions than individuals without mental illness. Moreover in studies sponsored by the NIMH it has been shown that by comparison with individuals without mental illness, persons with schizophrenia were more likely to have a greater number of conditions spanning several disease categories including cardiovascular, pulmonary, neurological, and endocrine diseases.

An estimated 30% of those with schizophrenia below 40 y.o already had three or more chronic physical health conditions. Clinical Depression [40] is now associated with a group of interconnected brain regions that fail to communicate properly. This organ failure is responsible for the sense of hopelessness, fatigue and inability to cope that are the outward hallmarks of depression. Mental health conditions are now increasingly dealt with as a biological problem, with medication for high blood pressure, heartburn, etc.

Our mental health upon which our cognition is based is dependent upon the health of organs in our brain AND our body i.e of the function, operability and interconnectivity of our component parts. It is beyond dispute that our mental health and our mental development, which affects our function, can be affected in the same way that our physiology can be affected by the various stress factors in our daily lives.

Within psychiatry [41, 42] there is debate e.g.

(1) whether the mental health of the patient could in part, or in whole, be due to physiological problems?
(2) whether the mental health patient patient has a brain which is unable to regulate its neurochemistry?
(3) does manipulating the already compromised system with drugs help or hinder its long term ability to function properly?
(4) by using a drug, do you prevent the body producing biochemicals which are essential for stability?
(5) by altering the level of one neurochemical using drugs, do we alter the level of other chemicals and hence create the possibility of other potentially more complex mental health problems in the future?
(6) by using drugs, do we affect the function of the brain waves in a manner which is damaging to the body/brain's physiological stability?

This is entirely consistent with the findings reported in this book and with the Theory of Brain Wave Synchronisation in which the function of the organs, their activity and interconnectivity are implicit aspects of brain function and hence of the psychology and physiology of the person.

Many of the symptoms which are dealt with by psychologists e.g.

- Depression and mood swings
- Shyness and social anxiety
- Panic attacks and phobias
- Cravings, obsessions and compulsions (OCD and related conditions)
- Chronic anxiety or worry
- Post-traumatic stress symptoms (PTSD and related conditions)
- Eating disorders (anorexia and bulimia) and obesity
- Insomnia and other sleep problems
- Difficulty establishing or staying in relationships
- Problems with marriage or other relationships you're already in
- Job, career or school difficulties
- Feeling "stressed out"
- Insufficient self-esteem (accepting or respecting yourself)
- Inadequate coping skills, or ill-chosen methods of coping
- Passivity, procrastination and "passive aggression"
- Substance abuse, co-dependency and "enabling"
- Trouble keeping feelings such as anger, sadness, fear, guilt, shame, eagerness, excitement, etc., within bounds
- Over-inhibition of feelings or expression

These are now demonstrated to be the psychosomatic traits which are characteristic of a person's physiology. We are who we are as a result of our genetic profile and of the accumulation of our past experiences and memories. Our physiology is not independent of our psychology. Nature and nurture are both relevant. One cannot be separated from the other. Together they make up who we are.

We cannot erase our past memories but we can resolve these ailments (which have arisen as a result of past stress events). Virtual Scanning is one of a number of therapies such as cognitive behavioural therapy, psychotherapy, hypnosis, medication, virtual scanning therapy, etc; which can be used to address these psychological ailments.

## 6.12  Industry

*How would industry benefit if we could reduce the costs associated with sickness and absenteeism?*

The cost to British Industry 43 of stress-related sickness is estimated to be £1.24BN pa according to a recent survey of managers.

The impact of illness upon UK business is an estimated £1.25Bn pa according to a recent survey of industry managers in the UK. Of the 700 managers polled stress was considered to lower productivity and 60 percent blamed it for higher rates of staff turnover.

Of the data provided by the 581 employers who responded with data, c1.5M days were lost to stress which suggests that c11% of the UK's total sickness absence was due to stress.

Apart from the obvious indications of absenteeism and illness the effect of stress creates inter-personal tensions which affects the working environment, reduces productivity, increases job dissatisfaction. In the most extreme cases results this may have implications, perhaps through alcoholism, drug-taking, impaired sleep, etc; which affect a worker's performance and their safety in the work environment.

Stress in the workplace carries a cost:

- of increased staff turnover and increased recruitment costs

- of loss of key employees, lost expertise, and potentially loss of order

- the time and cost of mistakes

- of long-term absenteeism, the need to recruit temporary employees, and of increased insurance premiums
- of lost productivity due to internal strife

- of lost productivity due to accidents

- of the need to pay higher wages

Virtual Scanning provides a means of monitoring the psychological and physiological profile of an employee and hence is able to monitor the effect of stress upon a person's behaviour.

In addition, by treating the psychosomatic effects of stress using Virtual Scanning Colour Therapy it is possible to reduce the effect of stress on the employee and hence improve their ability to function which lessens their negative effect upon their colleagues in the workplace.

The modern society is based upon achievement of a lifestyle which offers perceived benefits. Success is considered to bring the benefits of an improved lifestyle, of greater levels of comfort, and of greater **self-esteem** yet we cannot all be successful. There is a wide gap between the rich and poor in society which affects our perceived self-esteem from work but self-esteem is not solely based upon achievement in the work environment. It is also based upon our perceived value in society.

Low self-esteem is considered to be a factor in behavioural problems. Insufficient outlets for our energies and for our ability to achieve at something damage our self-esteem and self-confidence. **Our society is growing and yet the outlets for someone to differentiate themselves are not growing.** The competition for our perceived sense of achievement upon which self-esteem is based is becoming greater. Our teenage children seemingly have insufficient pride, lack self-restraint, dress to reflect their low self-esteem, and conceivably lack the personal self-confidence which is required to pursue personal objectives. Perhaps their lives lack the spectrum of activities which are essential for their personal development.

For some, pursuit of the quick buck has overtaken the need for discipline, dedication, persistence and hard work. The 'big brother' syndrome illustrates how fame is sought by individuals, often by many who lack talent but who seek an identity i.e. who have low self-esteem.

Society is the big loser because, as a result, the pool of skilled labour is low, the workforce lacks incentives and pride, we have high levels of alcoholism, drunkenness, obesity and violent behaviour which has to be financed from taxation. As a result those with strongly held religious viewpoints and who treasure family values are appalled by the behaviour of youth in western societies.

Amongst the consequences – we eat to excess, we drink alcohol without moderation, and eventually we pay the penalty.

Businesses suffer because this lack of self-esteem equates to a lack of demand for the better things in life e.g. suits, fashion clothing, etc; which are produced by indigenous companies and hence which required skilled labour - whereas by contrast society is now supplied by the cheap mass produced items.

There are lessons to be learned.

## 6.13  Beauty and Wellbeing

*What benefits would Virtual Scanning bring to the Beauty Industry?*

Beauty and wellbeing can be used to describe our outer beauty and our inner beauty i.e. the beauty of our physical form and the beauty of our inner form.

Cosmetics and perfumes have been used for thousands of years to make a woman more alluring to a man and in recent years this has become a multi-billion dollar industry yet like the medical industry this approach has distinct limitations because it only disguises the person's exterior. Beauty is not just about the physical form but is also about demeanor, vitality, energy, poise, presentation, warmth and wellbeing.  If you are not well how can you be beautiful?

### Light up your Life

Virtual Scanning gives the person an option for improvement of their health and hence to improve the condition of their skin, health, self-confidence, energy levels, mental clarity, and their feelings of wellbeing.

For example:

- By stimulating the systems which regulate blood flow Virtual Scanning is able to improve skin texture and treat issues which affect appearance e.g. psoriasis, eczema, etc.

- By stimulating the systems which regulate blood flow to the brain Virtual Scanning is able to improve mental clarity.

- By stimulating the systems which regulate our endocrine system Virtual Scanning is able to relieve depression, improve energy levels and improve a person's quality of life.

- By stimulating the systems which regulate our sexual function Virtual Scanning is conceivably able to improve sexual performance and reproducibility.

- By simulating the systems which regulate blood flow to the spinal chord and skeletal structure Virtual Scanning is conceivably able to improve poise, presentation and mobility.

## 6.14 How can we use this information to improve the quality and quantity of our lives?

Virtual Scanning is not a miracle therapy. It just explains a phenomena which has hitherto not been understood. Arising from this therapy we are able to recognise the importance of a number of health-related issues which have, perhaps, become less valued in society over the last 50 years.

No medical text would be complete without some recommendations about how to maintain or improve your health. These are, unsurprisingly:

- The importance of sufficient good quality sleep

- The need to eliminate stress and the importance of periods of rest and relaxation in our lives
- The importance of a good quality diet with sufficient protein, appropriate fatty acids, et al
- The importance of appropriately sized food portions for male and female, young and old.
- The need for regular exercise

- The need for adequate sensory stimulus through colour, music, play, etc

- The value of a safe, secure and happy home when raising children i.e. stress-free environment

And, by contrast, we caution

- excessive exposure to television and late viewing (to differing degrees by children and adults)
- the adverse effect of alcohol upon the quality and quantity of sleep, and upon our psychoemotional stability
- the adverse and potentially irreversible consequences of recreational drugs

- the adverse influence of a fast food diet and of inadequate levels of protein in the diet
- the adverse influence of soft drinks containing caffeine, phosphoric acid and perhaps also of artificial sweeteners
- the adverse influence of inadequate levels of exercise

- too much emphasis upon the use of computer games which improve short-term response at the expense of long-term memory. Take the computers and televisions out of your child's room, put it in a study area.
- overuse of mobile phones

**What can we do to ward off the advancing years and to increase our longevity and quality of life?**

- Maintain the brain waves through mental and physical activity

- Avoid excessive habits and try and include change in your lives

- Select a diet which is appropriate for your age and your current state of health

- Adjust your weight to an appropriate level

- Seek out friendly contacts and avoid loneliness.

- Give yourself a purpose in life.

- Avoid stress

- Focus upon your future

# References:

1. *Scientific American* September 2003, A.Caplan

2. http://www.lifeprinciples.co.uk/downloads/Last.pdf

3. comments attributed to Dr Jeansok Kim of the University of Washington

4. *The Lancet,* 1998; 351; 637-641

5. http://www.infowars.com/articles/science/autism_none_for_unvaccinated_amish.htm;

6. http://en.wikipedia.org/wiki/Autism_(incidence); http://en.wikipedia.org/wiki/Dan_Olmsted

7. http://www.ssi.dk/sw4252.asp;

8. http://www.usatoday.com/news/opinion/editorials/2005-07-05-oppose_x.htm

9. http://www.ncbi.nlm.nih.gov/entrez/query.fcgi?cmd=Retrieve&db=pubmed&dopt=Abstract&list_uids=12949291

10. *Journal of Pediatrics* 2003 Sep;112(3 Pt 1):604-6; Thimerosal and the occurrence of autism: negative ecological evidence from Danish population-based data; Madsen K.M, Lauritsen M.B, Pedersen C.B, Thorsen P, Plesner A.M, Andersen P.H, Mortensen P.B.

11. bird flu vaccine ineffective

12. *FDA web site*

13. TAMIFLU-Guillain Barre link

14. *FDA web site*

15. *Pediatrics*, 2006; 117: 620-5

16. http://www.cancer.gov/cancertopics/factsheet/Risk/HPV

17. The rate of occurrence is typically 3-4 per 100,000 and the occurrence of cervical cancer happens typically 20-50 years after infection

18. Duesberg.P and Schwartz.J, Progress in Nucleic Acid Research and Molecular Biology 43:135-204, 1992 **Latent Viruses and Mutated Oncogenes: No Evidence for Pathogenicity**

19. www.redflagsweekly.com/second_opinion/2002_nov25.html

20. *New England Journal of Medicine* 347:1645-1651 A Controlled Trial of a Human Papillomavirus Type 16 Vaccine, Koutsky.L.A., et al

21. Munoz N, Bosch FX, de Sanjosé S, et al. Epidemiologic classification of human papillomavirus types associated with cervical cancer. *New England Journal of Medicine* 2003; 348(6):518–527.

22.     Castle PE, Wacholder S, Lorincz AT, et al. A prospective study of high-grade cervical neoplasia risk among human papillomavirus-infected women. *Journal of the National Cancer Institute* 2002; 94(18):1406–1414.

23.     www.ahrp.org/cms/content/view/263/28/;

24.     comments attributed to Barbara Loe Fisher, President, National Vaccine Information Centre

25.     pcv vaccine as reported in wddty

26.     Dr Vera Scheibner, "Vaccination: The Medical Assault on the Immune System" pub.....

27.     Biological causes of deviant behaviour:  Moir, Anne & David Jessel, "A Mind to Crime", (London: Signet Books, 1995).

28.     U.S. Department of Justice, Bureau of Justice Statistics June 2002

29.     *Office of Juvenile Justice and Delinquency Prevention 1994 and U.S.Department   of Justice, Bureau of Justice Statistics 1995*

30.     http://www.dyslexia-parent.com/mag50.html

31.     Alpha-theta biofeedback was pioneered in the '70s by Elmer and Alyce Green of the Menninger Clinic in Topeka, Kansas -- still a leading center for biofeedback research -- and Joe Kamiya, a researcher in San Francisco.

32.     Eugene Peniston, a clinical psychologist then of Fort Lyon Veterans Affairs Medical Center in Fort Lyon, Colorado

33.     Legwold.G., Colour boosted energy: How Light Affects Muscle Action, *American Health*, May 1988.

34.     *Journal of  Cell Metabolism*, March 2007, Enriori. P, Cowley. M, et al

35.     *British Medical Journal* 2007, 334: 164-5

36.     *American Journal of Clinical Nutrition*, 2006, 84, 3, 475-482, Wolfe R.R.

37.     'A Dose of Sanity' Dr. Sydney Walker, (former director of Southern California's Neuropsychiatric Institute), pub: John Wiley & Sons Inc., 1996

38.     *Journal of General Internal Medicine*, November 2006

39.     Caroline Carney Doebbeling, M.D., M.Sc., associate professor of psychiatry and medicine at the Indiana University School of Medicine and a research scientist at the Regenstrief Institute, Inc. Co-authors of the study are Laura Jones, M.Sc., of the University of Iowa, and Robert F. Woolson, Ph.D., of the Medical University of South Carolina. The research was funded by the National Institute of Mental Health.

40. http://mednews.stanford.edu/stanmed/2005fall/brain-main.html

41. review of the EEG and depression, see Pollack, V.E. & Schneider, L.S., *Journal of Biological Psychiatry*, Vol. 27:757.

42. http://www.greatbrain.com/thesamscenter_006.htm

43. reported in *Personnel Today* magazine

44. Psychosocial Genomics

45. Critser.G., How Americans became the Fattest people in the World" pub Houghton Mifflin, NY   www.newstarget.com/004416.html

46. "Soft Drinks Undermining Americans Health" op cit  Jackobson.M.F, 1998

47. *Journal of Dyslexia* 11:61-77 (2005), An Evaluation of a Visual Biofeedback Intervention in Dyslexic Adults, Liddle.E, Jackson.J, Jackson.S

48. Norvikov VS. "Psycho-physiological Support of Combat Activities of Military Personnel". *Military Medical Journal.* 1996; No. 4, P 37-40.

49. *Novikov.VS, Sharmin IA, Bornovsky VN 1992 A trial of the Pharmacological Correction of Sleep Disorders of Sailors during a  Voyage , Military Medical Journal 8, 47-49*

50. Delong.R,  In Live Viral Vaccine, Biological Pollution, (Carlton Press, New York, 1996).,

51. Mirko D Grmek, *Histoire du SIDA*, Payot, 1989, p. 261

52. *Medical Practice* (No 467) Lépine.

53. *The Dayton Times*, 28 May 1993, published details from a study by the *Department of Health*

54. *Le Concours Médical*, No 8, 1993 (Vol 115) by Sicot.C

55. Shirakawa.T, *Science*, Vol 275, 3 Jan 1997.

56. 'La Poliomyélite: quel vaccin? quel risque?', *L'Aronde*, 1997, Pilette.J

57. 'Vaccination  : Social Violence and Criminality' (North Atlantic Books, Berkeley, 1980), Coulter.H

58. *Science*, Vol 29, 19 July 1985

## Further reading

59. Linder, M., Habib, T., & Radojevic, V (1993). A controlled study of the effects of EEG biofeedback on the cognition and behavior of children with attention deficit disorders and learning disabilities. Manuscript submitted for publication.

60. Lubar, J. F. Psychophysiology and biofeedback treatment for attention deficit hyperactivity disorder. Handout administered by Dr. Lubar.

61. Lubar, J. F (1991). Discourse on the development of EEG diagnostics and biofeedback treatment for attention deficit/hyperactivity disorders. *Biofeedback and Self-Regulation*, 16, 201-225.

62. Lubar, J. F., & Shouse M. N. (1976a). EEG and behavioral changes in a hyperkinetic child concurrent with training of the sensorimotor rhythm (SMR): A preliminary report. *Biofeedback and Self Regulation*, 3, 293-306. 1

63. Lubar, J. F., & Shouse M. N. (1976b). Use of biofeedback in the treatment of seizure disorders and hyperactivity *Advances in Clinical Child Psychology*, 1, 203-265.

64. Mann, C. A., Lubar, J. F, Zimmerman, A. W., Miller, B. A., & Muenchen, R. A. (1992). Quantitative analysis of EEG in boys with attention deficit/hyperactivity disorder. A controlled study with clinical implications. *Pediatric Neurology*, 8, 3036.

65. Tansey, M. A., & Bruner, R. L. (1983). EMG and EEG biofeedback training in the treatment of a 10-year old hyperactive boy with a developmental reading disorder. *Biofeedback and Self-Regulation*, 8, 25-37.

66. *Journal of Neurotherapy*: Reprint (1-2)3 EEG Biofeedback: A New Treatment Option For ADD/ADHD, Marabella A. Alhambra, M.D., Timothy P. Fowler, and Antonio A. Alhambra, M.D.

    Attention Deficit Disorder is commonly treated with stimulant medications such as Ritalin (methylphenidate). However, this medication has short-term effects and numerous undesirable side effects including insomnia and loss of appetite. This study explores using EEG biofeedback, with its minimal side effects and long-term results, as an alternative to pharmacological treatments for ADD.

67. *Pediatric Neurology*, Vol. 21, No. 3, 633-637. ... Lubar, Joel F, and Judith O. Lubar. (1999). Neurofeedback Assessment and Treatment For Attention

68. White, J. Noland Jr., M.S., Joel F. Lubar, Ph.D., M.O. Swartwood, Ph.D., & J.N. Swartwood, Ph.D. (1999). Relationships between T.O.V.A. Measures and Age-dependent QEEG in ADHD Boys. *Presented at the Annual Meeting of the National Academy of Neuropsychology*, San Antonia, TX, November 1999.

69. Lubar, Joel F. (1997). Neocortical Dynamics: Implications for Understanding the Role of Neurofeedback and Related Techniques for the Enhancement of Attention. *Applied Psychophysiology and Biofeedback,* Vol. 22, No. 2, 111-126.

70. Lubar, Joel F., PhD, J. Noland White, Jr, MS, Michie O. Swartwood, PhD, & Jeffery N. Swartwood, PhD. (1999). Methylphenidate Effects on Global and Complex Measures of EEG. *Pediatric Neurology,* Vol. 21, No. 3, 633-637.

71. Lubar, Judith O., Joel F. Lubar. (1984). Electroencephalographic Biofeedback of SMR and Beta for Treatment of Attention Deficit Disorders in a Clinical Setting. *Biofeedback and Self-Regulation.* Vol. 9, No. 1, 1-23

72. White, J. Noland , Joel F. Lubar. (1999). Effects if Methylphenidate on Global and Complex Measures of EEG. Citation Poster, 194-196.

73. Hoffman, Daniel A., M.D., Joel F. Lubar, Ph.D., Robert W. Thatcher, Ph.D., M. Barry Sterman, Ph.D., Peter J. Rosenfeld, Ph.D., Sebastien Striefel, Ph.D., David Trudeau, M.D., and Steve Stockdale, Ph.D. (1999). Limitations of the American Academy of Neurology and American Clinical Neurophysiology Society Paper on QEEG. *Journal of Neuropsychiatry Clinical Neuroscience.* Vol. 11:3, 401-407.

74. Lubar, J.F., PhD, K.J. Bianchini, BA, W.H. Calhaun, PhD, E.W. Lambert, PhD, Z.H. Brody, MA and H.S. Shabsin, PhD. (1985). Spectral Analysis of EEG Differences Between Children With and Without Learning Disabilities. *Journal of Learning Disabilities.* Vol. 18, No. 7, August/ September, 403-406.

75. Timmermann, DeAnna L., Joel F. Lubar, Howard W. Rasey, Jon A. Fredrick. (1998). Effects of 20-min audio-visual stimulation (AVS) at dominant alpha frequency and twice dominant alpha frequency on the cortical EEG. *International Journal of Psychophysiology.* Vol. 32, 55-61.

76. Rasey, Howard W.,B.A., Joel F. Lubar, Ph.D., Anne McIntyre, Ph.D., Anthony C. Zoffuto, B.S., and Paul L. Abbott, B.A. (1998). EEG Biofeedback for the Enhancement of Attentional Processing in Normal College Students. *Journal of Neurotherapy.* Vol. 1, No. 3, 15-21.

77. Benham, Grant,B.Sc., Howard W. Rasey, B.A., Joel F. Lubar, Ph.D., Jon A. Fredrick, M.S., and A. Charles Zoffuto, B.S. (1997). EEG Power- Spectral and Coherence Differences Between Attentional States during a Complex Auditory Task. *Journal of Neurotherapy.* Fall/Winter, 1-9.

78. Swartwood, Michie O., PhD, Jeffrey N. Swartwood, PhD, Joel F. Lubar, PhD, DeAnna Timmermann, BS, Andrew W. Zimmerman, MD, and Robert A Muenchen, MS. (1998). Methylphenidate Effects on EEG, Behavior, and Performance in Boys with ADHD. *Pediatric Neurology.* Vol. 18, No. 3, 244-250.

79. Lubar, Joel F, and Judith O. Lubar. (1999). Neurofeedback Assessment and Treatment For Attention Deficit/Hyperactivity Disorders. Introduction to Quantitative EEG and Neurofeedback. Academic Press. P 103-143.

80. Rasey, H. W., Lubar, J. E., McIntyre, A., Zoffuto, A. C., & Abbot, P.L. (1996). EEG Biofeedback for the enhancement of attentional processing in normal college students. *Journal of Neurotherapy*, 1, 15-31.

81. Lubar, J. F., Swartwood, M. O., Swartwood, J. N., & O'Donnell, P. (1995). Evaluation of the effectiveness of EEG neurofeedback training for ADHD in a clinical setting as measured by changes in T.O.V.A. scores, behavioral ratings, and WISC-R performance. *Biofeedback and Self-Regulation*, 20, 83-99.

82. Lubar, J. F., Swartwood, M. O., Swartwood, J. N., & Timmermann, D. L. (1995). Quantitative EEG and auditory event-related potentials in the evaluation of Attention-Deficit/Hyperactivity disorder: Effects of methylphenid ate and implications for neurofeedback training. *Journal of Psychoeducational Assessment* (Monograph Series Advances in Psychoeducational Assessment) Assessment of Attention-Deficit/Hyperactivity Disorders, 143-204.

83. Mann, C. A., Lubar, J. F., Zimmerman, A. W., Miller, B. A., & Muenchen, R. A. (1992). Quantitative analysis of EEG in boys with attention deficit/hyperactivity disorder (ADHD). A controlled study with clinical implications. *Pediatric Neurology*, 8, 30-36.

84. Lubar, J. F., Mann, C. A., Gross, D. M., & Shively, M.S. (1992). Differences in semantic event related potentials in learning disabled, normal, and gifted children. *Biofeedback and Self-Regulation*, 17, 41-57.

85. Lubar, J.F. (1983) *Electroencephalographic Biofeedback and Neurological Applications. In J.V. Basmajian (Ed.)*, BIOFEEDBACK:PRINCIPLES AND PRACTICE. Baltimore, MD: Williams and WIlkins Publishers.

86. Lubar, J.F. (1985) *Changing EEG activity through biofeedback applications for the diagnosis and treatment of learning disabled children.* THEORY INTO PRACTICE, Ohio State University, 24, 106-111.

87. Lubar, J.F.(1989) *Electroencephalographic biofeedback and neurological applications. In J.V. Basmajian (Ed.)*, BIOFEEDBACK:PRINCIPLES AND PRACTICE (3rd Ed, pp67-90), Baltimore, MD: Williams and Wilkins Publishers.

88. Lubar, J.F.(1991), *Discourse on the development of EEG diagnostics and biofeedback treatment for attention deficit hyperactivity disorders. Biofeedback and Self-Regulation* 16, 201-225.

89. Lubar, J.F., Swartwood, M.O., Swartwood, J.N., & Timmermann, D.L. (1995). *Quantitative EEG and auditory event related potentials in the evaluation of attention deficit disorder: Effects of Methylphenidate and implications for neurofeedback training. JOURNAL OF PSYCHOEDUCATIONAL ASSESSMENT* ( Monograph series, Special ADHD Issue), 143-160

90. Monastra, V.J., Lubar, J.F.,& Linden, M.K. (2000). *The development of a QEEG scan for ADHD: Reliability and validity studies. NEUROPSYCHOLOGY*

91.  Monastra, V.J., Lubar, J.F., Linden, M., VanDeusen, PL, Green, G., Wing, W., Phillips, A., & Fenger, T.N. (1999). *Assessing attention deficit hyperactivity disorder via quantitative electroencephalography: An initial validation study.* *NEUROPSYCHOLOGY*, 13, (1), 19-25.

92.  Rasey, H.W., Lubar, J.F., McIntyre, A. Zoffuto, A.C., & Abbott, P.L. (1996). *EEG biofeedback for the enhancement of attentional processing in normal college students.* *JOURNAL OF NEUROTHERAPY* 1, 15-21

93.  Dyslexia and Delinquency: A New Dyslexia Screening Test
Rizzot *Int J Offender Ther Comp Criminol.*1975; 19: 164-177

94.  http://sportsinjurybulletin.com/archive/lack-sleep-cardiovascular.html

95.  *Strength and Conditioning Journal*; **Vol 24 No 2, pp 17-24**

96.  Peak Performance: Mental Training Technique of the World's Greatest Athletes, Charles Garfield and Hal Bennett

97.  The Effect of Repetitive Audio/Visual Stimulation on Skeletomotor and Vasomotor Activity, Dr. Norman Thomas, David Siever, 1988, *Hypnosis* - The Fourth European Congress at Oxford

98.   http://www.transparentcorp.com/products/np/learnmore/sports_performance.php

99.  http://www.staplethorne.co.uk/Alpha_Active_IEE_2005.pdf

100.  *Using Light And Sound Technology To Access "The Zone" In Sports And Beyond*, Thomas Hawes, M.ED., ED.S.

101.  *Circulation*, published online, March 26, 2007

# Chapter 7

# In Summary

## Why Virtual Scanning is a world-leading technology

by

**Graham Ewing**

Virtual Scanning, based upon the principles outlined in this text, enable us to define the role that light and colour plays in the regulation of our mental and physical health.

Civilisations, existing for thousands of years, have appreciated the therapeutic value of sunlight e.g. Aztecs, Incas, Egyptians, ancient Picts, Indian, Tibetan, etc. The use of colour has consequently become an implicit component in various ethnic or complementary health technologies.

Eastern medicine considers that consciousness precedes reality. By contrast, western medicine considers that consciousness is the result of brain function. Is it simply, that consciousness, emotions and spirituality are merely the inevitable consequence of our biological function – arising from the processing of sensory data? Does the western viewpoint overlook fundamental concepts, related to spirituality, which have yet to be researched?

By the beginning of the 20th century the value of light in medicine had become sufficiently well appreciated that researchers established how light could be used to treat a number of ailments including hyperbilirubinema – for which the Nobel Prize for Medicine was awarded.

By the early-mid 20th century there was intense research into the therapeutic power of sunlight. By this time it was known as 'photic stimulation'. The advent of sulpha drugs and penicillin in the mid 30's resulted in a much greater emphasis in biomedical research to the detriment of 'photic stimulation' and other forms of light-based research.

By the 1960's research had established that over 100 medical conditions respond positively to the therapeutic effect of light and colour although the results lacked precision and reproducibility. Since then there has been a resurgence of interest into other forms of 'biofeedback' involving sound, light, lasers, etc. Each claiming to offer some therapeutic benefit but again lacking precision, reproducibility and a theoretical justification. Some of these 'flashing light' techniques have been introduced to treat skin conditions, migraines, dyslexia and related disorders, although they are empirically-based and considered to be controversial and expensive.

It has taken the application of sophisticated mathematics and the phenomenal processing power of modern computers to enable researchers to establish the essential relationships between sensory processing and physiology. These findings have facilitated the development of a technology which is conceivably more valuable to the medical processes - of diagnosis and treatment - than any previous technology.

- It can provide a complete psychological and health assessment for a mere fraction of the cost of conventional diagnostic tests and procedures.

- It can provide an effective non-drug therapy for any medical condition which is predominantly psychosomatic and hence is not chronic and irreversible.

Virtual Scanning offers a means of dealing with human fallibility which is the most significant cause of misdiagnosis and errors in treatment in the medical industry.

- It fulfills the requirements set out in the NHS plan for better ways of working, providing a patient health report, better means of diagnosis and treatment, etc.

- It conceivably improves the efficiency of diagnosis and treatment of a wide range of medical disorders.

- It reduces the cost of a medical consultation.

The significance of these findings places doubts around a generation of medical research which is based upon the fundamental assumptions. For example, that a specific part of the anatomy functions in a simplistic manner independent of all other organs or, that the existence of a single organism is responsible for a medical condition. For a bacterial infection it is entirely logical to kill the invading bacterium [1-3] because this is the fundamental cause of the ailment but this does not necessarily apply to every, apparently similar, case.

For example

- the eye has two mechanisms which affects its function: (1) the primary function of the retina - rods, cones and photopsins [4-6] - convert the visual stimulus into a biochemical response; and (2) the secondary function of the eye is influenced by the autonomic nervous system which affect the mechanisms of transduction in the retina.

- the existence of a single organism may not necessarily the cause. It may be a symptom of the condition e.g. in a duodenal ulcer the prevalence of helicobacter pylori [7-9] in the digestive tract is often, but not always, the problem. This results from the destabilisation of the physiological systems and hence affects localised conditions which are conducive to the growth of helicobacter pylori. Most people have helicobacter pylori in their gut but relatively few go on to develop ulcers.

- the organs function in a manner which is unrelated to overall health and can be excharged like parts in a car when it is the regulation of the physiological systems, of which the organ is a part, which has led to its malfunction. Whereas it is considered that an organ is no longer functioning and may have to be replaced it may be possible to stimulate the organ to regain its proper function.

- MRI scans claim to be able to determine the precise locations in the brain that are responsible for brain function, emotions, memories, etc. This disregards that every brain is different and that each of us reacts to sensory stimulus in an entirely different way. Accordingly such a simplistic and naïve approach will inevitably lead to over-simplistic conclusions when considering, by comparison, that the human physiology function in a highly complex and sophisticated manner.

383

It also places a fundamental questionmark

- over the use of biomarkers to determine the levels of specific medical conditions.

  This technique is based upon the fundamental assumption that the body acts in a simplistic manner when by contrast the body is actually a highly complex system. Such assumptions lack precision in complex systems therefore the use of biomarkers will inevitably lead to erroneous conclusions and misdiagnosis.

- over the way in which illnesses are categorised.

  The diagnosis of medical conditions can be complicated by the existence of a range of factors which exist at differing degrees of severity. Whereas there are many medical conditions which arise from infection by a bacterium, by contrast there are a number of medical conditions which have a complex nature and hence are the sum of a number of medical conditions. The combined effect of these indications will inevitably lead to differences of opinion between physicians and hence to misdiagnosis.

- over the assumption that many categories and types of illness and of the degree of severity are untreatable.

  There are clearly mechanisms which if stimulated can lead to improved health - often when conventional opinion is that there is little hope of recovery. The biomedical approach deals with the processes of pathology and disregards the mechanisms which under normal circumstances regulate our health and wellbeing.

- over the segregation which exists between mental and physical health.

  There are clearly mental health problems which arise as a result of problems with physical health which are induced by stress.

- how drugs disturb the function of the physiological systems and hence the function of the organs and of biochemistry at the cellular and molecular levels.

  By acting upon pathology drugs may in fact be depressing the mechanisms which regulate our health. For example (1) steroids depress the immune system which is in contrast to the need to regulate immune system function, (2) anticancer drugs act upon the processes related to the growth of a tumour but also alter brain wave function and hence the stability of the body's physiological systems, (3) anti-depression drugs alter the brain waves and hence affect the stability of the body's physiological systems.

All aspects of our function are related to our biochemistry. There is no other way in which our thoughts, emotions and behaviour can be processed. Our health comprises genetic aspects ascribed to our inherited profile – the accumulation of experiences and of evolution – and of our exposure to stress-related experiences during our lifetimes.

Our decision-making traits can therefore be defined in terms of (1) rational and (2) emotional, i.e. that our genetic predisposition is responsible for a rational decision-making process which is determined by our inherited epigenetic character. This process is also significantly influenced by the experiences which have shaped our personality since birth.

All aspects of our health, mental or physical, are therefore the direct reflection of our biochemistry and hence of our genetic profile and stress-related experiences. The only exceptions are where physical injury, genetics or chronic conditions (of an irreversible nature) resist the body's natural ability to heal itself – thereby fuelling the long-standing debate between Nature versus Nurture, Psychology versus Physiology, Mind or Body, Complementary Health versus Conventional - and illustrates how these converge.

There is a substantial amount of evidence which illustrates the subjective nature of the relationship between

1.  psychology and cognition

2.  psychology and health

3.  health and cognition

and

4.  how stress affects the function of the autonomic nervous system and hence affects sensory function,
5.  how our health is governed by the body's physiological systems,

6.  how the brain waves regulate the body's physiological systems,

7.  how one person's health affects another person's psychology.

The inevitable conclusion is therefore that our receipt of sensory data, mental processes and brain waves, regulate the function of the body's physiological systems, organs and the levels of the body's biochemistry.

The body functions in a manner which is more sophisticated than mere belief. For the body to recover, especially in the most extreme life and death situations, there has to be a neural stimulus which improves the function of our body's physiological systems. The end-effect regulates the physiological processes and organs, stimulates our immune system, and stabilise the overall levels of our biochemistry.

Biomedical research considers that the body has clearly defined pathologies yet apparently fails to consider that the body's biochemistry is regulated by the brain's function and in particular by the brain waves. This includes the processes which replenish and maintain our immune system, the levels of proteins, etc.

Biomedical research in the 21st Century is now increasingly devoted to the study of the brain. Huge amounts of research are being invested by the US government as part of their efforts to establish the mechanisms of brain function. Consequently researchers now understand that the functions of mind and body are inextricably linked.

- The mind is not just a function of the brain. It also involves the interaction of the brain with the body. Differing levels of biochemicals affect the function of the organs which in turn affect the function of the brain.

  There is evidence that the brain and body communicate - that peptides found in the brain, stomach, muscles, glands, and organs - send messages back and forth. Messenger peptides carry messages from the brain to receptors in other parts of the body.

- What emerges is a strengthening body of evidence which illustrates that memories are not stored in individual neurons in compartments of the brains. This does not explain the available evidence. Memories appear to be stored as networks of neurons which are located throughout the brain and body.

  Accordingly the prevailing reductionist viewpoint on which NeuroScience appears to be based ignores the emerging body of evidence which illustrates that the brain and body work together in a synergistic manner.

- Emotion and Personality are biochemical constructs which share memory (mirror neurons) events with the levels of biochemical components. The low levels of biochemicals reduces our level of wellbeing which simultaneously are associated with specific memory of events which are associated with negative issues such as death, loss, damage, coldness, wetness, etc. Our exposure to emotional events, combined with our genetic profile, defines our personality.

  Good health, wellbeing and enjoyment are associated with elevated levels of endorphins and our general biochemistry. Similarly poor health, lower levels of wellbeing and diminished 'joie de vivre' are associated with inhibited function of the immune system, etc.

  Our rational thinking and hence of 'unexpressed emotions' are directly related to our biochemistry whilst 'expressed emotions' are related to our biochemistry and the mirror neurons which have recorded the pleasurable and stress-related experiences in our lives. There is not therefore an emotional centre in the brain. The whole organism, comprising brain and body, is our emotional centre.

- The brain scans continuously but does not take a series of pictures or build up what we would regard as a holographic image. The brain's ability to scan and absorb information takes place continuously. This is regulated by the brain waves and in particular by the beta-wave which regulates our absorption of sensory data.

  The implications are that the brain identifies an image, and its spatial representation, in terms of data which is processed by the brain. It does not and cannot record each and every image but instead records changes to images e.g. if we walk our dog in the same field each day we do not record in our brains repeated images of the field. We record only the significant changes which we have seen, or heard, etc.

The existence of Virtual Scanning revolutionises our understanding of how the mind and body function It illustrates how relationships, hitherto considered to be subjective, are in fact objective, precise and can be mathematically modelled to provide an unprecedented amount of information about mental and physical health. It also illustrates how these findings can be used as the basis of an effective and reliable non-drug therapy able to treat mental and physical disorders. It illustrates how new technology bridges the gap between complementary and conventional medicine and how it can be used to advance the understanding of medical conditions. New technologies bring new levels of understanding.

Modern medicine is required to comply with the requirements for an evidence-based conclusion yet is based upon assumptions which have significant limitations. Virtual Scanning addresses this technology deficit.

It also illustrates that changes to the body's stability are primarily due to stress and that it is possible to re-establish good health (homeostasis) by treating with light and colour. As a result we are able to conclude that the body is a complex holistic organism with signals passing to and from the brain and organs .

The existence of Virtual Scanning, and its apparent world-leading significance for modern medicine, is unprecedented for many reasons:

1. It considers the human as a data processing entity rather than a biochemical entity. This illustrates that cognitive function directly relates to health.

2. It establishes the significance of the sensory mechanisms and physiological systems which are used to regulate the systems, organs and cells of the body.

3. It precisely defines the nature of the body's physiological systems and that these systems are regulated by the delta waves. This defines the need for an organ which has huge processing capability and regulates the limits for each of the body's physiological systems i.e. the cerebellum.

4. It applies mathematical modelling to the human physiology.

5. It identifies the holistic nature of the human physiology. These signals are indicative of the processes of pathology and the body's natural compensatory responses.

6. It relate our psychological and psycho-emotional profiles to our health profile i.e. it relates our mental function to our health and vice versa.

7. It provide a full diagnosis of every system and organ of the body, providing:

   • The psychological and psycho-emotional profile

   • The health profile defined in terms of

      (1) the most destabilised physiological system

      (2) the most destabilised organ

      (3) the precise medical conditions (reported in precise medical terms) for each organ
      (4) the morphology of each organ

8. It is able to diagnose the causal factors responsible for a range of medical conditions which are not able to be diagnosed by conventional procedures including migraine; chronic fatigue, chronic fatigue syndrome, fibromyalgia and depression; stroke; irritable bowel syndrome and digestive system disorders; dyslexia, etc.

9. It can selectively and effectively treat the physiological system or organ, OR the psychological profile of a patient using a non-drug therapy.

10. It explains the placebo effect in precise mathematical terms. The implications are that this can be used to assess and treat the psychology of groups of people.

Intriguingly Virtual Scanning is a complementary health technology for a number of reasons. It is based upon an appreciation of the most natural of phenomena - of light and colour - and hence has fundamental similarities to Colour Therapy, Chromotherapy, Kinesiology and Ayurvedhic medicine which are widely recognised as complementary health techniques. It differs only in that it involves the mathematical modelling of cognitive measurements and hence is related to psychology and neuroscience – of which cognition is an integral part. It is completely non-invasive and does not provide any exposure to radiation or drugs. It's application – it is a software programme - is no different to a computer game or a television program which offers an intriguing insight into the future evolution of medicine.

By providing a precise colour therapy as indicated in this text it is possible to enhance a person's health. The precise understanding of how the brain functions and in particular how it absorbs colour can be used to massively increase the effect of exposure to colour and hence to stimulate the function of the physiological systems which regulate our health and wellbeing.

Accordingly it can be used to justify complementary health technologies but also to identify their inherent limitations.

Whereas conventional diagnosis is constrained by the time and cost of each diagnostic test – which places subsequent constraints upon the diagnosis of medical disorders which have a complex nature – Virtual Scanning is able to provide a precise assessment of the health of each physiological system and organ and of any medical disorders affecting their function. The consequences arising from the introduction of this technology are of better, cheaper and faster diagnosis and for greater understanding of complex medical issues which will lead to improved methods of treatment.

This is the first time that I have attempted to compile a book. The need to write it is to ensure that this technology gets known and the issues, which are associated with this technology, debated fully. For the more open and broad-minded this technology is the evolution of medical research whilst for others it will be too revolutionary. Like so many new technologies it will have those who are seeking newer and better ways of working and it will have its detractors.

For it to be adopted by the medical profession it is necessary to get government approval, the support of the public, and the acknowledgement of this technology by academics, medical researchers and the medical establishment.

The concept is simple: that our cognition (of which visual perception is a part) is the direct reflection of our biochemistry. It is astonishingly simple and logical. The ability to process data is the fundamental reason for our existence.

The content is entirely based upon (1) the genius of Dr Grakov's research and development, (2) the work of medical practitioners in Russia who have made available the results of their work, (3) the work of many biomedical researchers who though their work have contributed to this compilation of evidence, and (4) of the experience of Dr Elena Ewing with this technology.

I have merely taken their work and woven it into a tapestry which I hope will be of interest to you and can be of value in the diagnosis and treatment of disease. It should, I hope, make you pause and reflect upon issues which have far-reaching implications for the way in which we wish to conduct our lives in future.

Inevitably there will be questions about the precise methodology employed by Dr Grakov in the computation and processing of data. What is the nature of the mathematical concepts which have been involved? How has he been able to use algorithms to elucidate the data? Regretably it is not possible to patent software in the EU and hence it is not possible to protect the intellectual property. Accordingly Dr Grakov has adopted the only commercial avenue available i.e. to protect his IP by non-disclosure.

I hope to have given you a glimpse of the future of medicine.

Graham Ewing

**References**

1.    Nobel Laureates Sir Alexander Fleming, Howard Florey and Ernst Chain

2.    http://www.iah.bbsrc.ac.uk/schools/scientists/fleming.htm

3.    http://topics.nytimes.com/top/news/health/diseasesconditionsandhealthtopics/anti
      biotics/index.html?inline=nyt-classifier

4.    http://en.wikipedia.org/wiki/Retina

5.    Nobel Laureates Ragnar Granit, Haldan Keffer Hartline **and** George Wald.

6.    http://en.wikipedia.org/wiki/Ragnar_Granit

7.    http://www.madsci.org/posts/archives/may97/863468915.Me.r.html

8.    The helicobacter foundation: **http://www.helico.com/h_epidemiology.html**

9.    Blaser MJ. Not all Helicobacter pylori strains are created equal: should all be
      eliminated? *The Lancet* 1997; 349: 1020-2.

# APPENDICES

## APPENDIX A

THE SOURCE OF THE ORIGINAL ENGLISH TRANSLATION IS KNOWN AND CERTAIN CHANGES OF VOCABULARY HAVE BEEN MADE BY MONTAGUE DIAGNOSTICS LIMITED IN THE INTERESTS OF CLARITY. IN ANY REPRODUCTION OF TEXT, PLEASE ALSO INCLUDE THIS ATTRIBUTION STATEMENT TO PRESERVE THE AUDIT TRAIL OF PROVENANCE.

## Professor Vysochin Yuri Vasilievich

The Vice-Rector in Academic and Research Work of the International University of Fundamental Studies; Director of the International Scientific-Research Institute "Health and Sport", International University of the Fundamental Studies; the Professor of the Pulpit of Physical Culture and Sport at Sankt-Petersburg State University; the Doctor of the Medical Sciences; the Professor, Member of the Scientific Council and Problem-Solving Commission on Physiologies of Extreme Conditions in the Russian Academy of Science; the Member (the academician) of the International Academy of Information; the Member (the academician) of the International Academy "Information, relationship, management in technology, nature, society".

Grande-Master 10 Dan in Gong-Fu; the leader of the sanitary direction athletic-combat in Europe; the member of the Presidium Intercontinental Athletic Alliance; the Member of the Presidium International qualifying committee in athletic-combat; the Golden Laureate of the International contest 1999 on the best sanitary technology in combat art; The Expert of the Council to National Safety of the State Parliament of Russian Federation.

The Specialist in the field of Physiologies, Sport Medicine, Sport Traumatology, the latest athletic-sanitary and preventive technology. The Main developer and leader of the State of Russian Federation "Health of the Nation" Programme. The Author 250 scientific works (including 3 monographs and 8 scholastic allowances) and has prepared 9 candidates of the sciences and 10 doctors of the sciences.

The Awards: Medal USSR "For labor" - for successes in scientifically-methodical provision of preparing the USSR team to Olympic games 1980 in Moscow. The State award (Russian Federation) "Well-earned figure of the science in Russian Federation" - for prominent scientific achievements. The Order "Saint Russia". The International order "Tsialkovsky's Star". The International Order "North Star". The Medals of the name Y. A. Gagarin and S. P. Korolev from Federation of Astronaut's of Russia for achievements in astronautics. Memorable sign "For Courage and Love of Country". The Honourable Award "For Special Achievements in Science". The Golden Cup Grande-Master from International Athletic Alliance. The Memorable Silver Sign from the Government of Germany. The Golden Medal from International College of Martial Art (USA). The Memorable Board of the Laureate Athletic Glory (USA). The Honourable Laureate's

Certificate in nomination "High scientific achievements" from International Alliance Karate (Japan - USA).

The Thanksgiving letter from the Council of National Safety of the State Parliament of Russian Federation "For development and introducing the State Program of Russia "Health of the Nation".

The telephone: (8-812) 314-19-84; E-mail: vysochin@comset.ru

10.12.2003                                                          Yu. V. Vysochin.

STATE COMMITTEE OF RUSSIAN FEDERATION IN PHYSICAL
TRAINING, SPORTS AND TOURISM
State Scientific Research Institute of sport-invigorative technologies of St-Petersburg
State P.F. Lesgaft Academy of Physical Training

«УТВЕРЖДАЮ»
Директор ГНИИ СОТ
СПб ГАФК им. П.Ф. Лесгафта
Ю.В. Высочин
"15 " августа 2002 г.

O  REPORT

about the Research in 2001-2002

**Problem 01.02.00:** Methodology and Technology of invigoration of different population
orders.

**Subject 01.02.06:** Development of mass sport-invigorative technologies for the
establishment of the Russian Federation "Health of the Nation" program  and for the
invigoration of different age and sex population groups.

**Particular Subject:** The research of the universal computer medical-diagnostic and
prophylactic program "Virtual Scanner" efficiency (1) for the establishment of the
Russian Federation "Health of the Nation" program and (2) for the invigoration of
different population groups.


Issue Supervisor:
Honoured Scientist of RF,

Doctor of Medical Science of RF,                              Professor **Yu.V. Vysochin**

# CONTENT

# EXECUTORS' LIST

1. Head of SSRI SIT, HS of RF, DMS .............................……............ Yu.V.Vysochin

2. Branch Manager, Candidate of Science,......…………………….….. V.V. Lukoyanov

3. Senior Staff Scientist, Candidate of Medical Science........................ I.K. Yaichnikov

4. Senior Staff Scientist, Candidate of Medical Science.....................… M.I. Tkachuk

5. Senior Staff Scientist, Candidate........................................... V.A. Chyev

6. Senior Staff Scientist.................................................... V.V. Yemelyanenko

7. Research Assistant, Graduate student................................... Yu.V. Gordeyev

8. Research Assistant, Graduate student..............................…… N.V. Tsitsenova

9. Research Assistant, Candidate............................................ L.K. Kaplina

10. Free-lance Research Assistant, Candidate of Biological Science,     Ye.G. Vashchillo
    working for doctor's degree………...............................................

11. Free-lance Research Assistant, Candidate of Biological Science,     Yu.P. Denisenko
    working for doctor's degree………...............................................

12. Free-lance Research Assistant, Programmer .................................. M.A. Konstantinov

# REPORT

Scientific report: "Research into the efficiency of the universal computer medical-diagnostic and prophylactic program "Virtual Scanner" for the establishment of the Russian Federation "Health of the Nation" program and for invigoration of different population groups" according to the Problem 01.02.00: "Methodology and Technology of invigoration of different population orders" of Consolidated 5-years Research Plan of Physical Training, Sports and Tourism State Committee of Russian Federation, is set out in 23 pages of typescript, consists of 2 Chapters, 6 Tables, 4 figures, Conclusion and Finding.

To succeed in the main Research object "Research of the efficiency of the universal computer medical-diagnostic and prophylactic program "Virtual Scanner" for the establishment of the Russian Federation "Health of the Nation" program and invigoration of different population groups during 2001-2002 period, the following main tasks were accomplished:

- Analysis and review of scientific literature data about computer and medical technologies.
- Research of diagnostic and therapeutic "Virtual Scanner" system efficiency.

- Research of "Virtual Scanner" therapy upon the functional condition of different organism systems and upon the physical activity of almost healthy people.

To cope with all those tasks special research took place with the help of 20 almost healthy volunteers, each of them passed fivefold complex check-up using electroencephalography, polymyography, cardiovascular, ergometry, clinical and statistic methods. There were 2,800 total measurements taken, and 105,440 initial and calculated parameters were received and analysed, which characterize the functional condition of different organism systems.

On the basis of those researches the following important results and conclusions were obtained:

1. Clinical research, carried out with a significant number of patients (370 people – diagnostics; 1,672 people – treatment), **proved the high degree of accuracy of diagnosis (on average 82.4% of coincidences with clinical diagnosis) and high efficiency of treatment (on average 93.2% of recovery cases and considerable improvements)** with the help of "Virtual Scanner" system.

2. According to the data of electroencephalographical and polymyographical research it was established **that "Virtual Scanner" therapeutic sessions lead to the fast recovery and essential increase** Development Rate and the force of Inhibiting processes (DRI) (for 18.8%: $D < 0.001$), functional Activity of Inhibiting Systems (AIS) for 15.2% ($D < 0.01$), substantial progress of Balance of Nerve Processes (BNP) toward inhibiting (for 19.4%: $D < 0.001$) accordingly,

increase of inhibiting control by Central Nervous System, which is one of the most important conditions for the establishment of control of the regulating functions of the cerebrum.of adaptability (for 20.5%: P < 0.001) and percentage of alpha-rhythm (for 31.6%: D < 0.001) in summary electroencephalography (EEG), and also to the improvement of general functional condition of Central Nervous System (for 7.2%: D < 0.001) due to increase of

3. **Increase of control and regulating functions of cerebrum activity** under the influence of "Virtual Scanner" therapeutic sessions leads to the substantial increase of stress rate (for 33.7%: D < 0.001), the maximum force (for 27.6% D < 0.001), relaxation rate (for 30.4%: D < 0.001) and general functional condition of NMS (for 30%: D < 0.001).

4. The **pronounced positive changes in Central Nervous System and NeuroMuscular System entailed with the same pronounced positive dynamics of physical activity and functional condition of the cardiovascular system.** After 20 sessions of "Virtual Scanner" therapy by comparison to the Initial Data, the Frequency of Cordial Clonus in quiescence decreases considerably (FCCq) for 8.9% (D < 0.001), and in period of rehabilitation (FCCr) – for 5% (D < 0.01). Efficiency and high-speed endurance increase to 13.2% (D < 0.001) and 12.8% (D < 0.01) accordingly. Heart Activity Efficiency Factor (HAEF), Pulse Recovery Rate (PRR) and General Efficiency (GE) of organism systems increase accordingly for 15.6% (D < 0.001), 20% (D < 0.001) and 17.5% (D < 0.001).

5. After 5, 10 and 20 "Virtual Scanner" treatment sessions the substantial decrease of the characteristic, which shows the Possibility of Injury (IP) and Musculoskeletal system diseases, and also the heart overstress accordingly for 15% (D < 0.001), 16.8% (D < 0.001) and 18.1% (D < 0.001). **That allows concluding that "Virtual Scanner" therapeutic sessions can become an effective overstress, injury and musculoskeletal system diseases preventive measure, and also of cordial overstresses at hard physical and psycho-emotional load.**

6. **Considerable improvement of retractive and relaxation muscle characteristics, increased physical activity, heart functioning efficiency, coordination in different organs and systems activity, which limit physical efficiency and also the reduction of Injury Possibility, musculoskeletal system diseases and cordial overstresses is explained by improvement of overall condition of the functional Central Nervous System** and, accordingly, of its control and regulator functions under the influence of "Virtual Scanner" sessions.

7. The "Virtual Scanner" is a high-performance system and absolutely suitable for wide application not only in public health service (for treatment and prophylaxis of different pathological processes), but in any kinds of sport or professional human activity that requires effective correction of psychofunctional abnormalities, normalization of regulator systems control functions, improvement of inhibition of Central Nervous System control, increasing of retractive and

relaxation muscle characteristics, economy and effectivity of CardioVascular System activity, mental and physical activity, stress stability and human survival rate in complex and extreme conditions of activity or environment.

8. Taking into account the minimal time spent for all-around diagnosis (less than 10-15 minutes) and treatment (or so called informational correction) (session lasts 15-20 minutes), and also the main object of informational correction – normalization of regulator and management of cerebrum functions, it is expected the "Virtual Scanner" system to find in the nearest future the deserved application in all areas of human activity concerned with hard physical and psycho-emotional load, increased requirements to regulating and movement coordination systems, physical efficiency, endurance, stability to different stress-generative or confusing factors (sport, choreography, ballet, rescuers, firemen, landing troops, emergency platoons, aviation, cosmonautics and others).

# 1. Analysis of "Virtual Scanner" System Medical-Diagnostic Efficiency

Many years' of science research including practical results show that the Virtual Scanner reveals not only the formed but also the earliest signs of regulation and control of cerebral function abnormalities, failures in operation of different functional systems, organs and tissues, i.e. to carry out fast (in 10-15 minutes) and exact diagnosis of pre-pathological conditions at the pre-clinical level, when the human being doesn't feel any sign of one or another disease.

Here is the data of Medical Department National Enterprise "Moscow Mint" (N.P. Skvortsova and others, 1999) and of "Metallurg" Sanatorium (V.P. Yerkhov and others, 2001), combined in the Table 1. The investigation of accuracy rating and diagnostics efficiency of "Virtual Scanner" system was carried out with the help of plenty of patients.

## Table 1: Diagnostic Efficiency of "Virtual Scanner"

| № | Diagnosis | № of Patients | Confirmed | Effectiveness |
|---|---|---|---|---|
| 1 | Vegetative-vascular Distony | 14 | 10 | 71,4 % |
| 2 | Encephalopathy | 4 | 4 | 100,0 % |
| 3 | Cerebrovascular Disorders | 28 | 22 | 78,6 % |
| 4 | Acute Bronchitis | 12 | 10 | 83,3 % |
| 5 | Chronic Bronchitis | 11 | 9 | 81,8 % |
| 6 | Acute Rhinitis | 16 | 13 | 81,5 % |
| 7 | Tonsillitis | 13 | 11 | 84,6 % |
| 8 | Chronic Otitis | 3 | 3 | 100,0 % |
| 9 | Ankilosing Spondilitis | 6 | 5 | 83,3 % |
| 10 | Vertebral Osteoarthrosis | 34 | 30 | 88,2 % |
| 11 | Intercostal Neuralgia | 11 | 8 | 72,7 % |
| 12 | Polyneuropathies | 11 | 9 | 81,8 % |
| 13 | Ischaemic Heart Disease | 9 | 7 | 77,8 % |
| 14 | Hypertension | 33 | 27 | 81,8 % |
| 15 | Chronic Pyelonephritis | 6 | 5 | 83,3 % |
| 16 | Nephrolithiasis | 11 | 9 | 81,8 % |
| 17 | Chronic Gastritis | 29 | 24 | 82,8 % |
| 18 | Peptic Ulcer Diseases | 22 | 19 | 86,4 % |
| 19 | Chronic Pancreatitis | 16 | 12 | 75,0 % |
| 20 | Chronic Hepatitis | 5 | 4 | 80,0 % |
| 21 | Chronic Cholecystitis | 46 | 39 | 84,8 % |
| 22 | Cholelithiasis | 13 | 10 | 76,9 % |
| 23 | Diabetes Mellitus | 17 | 15 | 88,2 % |
| | Всего | 370 | 305 | 82,4 % |

To evaluate the compliance of the revealed pathology by "Virtual Scanner" to the official clinical diagnosis the patients were submitted for laboratory, biochemical, cardiology, functional, roentgenologic and ultrasonic tests. **Due to the findings the authors make the conclusion that "Virtual Scanner" system is more informative and able to identify and reveal disease, especially of the pre-pathological conditions, than the existing clinical diagnostic methods.**

In this case we could talk about the so-called hyper-diagnostics or the excessive diagnostics. However the conclusions of these authors are proved with data of other researchers, who gave plenty of examples when the diagnosis, diagnosed with the help of "Virtual Scanner" system, was revealed by clinical methods only after several weeks or even months. **It means that the virtual scanner really diagnoses the pre-pathological conditions and diseases at the earliest pre-clinical stage, when only some abnormalities of control and regulatory functions exist that can't be determined by current clinical methods.**

Fundamentally the new approaches are laid in construction of functional abnormalities correction system and also by treatment of different diseases with the help of "Virtual Scanner" system. The main methodological principle of virtual scanning is based on the principles of outer world and internal environment reflecting adequacy by the cerebrum functions. At that the cerebrum builds two groups of matrixes or images: images, describing and detailing the outer environment, i.e. the outer world; and images, describing and detailing the internal environment, i.e. the human organism, in fact. Coordination of these matrix groups is fulfilled by cerebral functions that are able to define the mutual relations of matrixes to each other and always find matrixes the most close to each other in characteristics depending on requirements of one or another situation.

During the diagnostic process the "Virtual Scanner" system analyses the fulfillment of special test by the patient on the computer simulator. The task is the following. At first the patient is presented the image (the picture) on the monitor for several seconds, and he has to remember it. Then the colour spectrum is fully broken and the patient has to restore it. During diagnostics in automatic mode one can see usually from 3 to 5 images one after another. The speed and reproduction quality of images by the patient lets to evaluate the main cerebrum functions and then to create the biomathematics model of the patient similar to the body scheme, built by the cerebrum.

The Virtual Scanner reproduces the set of matrixes in the computer, which are typical for the investigated patient. This process is called the Personal Biological Modelling. The basis of the virtual technology is the evaluation and comparison of matrixes, the same way as the cerebrum does, and, also, the transfer of received data to the standard medical terms.

During treatment the virtual scanning technology lets to correct the signals and, accordingly, the cerebral functions, brings them up to the evolutionary standard. The correction is fulfilled by the purposeful generating and presenting to the patient on the monitor of individually calculated colour sets in the delta-rhythm range, that are presented in the changing colour tints, coming to the Central Nervous System via visual analyser. In that way, by means of **Virtual Reality Technology** it is possible to reproduce the required characteristics of one or another matrix, and the cerebrum can be quickly tuned to these characteristics and restore its management functions. As a result there is a unique possibility of the natural non-medicinal influence on the pathological process/source and treatment of diseases which are caused by failures in the function of higher regulatory systems.

Efficiency of treating different diseases with the help of the "Virtual Scanner" system is shown in Table 2, where the research materials of some large sanatoriums, medical-diagnostic centres and hospitals, such as Kislovodsk Central Sanatorium of Ministry of Defence of RF, Orenburg Regional Clinic, Kislovodsk Mud-bath Clinic/Health Spa, Krasnoyarsk City Ambulance Hospital, Novosibirsk Regional Centre of Medical Prophylaxis, Novosibirsk Musical College, Medical Centre of "Drujba" Oil-trunk Pipeline Corporation, Pyatigorsk Sanatorium "Rodnik", Moscow Molecular Technology Laboratory "Mirra-Lux", Nalchik Medical Centre "Aesculapius", Odessa Medical Centre "Gigiya", Yessentuki Sanatorium "Metallurg" (and others) are summarised.

## Table 2: Therapeutic Efficiency of "Virtual Scanner"

| № | Diagnosis | № of patients | № of therapy courses | Effectiveness |
|---|---|---|---|---|
| 1 | Chronic Fatigue Syndrome | 43 | 1 | 97,7% |
| 2 | Depressive and Anxiety Disorders | 54 | 1-2 | 96,3 |
| 3 | Organic Disorders/Diseases of CNS | 26 | 1-2 | 95,0% |
| 4 | Vegetative-vascular Distony | 96 | 1-2 | 85,0% |
| 5 | Cerebrovascular Disorders | 46 | 1+ massage | 97,8% |
| 6 | Spinal Circulation Disorders | 57 | 1+ massage | 100% |
| 7 | Cerebral Palsy | 12 | 1+ medications | 100% |
| 8 | Chronic Bronchitis | 37 | 1-2 | 100% |
| 9 | Bronchial Asthma | 12 | 2 | 91,7% |
| 10 | Chronic Tonsillitis | 7 | 1 | 100% |
| 11 | Chronic Otitis | 8 | 1 | 100% |
| 12 | Ischaemic Heart Disease | 63 | 1-2 | 90,5% |
| 13 | Chronic Cardiac Insufficiency | 11 | 1-2 | 81,8% |
| 14 | Cardiac Arrhythmias | 12 | 1-2 | 83,0% |
| 15 | Myocarditis | 30 | 1-3 | 93,3% |
| 16 | Hypertension | 120 | 1-2 | 87,5% |
| 17 | Chronic and Acute Gastritis | 105 | 1-2 | 98,1% |
| 18 | Chronic Duodenitis | 29 | 1 | 100% |
| 19 | Peptic Ulcer Diseases | 75 | 1-2 | 100% |
| 20 | Chronic Hepatitis | 53 | 1-2 | 92,5% |
| 21 | Chronic Cholecystitis | 58 | 1-2 | 98,3% |

| 22 | Dyskinesia Biliary Ducts | 52 | 2 | 100% |
|---|---|---|---|---|
| 23 | Cholelithiasis | 15 | 1-2 | 86,7% |
| 24 | Chronic Pancreatitis | 49 | 1 | 85,7% |
| 25 | Nephrolithiasis | 42 | 2 | 86,5% |
| 26 | Pyelonephritis | 26 | 2 | 84,6% |
| 27 | Hydronephrosis | 2 | 2 | 100% |
| 28 | Cystitis | 12 | 3 | 83,0% |
| 29 | Prostatitis | 70 | 2 | 94,3% |
| 30 | Disorders of Thyroid Gland | 73 | 1 | 93,2% |
| 31 | Hypofunction of Adrenal Cortex | 21 | 1-2 | 61,9% |
| 32 | Ovarian Cyst | 14 | 1 | 86,0% |
| 33 | Mastopathy | 18 | 2-3 + medications | 83,0% |
| 34 | Gynaecological Diseases | 40 | 1 | 100% |
| 35 | Diabetes Mellitus | 31 | 1-2 | 100% |
| 36 | Musculoskeletal System Disorders | 19 | 1 + medications | 100% |
| 37 | Vertebral Osteoarthrosis | 168 | 1-3 | 93,5% |
| 38 | Gout | 26 | 1 | 100% |
| 39 | Ankylosing Spondilitis | 40 | 1-2 | 95,0% |
| | | 1678 | | 93,2% |

Totally one (1s.), two (2s.) or three (3s.) treatment courses were taken by 1672 patients with the help of "Virtual Scanner" system. Some of them received additional kinds of treatment (+ therapy), including massage, pharmacological medications and so on. **Treatment was considered as effective in case if the patient condition after the full course of treatment was diagnosed as fully recovered, considerably improved and improved.** The research, given in Table 2, showed the high effectivity of "Virtual Scanner" treatment sessions. The therapy effect was observed on average in 93.2% cases out of 1672 patients. And, as most specialists will notice, the positive changes for better in the state of health appeared after the first 4-5 treatment sessions. Negative consequences and deterioration of patient's state of health were not discovered.

Interesting enough are the examples of some individual cases of diseases and the results of their treatment, carried out by the specialists of Orenburg Regional Clinic (V.I. Voynov, 2000):

1. Dudakova Masha, 16 years old, was observed at endocrinology department with the diagnosis: Diabetes, 1 type, heavy form, labile process. Diabetic encephalopathy, polyneuropathy, retinopathy; concentration of sugar in blood was up to 28.4 mmol/l; she got insulin – 24 units of prolonged and 28 units of simple one. She passed the colour therapy for the cerebrum. As a result, after 5 sessions the level of sugar in the blood lowed to the 7-9 mmol/l.

2. Rekhviashvili S., 23 years old, was observed at endocrinology department with the diagnosis: Diabetes, 1 type, heavy form. Diabetic encephalopathy, polyneuropathy, microangiopathy. Narcotic dependence, concentration of sugar in blood was up to 10-

17 mmol/l, he got insulin up to 40 units per day. After 5 sessions of colour therapy the level of sugar in the blood lowed to 5 mmol/l, and it was accompanied by hypoglycaemia, and then it was set at level of 7-8 mmol/l. It let to low the insulin dose. The abstinent syndrome decreased.

3. Mamayev Alesha, 9 years old. Diagnosis: Enuresis (involuntary urination 3-4 times per night). The boy got treatment for the cerebrum and urinary bladder. After the fourth session the involuntary urination was observed once in 4 days.

4. Brekhova Natasha, 14.5 years old. Complaints for absence of menstruation during 1.5 years against the background of nervous anorexia, hypothyroidism. After 2 series of cerebrum treatment the menstruation was recommenced in 3 weeks.

5. Patient M., 23 years old. Complaints about repeated sexual weakness against the background of narcotic dependence at the stage of remission, abstinent disorder was reasonably expressed. After cerebrum course of treatment the libido and potency were restored, abstinent disorder decreased.

6. Vinkova Ye.M., 50 years old. She was observed at the physician with the diagnosis: Myocardious myocardic cardiosclerosis with rhythm disorders: extrasystoly, sino-tachycardia. During the diagnostics with the help of "Virtual Scanner" system the data was confirmed, and besides that the calcium deficit was revealed. After cerebrum, heart and the microelements metathesis course of treatment the patient condition noticeably improved, the heart rhythm disorders fully disappeared.

7. Pikaleva O.V., 45 years old. In the result of diagnosis with the "Virtual Scanner" system the pathologic signals from liver and gall bladder were obtained. During the ultrasonic investigation the gallstone disease and calculus cholecystitis were diagnosed for the 1st time.

8. Brekhova O.V., 37 years old. After testing with the help of "Virtual Scanner" system the thyroid gland pathology was revealed, and also the Diabetes. Laboratory methods confirmed the diagnosis. With the help of that system the Diabetes and lowering of the thyroid gland functioning was revealed for the first time.

Treatment with the help of "Virtual Scanner" system of so-called difficult diseases such as disseminated sclerosis, concomitant mental disorders, vegetative syndromes at organic lesion of cerebrum and some other diseases, the treatment of which didn't lead to the positive results with the help of usual treatment methods, is of special interest.

1. Patient S., 42 years old. Endogenous depression, 2 group of disablement, doesn't work, doesn't do even simple house work. During 8 months he took 2 courses of informational colour therapy for the cerebrum. Patient began working not only at home, but also, at the state farm. The suicidal tendencies fully disappeared.

2. Patient Ts., 54 years old. Diagnosis: disseminated sclerosis, 1 group of disablement. Complaints: general weakness, shaky walk, moved only with the help of others, irritability, disturbed sleep, bad appetite, weight deficit, depression. After the first course of general informational correction he began walking without any help, put on weight (2kg in 1 month), had good appetite and normal sleep. After the second course of cerebrum treatment he began doing simple work at home.

3. Patient K., 60 years old. Diagnosis: neuritis of facial nerve and of the second branch of trifacial nerve. Complaints for skin desensitisation of the right face part, speech infringement, and headaches. After the forth session of the general informational correction the speech became better, and at the end of treatment course it was fully restored, headaches disappeared.

Wide use of "Virtual Scanner" system at all levels of the educational institutions is being implemented now and in future programmes. **Application of this system in the medical practice by institutions and clinics greatly increases the quality of medical care due to the complex system of check up and treatment, which significantly reduces the time of data processing, and also gives the possibility to do screening-check up in an efficient, versatile manner which enables the deep analysis of findings both at the diagnostic and treatment stages.** More than 100 psychosomatic nosological diseases can be treated by the "Virtual Scanner" system. In some publications the special effect upon the treatment of gynaecological disorders is recorded. There were stated some cases when informational correction helped to overcome the narcotic dependence, to get rid of skin diseases (psoriasis, eczema, neurodermatitis), which are difficult to treat by the traditional means of treatment. **In many publications it is noticed that informational correction gives more effective and quick result than usual technologies.** Special effect is noticed at their combined use. It should be noted that regardless of the reason of the Virtual Scanner treatment that practically all patients experienced an improvement of their state of health, normalised sleep patterns and appetite, improved mental and physical activity, and loss of "chronic tiredness" syndrome.

Based on the abovementioned the high effectiveness of "Virtual Scanner" system and its absolute adaptability to the wide use in public health service is clearly evident.

## 2. Pilot Research of "Virtual Scanner" System Efficiency for Improvement of Physical Activity and Functional Condition of Different Organism Systems

### 2.1. Basis of working hypothesis, definition of object and research tasks

Complex population situation, existing in Russia during the last 10-15 years, requires the development of new and high-performance diagnostic, medical and prophylactic technologies, suitable for mass use and capable to fulfil powerful breakthrough in solving and improving the problems of the nation's health. The universal computer system "Virtual Scanner" is the neo-technology, designed by I.G. Grakov (1998, 2000, 2001) on the base of the concept about natural biological answer to the wave influence (Grakov B.S., Grakov I.G., 1985), and also on the base of the modern scientific conception about the leading role of higher regulator systems, cerebrum in particular (Bekhtereva N.P., 1974, 1980, 1997), and inhibiting-relaxation processes (Vysochin K.V., 1988) in the most important display of the whole organism vital activity, such as adaptation, work capacity, stability to the extreme environmental influences and etiopathogenesis of different pathological conditions, injuries and diseases.

Today, due to the wide experimental and theoretical researches (Anokhin P.K., 1975, 1979; Sudakov K.V., 1971; Medvedev V.I., 1982; Vasilevskiy N.N., 1979) the statement is proved that adaptation mechanisms are provided with both rigid and flexible programs of function regulation. According to Vasilevskiy N.N. (1984) adaptation mechanisms are to be studied as combined control systems with rigid and flexible programs, and also as tracing systems, necessary for generating of starting signal and extracting of certain sequence of signals and programs, forming the flexible regulation group. **Exactly the abnormality of regulation role of Central Nervous System and the hormonal system that is under its control, that the numerous experiments show (Gorizontov P.D., 1973; Medvedev V.I., 1982; Sapov I.A., Novikov V.S., 1984; Vasilevskiy N.N., 1984), can be the main reason for weakening of protecting mechanisms and pathological development.** The researches of Bekhtereva N.P. (1974, 1980) played an important role in understanding of neuropathalogical processes essence. She stated the conception of steady pathological condition while cerebrum lesion. Under existing conditions not only the completion of lesion structures takes place, but producing of new intra-central relations, fixed in the corresponding long-time memory matrix, and that makes that new (pathological process) stable and steadiness. On the basis of these ideas Kryjanovskiy G.N. (1980, 1984) developed the idea of pathological Functional System as one of the most prevalent mechanisms, constituting the basement for many kinds of Central Nervous System pathologies. In contrast to the physiological Functional System, described in details by Anokhin P.K., pathological Functional Systems are such nerve organisations, the result of which activity has not the adaptive but, on the contrary, disadaptive meaning. It appears in the fact that the activity of pathological Functional System doesn't correspond neither to the active irritant nor to the changing of situation, neither motivating reasons of human or animal behaviour, nor organism requirements. Moreover, the result of pathological Functional Systems activity can have the direct pathogenic effect, causing the following development of present or new pathological process. Pathological Functional Systems, also, cause the inhibiting of other systems, especially of those that are in interfering relations with them. That effect has an important pathogenetic significance, because it is connected to the disintegration of Central Nervous System activity in the pathologic conditions and to the suppression of compensating and recovery mechanisms.

A special place among physiological Functional Systems is devoted for the General, nonspecific Inhibiting-Relaxation Functional System of urgent organism adaptation and Protection (IRFSP) from extreme influence of physical hypoxia, hypothermal and other stresses that lead to the serious abnormalities of homeostasis and, first of all, to the Oxygen and carbon dioxide ratio distortion in the organism. The principle of IRFSP functioning is the following. Along with the hypoxia and homeostasis abnormalities, the activation of inhibiting processes, excitability decrease, normalization of nerve processes and improvement of Central Nervous System regulation functions take place. And at the periphery all that results in considerable (sometimes up to 70%) increasing of speed of voluntary simultaneous weakening of all skeletal muscles. IRFSP activation, e.g. together with hard physical load, is accompanied by a mix of psychoemotional tension and muscle hypertonus, considerable improvement of regulation and movement coordination; the increase of economy and effectivity of Central Nervous System, nerve-muscle, cardiovascular, respiratory, neuro-endocrine and other systems; improvement of muscle blood-delivery and of energy-supply for muscular activity; increase of recovery processes rate and of energy resources resynthesis; and finally, to the normalization of homeostasis and to effect of extraordinary increase of physical activity or the "second wind" phenomenon (Vysochin Yu.V., 1983, 1988, 2000).

**"Virtual Scanner" system, realised on the base of original virtual scanner technology, fulfils the on-line and complex diagnostics, treatment and prophylaxis of various functional abnormalities or any organ or system diseases due to the normalisation of control and regulation of cerebral functions (Grakov I.G. and others, 2000).** It has no weak points, which are inherent to the most of methods, used in medicine and physiology (which let us only to estimate the structure or function of single organ, tissue or system, but they don't inform us about regulatory aspects of object under test activity and its mutual relations with other organs and systems). Virtual Reality Technology gives us the possibility to investigate all levels of the whole organism organisation – from higher regulatory systems to the metathetical processes at the cellular level.

**The main methodological principle of virtual scanning is the principle of adequate reflection of outer world and internal organism environment by cerebral functions.** Any incoming cerebral signal has its own characteristics (energy, frequency and spatio-temporal). On the basis of that signal a certain image is made, or the matrix that has the corresponding characteristics. Set of all matrixes forms the "body scheme", i.e. the bio-mathematic organism model. Cerebrum brings the available "body scheme" into accord with sample one with the help of its main functions (sensing, imagination, associative thinking, memory, motivation, decision-making, and others), providing by that the homeostasis retaining and effective activity of all functional systems, organs and tissues.

Under the influence of different unfavourable factors and extreme influences, especially with the increased excitability or weakness of inhibiting Central Nervous System systems, there can appear the so-called operation errors, i.e. the temporary or steady abnormalities in higher regulatory systems activity. For example, the consequence of such failures in movement regulatory system, which lead to discoordination in work of muscles-antagonists, is the injury of musculoskeletal system (for sportsmen and ballet dancers), (Vysochin Yu.V., 1974, 1980, 1988, 2001). After long influence of unfavourable factors the cerebrum generates the invalid directive signal, which doesn't correspond to the "body scheme", as a result of which the pathological area is formed in some system, organ or tissue, and then the disease is developed. In turn, under the influence of afferent signals the areas of pathological excitation appear at the lesion areas of the corresponding parts of cerebrum, and then the pathological Functional System is formed. That way the exclusive vicious circle is formed, which turns the acute disease to the chronic one.

Taking into account the great therapeutic effect, attainable (as it was shown already) due to the normalization of control and regulatory cerebrum functions, it would be logical to assume that therapeutic sessions of "Virtual Scanner" system (judging from the results of our previous researches (Vysochin Yu.V., 1988 – 2000)) have to lead to the increase of functional activity of inhibiting systems and normalization of nerve Central Nervous System processes balance, improving of relaxation characteristics of neuro-muscular system and, as a result, to the increase of energy consumption economy, recovery processes rate and physical activity not only for the ill people, but, also, for the people with good health.

## 2.2 Organisation and Methods of Research

In order to check the working hypothesis the series of experiments were made with the help of 20 people in good health at the age from 20 to 60 years old with usual movement activity. Complex researches were made with the help of different physiological, neurophysiological and ergometric methods. Method of computer electroencephalography estimates the rhythm structure of electroencephalography (EEG) and the adaptability level (Soroko S.I. and others, 1995). Method of computer polymyography is based on the synchronous graphic registration of bioelectrical activity and muscles strain (quadriceps of both legs huckle) at their voluntary tension and relaxation in isometric mode. It help us to estimate the clonus rate, maximum force and relax rate of muscles under test, moving reaction rate at muscles strain and relax, development rate and the force of excitative and inhibiting Central Nervous System processes, balance of such nerve processes as excitation – inhibiting and other characteristics (Vysochin Yu.V., 1974, 1979, 1988). Method of computer veloergometry with the continuous registration of Heart Beating Frequency (HBF). With the help of these methods the dynamics of functional condition of Central Nervous System, neuro-muscular and cardiovascular systems, and also of the Physical Activity (PhA) under the influence of therapeutic sessions with the help of "Virtual Scanner" system.

After preliminary diagnostics with the help of "Virtual Scanner" system every tested person was prescribed to pass the individual therapy course (rhythmic colour correction) for the cerebrum. Complex tests of participants were held before (initial data), and also after 5, 10 and 20 therapeutic sessions with the help of "Virtual Scanner" system. Therapeutic sessions were 2 times a day, and their duration was 15-20 minutes. The remarkable feature of those therapeutic sessions was that all participants got the diskette with the prescribed therapy course and that they received the treatment at their work places at their PCs.

There were total 2800 measurements, and there were obtained and analysed 105440 of initial and calculated parameters, characterizing the functional condition of different organism systems. The research results were processed by methods of variation statistics. There were calculated the average values and average errors of every parameter. Precision of differences (distinctions) between average values of measures were estimated according to the T-criterion for the pairwise related variants.

## 2.3. Influence of therapeutic impact of computer treatment-and-diagnostic system "Virtual Scanner" on electroencephalography and polymyography characteristics of Central Nervous System functional condition

Among the new medical technologies, which have appeared during last years, the special place is devoted to the treatment-and-diagnostic computer system "Virtual Scanner" developed by Grakov I.G. (1998, 2000, 2001). "Virtual Scanner" system, developed on the basis of original Virtual Scanning Technology, enables to carry out operative complex diagnostics, treatment and prophylaxis of different functional abnormalities and of any organ and system diseases by normalisation of operating and regulatory cerebral functions (Grakov I.G. etc., 2000). The special clinical research, which have been carried out with the help of multiple patients (370 people-diagnostics; 1672 people-treatment), have proven high accuracy of diagnostics (average 82.4% of coincidences with clinical diagnoses) and high efficiency of treatment (average 93.2% of recovery cases and considerable improvement) with the help of "Virtual Scanner" system.

# Results of research

**Firstly, note the general state of health improvement of all people who passed tests. The improvement became apparent in decrease of HBF, normalization of arterial pressure and a psychological condition.** Many noted improved vivacity, reduced psycho-emotional intensity and irritability, increased calmness, steadiness, improved sleep, termination of headaches, improved sight, intellectual and physical activity.

*Two examinees got rid of chronic musculoskeletal system traumas. Two examinees (who had suffered from the myocardial infarction earlier) had the considerable state of health improvement and disappearance of any signs of heart discomfort.*

However the main attention in this experiment was given to the results of unbiased research. The analysis of research results (Table 3, fig. 1) has revealed the pronounced positive dynamics of a functional condition of Central Nervous System according to the electroencephalographic (EEG) parameters.

## Table 3: Dynamics of Central Nervous System functional condition - according to the EEG data after 5, 10 and 20 "Virtual Scanner" sessions

| Parameters | | ID | | After 5 sessions | | Distinctions | | |
|---|---|---|---|---|---|---|---|---|
| EEG | № | M | m ± | M | ±m | % | t | D |
| Adaptivity | 15 | 1.36 | 0.07 | 1.60 | 0.08 | 18.55 | 11.77 | 0.001 |
| Alpha rhythm | 15 | 37.00 | 1.97 | 47.13 | 3.09 | 26.81 | 8.03 | 0.001 |
| Beta rhythm | 15 | 35.27 | 1.08 | 29.13 | 2.39 | -18.22 | -3.22 | 0.05 |
| Theta Rhythm | 15 | 17.40 | 0.77 | 15.00 | 0.84 | -13.83 | -4.01 | 0.001 |
| Delta rhythm | 15 | 10.60 | 1.44 | 8.73 | 1.22 | -12.29 | -1.35 | - |

| Parameters | | ID | | After 10 sessions | | Distinctions | | |
|---|---|---|---|---|---|---|---|---|
| EEG | № | M | m ± | M | ±m | % | t | D |
| Adaptivity | 14 | 1.35 | 0.08 | 1.61 | 0.08 | 20.52 | 5.47 | 0.001 |
| Alpha rhythm | 14 | 36.71 | 2.10 | 48.29 | 3.59 | 31.64 | 4.35 | 0.001 |
| Beta rhythm | 14 | 35.36 | 1.16 | 25.93 | 1.86 | -25.67 | -4.57 | 0.001 |
| Theta Rhythm | 14 | 17.64 | 0.79 | 17.42 | 1.29 | -9.37 | -1.27 | - |
| Delta rhythm | 14 | 10.57 | 1.54 | 9.64 | 1.61 | -9.70 | -1.37 | - |

| Parameters | | ID | | After 20 sessions | | Distinctions | | |
|---|---|---|---|---|---|---|---|---|
| EEG | № | M | m ± | M | ±m | % | t | D |
| Adaptivity | 18 | 1.32 | 0.06 | 1.58 | 0.06 | 19.30 | 8.41 | 0.001 |
| Alpha rhythm | 18 | 37.00 | 1.66 | 46.78 | 2.37 | 27.07 | 6.01 | 0.001 |
| Beta rhythm | 18 | 34.78 | 1.01 | 28.17 | 1.27 | -17.33 | -3.55 | 0.01 |
| Theta Rhythm | 18 | 18.50 | 0.77 | 16.22 | 0.72 | -11.25 | -3.03 | 0.01 |
| Delta rhythm | 18 | 10.50 | 1.21 | 8.89 | 1.28 | -16.05 | -2.25 | 0.05 |

n.b. Names of parameters are stated in the text.

After 5 sessions already the statistically authentic increase of organism adaptability or flexibility was registered at the examinees (for 18.6% D < 0.001) and increase an alpha rhythm (for 26.8% D < 0.001), but decrease of beta (for 18.2% D < 0.05), theta (for 13.8% D < 0.001) and delta (for 12.3% D > 0.05) rhythms in summary EEG.

After 10 sessions even the greater increase of adaptability (for 20.5% D < 0.001) and of alpha rhythm (for 31.6% D < 0.001) was noticed, but, at the same time, the greater (for 25.7% D < 0.001) decrease of beta rhythm in summary EEG. Looking at the dynamics of theta and delta rhythms the distinction is not authentic.

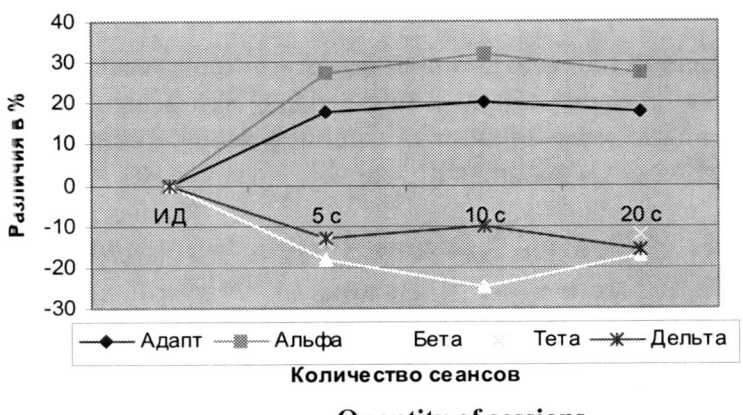

Quantity of sessions

Fig. 1. Dynamics of adaptability and EEG rhythms after 5, 10 and 20 "Virtual Scanner" sessions

(Distinctions Consistency Levels are: * - D 0.05; * - D 0.01; *** - D 0.001)

After 20 sessions, in comparison with 10 ones, the tendency to some decrease of adaptability and alpha rhythm and their returning to a level, achieved after 5 "Virtual Scanner" sessions, is noticed. **It means that peak efficiency of therapeutic influences of "Virtual Scanner" system on functional Central Nervous System condition was already achieved after the first 5 – 10 sessions, i.e. in 2.5 – 5 days with two sessions per day.**

Similar dynamics of functional condition of Central Nervous System is achieved, also, according to the data of PolyMyoGraphic (1PMG) research (Table 4, fig. 2). After 5 sessions already, in comparison with the Initial Level, an authentic improvement of the parameters describing the condition of inhibiting processes was registered: the rate of Motor Relaxation Reaction has increased (RMRR) for 5.1% (D < 0.05), Development Rate and force of Inhibiting processes (DRI) for 15% (D < 0.001), functional Activity of Inhibiting Systems (AIS) for 13.4% (D < 0.05).

411

**Table 4: Dynamics of functional Central Nervous System condition - according to the polymyography data after 5, 10 and 20 sessions of Virtual Scanner therapy.**

| Parameters | ID | | After 5 sessions | | Distinctions | | |
|---|---|---|---|---|---|---|---|
| | M | m $\pm$ | M | $\pm$m | % | t | D |
| RMSR | 3.30 | 0.151 | 3.25 | 0.100 | -1.52 | -0.44 | - |
| RMRR | 5.83 | 0.173 | 6.12 | 0.222 | 5.06 | 2.12 | 0.05 |
| DRE | 2.54 | 0.091 | 2.61 | 0.071 | 2.76 | 1.33 | - |
| DRI | 2.55 | 0.072 | 2.93 | 0.079 | 14.98 | 5.11 | 0.001 |
| BNP$_i$ | 0.98 | 0.044 | 1.13 | 0.036 | 15.52 | 4.76 | 0.001 |
| AIS | 9.61 | 0.724 | 10.9 | 0.588 | 13.42 | 2.31 | 0.05 |
| GFC$_{Central}$ Nervous System | 4.26 | 0.084 | 4.54 | 0.095 | 6.65 | 2.98 | 0.01 |

| Parameters | ID | | After 10 sessions | | Distinctions | | |
|---|---|---|---|---|---|---|---|
| | M | m $\pm$ | M | $\pm$m | % | t | D |
| RMSR | 3.25 | 0.068 | 3.30 | 0.065 | 1.39 | 0.75 | - |
| RMRR | 5.80 | 0.108 | 6.11 | 0.089 | 5.34 | 2.50 | 0.05 |
| DRE | 2.55 | 0.041 | 2.62 | 0.043 | 2.89 | 2.07 | 0.05 |
| DRI | 2.60 | 0.047 | 3.04 | 0.031 | 17.08 | 6.96 | 0.001 |
| BNP$_i$ | 0.99 | 0.03 | 1.16 | 0.020 | 17.17 | 6.43 | 0.001 |
| AIS | 9.65 | 0.401 | 10.99 | 0.317 | 13.89 | 3.40 | 0.01 |
| GFC$_{Central}$ Nervous System | 4.25 | 0.053 | 4.54 | 0.039 | 6.82 | 4.37 | 0.001 |

| Parameters | ID | | After 20 sessions | | Distinctions | | |
|---|---|---|---|---|---|---|---|
| | M | m $\pm$ | M | $\pm$m | % | t | D |
| RMSR | 3.24 | 0.057 | 3.29 | 0.044 | 1.50 | 0.67 | - |
| RMRR | 5.75 | 0.104 | 6.09 | 0.123 | 5.98 | 2.56 | 0.05 |
| DRE | 2.53 | 0.033 | 2.63 | 0.032 | 3.77 | 2.22 | 0.05 |
| DRI | 2.60 | 0.043 | 3.09 | 0.044 | 18.81 | 9.17 | 0.001 |
| BNP$_i$ | 1.00 | 0.024 | 1.19 | 0.024 | 19.44 | 6.57 | 0.001 |
| AIS | 9.67 | 0.332 | 11.14 | 0.373 | 15.20 | 3.98 | 0.01 |
| GFC$_{Central}$ Nervous System | 4.24 | 0.05 | 4.55 | 0.063 | 7.21 | 4.39 | 0.001 |

n.b. Names of parameters are stated in the text.

Consequently a considerable change of Balance of Nervous Processes (BNP$_i$) took place to the inhibiting side for 15.5% (D < 0.001). General Functional Condition of Central Nervous System (GFC$_{Central\ Nervous\ System}$) for 6.7% (D < 0.01) was authentically improved.

After 10 sessions even more improvement of all polymyographic characteristics was seen: increase of RMRR for 5.3% (D < 0.05), DRI for 17.1% (D < 0.001}, AIS for 13.9% (D < 0.001), change of BNP$_i$ to inhibiting for 17.2% (D < 0.001), increase of GFC$_{Central}$

Nervous System for 6.8% (D < 0.001). Rate of Motor Stress Reaction (RMSR) has also increased a little (inauthentically).

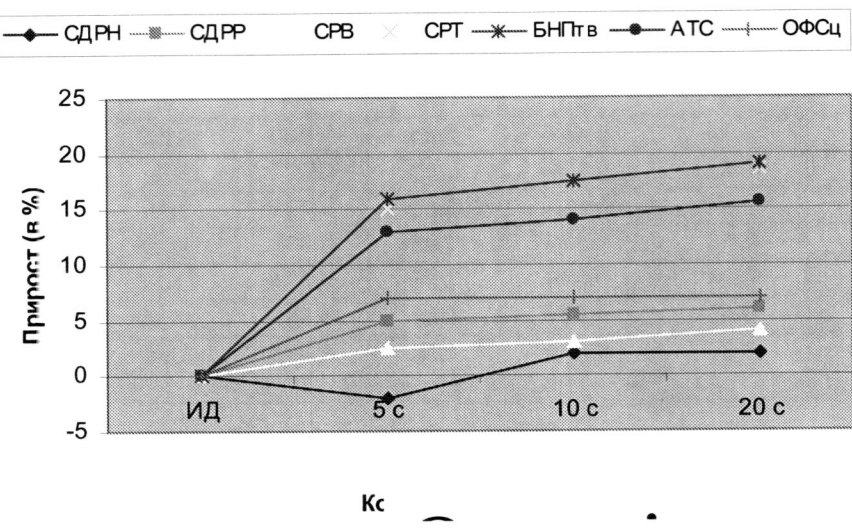

Fig. 2. Dynamics of functional Central Nervous System condition according to the polymyography data after 5, 10 and 20 sessions of "Virtual Scanner" system therapy.

(Distinctions Consistency Levels are: * - D 0.05; * - D 0.01; *** - D 0.001)

However the greatest increase in all polymyograhic characteristics of functional Central Nervous System condition is received after 20 sessions. The parameters, describing the excitative systems condition, have increased: the Rate of Motor Stress Reaction (RMSR) for 1.5% (inauthentically), Development Rate and force of Excitative processes (DRE) for 3.8% (D < 0.05). At the same time the parameters, describing functional activity of processes of Central Nervous System inhibiting, have increased even more – RMRR by 6% (D < 0.05), DRI by 18.8% (D < 0.001), AIS by 15.2% (D < 0.01). As a result, a considerable change of Balance of Nervous Processes took place to the inhibiting side (for 19.4% D < 0.001), and general functional Central Nervous System condition was, also, improved (for 7.2% D < 0.001). However, as well as in the previous observations, the biggest rates of all parameters growth were registered after the first 5 sessions.

**Summarising of these researches results allows concluding that therapeutic session with the help of "Virtual Scanner" system really results in fast and substantial improvement of functional Central Nervous System condition. And it happens mainly due to the increase of inhibiting systems functional activity, normalisation of BNP and, accordingly, increasing of inhibiting control, that is one of the most important conditions for the effective realisation of control and regulatory Central Nervous System functions.**

## 2.4. Influence of the Therapeutic Impact of Computer Medical-Diagnostic "Virtual Scanner" System on the Functional Condition of Neuro-Muscular System

The logical effect of functional Central Nervous System condition improvement was the increase of functional condition level and of nervous - muscular system that is under Central Nervous System control (Table 5, fig. 3).

## Table 5: Dynamics of Neuro–Muscular System (NMS) functional condition – after 5, 10 and 20 sessions of Virtual Scanner therapy

| Parameters | ID | | After 5 sessions | | Distinctions | | |
|---|---|---|---|---|---|---|---|
| | M | m ± | M | ±m | % | T | D |
| VSR | 5.63 | 0.246 | 6.04 | 0.335 | 7.32 | 1.71 | - |
| MVF | 5.59 | 0.27 | 5.79 | 0.292 | 3.54 | 0.97 | - |
| VRR | 4.58 | 0.179 | 5.72 | 0.268 | 24.92 | 4.44 | 0.001 |
| GFCm | 10.19 | 0.279 | 11.63 | 0.404 | 14.19 | 4.52 | 0.001 |
| CIAT | 1.2 | 0.082 | 1.05 | 0.072 | -12.85 | -3.85 | 0.01 |
| GFCcm | 6.71 | 0.201 | 7.96 | 0.327 | 18.64 | 4.74 | 0.001 |
| IP | 1.25 | 0.068 | 1.06 | 0.065 | -15.00 | -5.62 | 0.001 |

| Parameters | ID | | After 10 sessions | | Distinctions | | |
|---|---|---|---|---|---|---|---|
| | M | m ± | M | ±m | % | T | D |
| VSR | 4.97 | 0.19 | 5.8 | 0.192 | 16.64 | 4.26 | 0.001 |
| MVF | 5.23 | 0.151 | 5.8 | 0.183 | 10.84 | 5.98 | 0.001 |
| VRR | 4.74 | 0.133 | 6.17 | 0.113 | 30.08 | 8.63 | 0.001 |
| GFCm | 9.89 | 0.207 | 11.82 | 0.194 | 19.43 | 8.27 | 0.001 |
| CIAT | 1.17 | 0.049 | 0.98 | 0.035 | -16.10 | -6.17 | 0.001 |
| GFCcm | 6.73 | 0.146 | 8.86 | 0.389 | 31.65 | 5.23 | 0.001 |
| IP | 1.12 | 0.043 | 0.93 | 0.033 | -16.84 | -6.80 | 0.001 |

| Parameters | ID | | After 20 sessions | | Distinctions | | |
|---|---|---|---|---|---|---|---|
| | M | m ± | M | ±m | % | T | D |
| VSR | 4.36 | 0.225 | 5.83 | 0.269 | 33.74 | 7.94 | 0.001 |
| MVF | 4.92 | 0.167 | 6.27 | 0.192 | 27.59 | 7.97 | 0.001 |
| VRR | 4.8 | 0.115 | 6.26 | 0.095 | 30.41 | 13.01 | 0.001 |
| GFCm | 9.48 | 0.213 | 12.31 | 0.255 | 29.87 | 14.9 | 0.001 |
| CIAT | 1.14 | 0.049 | 0.94 | 0.03 | -17.54 | -7.31 | 0.001 |
| GFCcm | 6.75 | 0.127 | 8.93 | 0.245 | 32.25 | 9.16 | 0.001 |
| IP | 1.12 | 0.037 | 0.92 | 0.028 | -18.11 | -7.48 | 0.001 |

The note. Names of parameters are shown in the text

After 5 sessions already, in comparison with the initial level, the increase of Voluntary Stress Rate (VSR) for 7.3% (inauthentically), the Maximum Voluntary Force (MVF) for

3.5% (inauthentically), Voluntary Relaxation Rate (VRR) for 24.9% (D < 0.001) and the General Functional Condition of muscles (DFCm) for 14.2% (D < 0.001) was registered. The Classification Index of strategy of long-term Adaptation strategy Type (CIAT) for 12.9% (D < 0.001) was essentially improved and the probability of overstrain and Injury Possibility (IP) for 15% (D < 0.001) has decreased. The integrated parameter, characterized the general functional condition of Central Nervous System and NMS (GFCcm) for 13.6% (D < 0.001) has also increased.

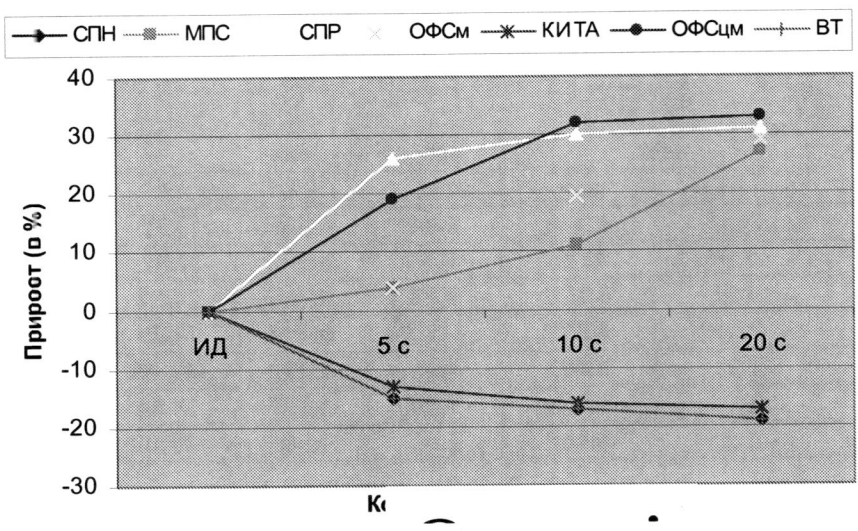

Fig. 3 Dynamics of functional NMS condition after 5, 10 and 20 sessions of system "Virtual Scanner" therapy (Distinctions Consistency Levels are: * - D 0.05; * - D 0.01; *** - D 0.001)

Even more expressed positive dynamics in all parameters, describing functional NMS condition, was noticed after 10 sessions of therapy. In comparison with the initial level, it is authentic (D < 0.001) that parameters VSR for 16.6%, MVF for 10.8%, VRR for 30.1%, GFCm for 19.4%, GFCcm for 31.7%, CIAT for 16.1% and TO for 16.8% were improved.

Further positive dynamics was kept for all parameters, but for some of them (such as VRR, GFCcm, CIAT, IP) the growth at the 20th session, in comparison to the 10th one, appeared small (no more than 1-2%). The general growth in all these parameters was, accordingly, – 30.4%, 31.7%, 17.5% and 18.1%. Stress rate, the maximum force and the general functional condition of muscles have increased in comparison with the initial level for 33.7% (D < 0.001), 27% (D < 0.001) and 30% (D < 0.001) accordingly.

## 2.5. Influence of therapeutic influences of computer medical-diagnostic system "Virtual Scanner" on physical activity and functional condition of cardiovascular system

The pronounced positive changes of functional Central Nervous System and NeuroMuscular System condition were accompanied by not less expressed positive dynamics of physical activity and functional condition of cardiovascular system (Table 6, fig. 4).

Table 6: Dynamics of the parameters, describing physical activity and functional condition of cardiovascular system - after 10 and 20 sessions Virtual Scanner therapy

| Parameters | ID | | After 10 sessions | | Distinctions | | |
|---|---|---|---|---|---|---|---|
| | M | m ± | M | ±m | % | t | D |
| FCCq | 74.44 | 1.06 | 69.71 | 1.46 | -5.99 | -4.67 | 0.001 |
| FCCm | 150.14 | 9.12 | 154.14 | 6.46 | 3.60 | 1.24 | |
| FCCr | 124.52 | 7.30 | 122.10 | 5.22 | -1.17 | -0.70 | |
| Np | 32.34 | 3.03 | 34.36 | 2.80 | 7.20 | 2.78 | 0.01 |
| HSE | 9.02 | 0.84 | 9.79 | 0.72 | 10.46 | 2.81 | 0.01 |
| HAEF | 8.77 | 0.89 | 9.34 | 0.90 | 7.04 | 5.30 | 0.001 |
| PRR | 8.00 | 0.85 | 8.59 | 0.81 | 8.75 | 5.42 | 0.001 |
| GE | 8.38 | 0.87 | 8.96 | 0.85 | 7.83 | 9.78 | 0.001 |

| Parameters | ID | | After 20 sessions | | Distinctions | | |
|---|---|---|---|---|---|---|---|
| | M | m ± | M | ±m | % | t | D |
| FCCq | 74.44 | 0.81 | 67.78 | 1.20 | -8.89 | -5.47 | 0.001 |
| FCCm | 142.78 | 6.83 | 142.89 | 4.85 | 1.23 | 0.03 | |
| FCCr | 121.19 | 4.81 | 114.74 | 4.24 | -5.03 | -2.87 | 0.01 |
| Np | 29.65 | 2.37 | 33.27 | 2.27 | 13.21 | 4.76 | 0.001 |
| HSE | 9.02 | 0.64 | 9.96 | 0.46 | 12.84 | 3.57 | 0.01 |
| HAEF | 8.23 | 0.63 | 9.50 | 0.69 | 15.59 | 6.02 | 0.001 |
| PRR | 7.46 | 0.60 | 8.82 | 0.61 | 19.97 | 5.36 | 0.001 |
| GE | 7.84 | 0.62 | 9.16 | 0.64 | 17.54 | 6.75 | 0.001 |

The note. Names of parameters are shown in the text.

After 10 therapeutic sessions frequency of Frequency of Cordial Clonus in quiescence decreases considerably (FCCq) for 6% (D < 0.001) and in period of rehabilitation (FCCr) – for 1.2% (inauthentically), that testifies to the increase of heart activity efficiency and pulse restoration rate. At that the work capacity ($N_p$) at veloergometre has considerably increased (for 7.2%, D < 0.01} and High-Speed Endurance (HSE) for 10.5% (D < 0.01). The special factors, calculated according to the ratio of work capacity and its pulse rate/cost, have considerably increased: Heart Activity Efficiency Factor (HAEF) – for 7.1% (D < 0.001), Pulse Restoration Rate (PRR) – for 8.8% (D < 0.001) and General Efficiency (GE) of organism systems – for 7.8% (D < 0.001), describing an efficiency of systems activity and energy-supply systems of muscular activity.

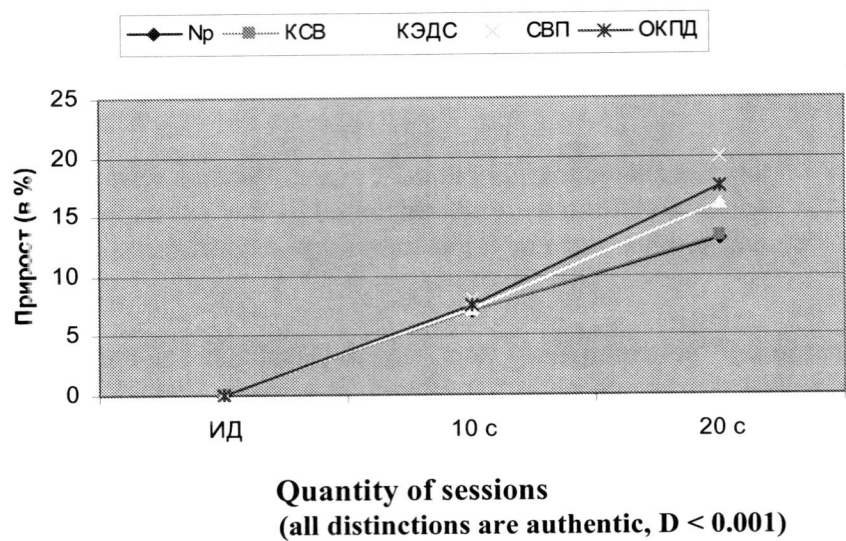

**Quantity of sessions**
**(all distinctions are authentic, D < 0.001)**

Fig. 4. Dynamics of the parameters, describing physical activity and a functional condition of cardiovascular system after 10 and 20 sessions Virtual Scanner therapy (all distinctions are authentic at D < 0.001).

Even more expressed positive dynamics of all parameters was registered after 20 sessions: $FCC_q$ and $FCC_r$ values have authentically decreased for 8.9% (D < 0.001) and 5% (D < 0.01) accordingly. Work Capacity and High-Speed Endurance have increased for 13.2% (D < 0.001) and 12.8% (D < 0.01). Heart Activity Efficiency, Pulse Restoration Rate and General Systems Efficiency of organism have increased for 15.6% (D < 0.001), 20% (D < 0.001) and 17.5% (D < 0.001) accordingly.

It is noteworthy that maximum FCC level during veloergometry performance ($FCC_m$) has remained at the initial level, though the work capacity has considerably increased (for 13.2%). That again testifies to the considerable increasing of organism systems activity, limiting physical activity and, also, about the lowered inquiries to the energy-supply systems of muscular activity, especially to the cardiovascular one.

# CONCLUSION.

## Discussion of research results

Computer system "Virtual Scanner" is developed on the basis of representations about laws of the biological answer to wave influence (Grakov B.S., Grakov I.G., 1985), the modern scientific concept about the leading part of the higher regulatory systems, the brain in particular (Bekhtereva N.P., 1974, 1980, 1997), and inhibiting-relaxation processes (Vysochin J.V., 1988) in the most important display of vital activity of the whole organism, such as adaptation, ability to work, resistance to extreme environmental influences and etiopathogenesis of various pathological conditions, injuries and diseases.

According to the research results, the therapeutic sessions of rhythmic colour correction with the help of "Virtual Scanner" system has resulted in considerable positive changes in all parameters characterising the functional condition of Central Nervous System, NeuroMuscular System and Cardiovascular System, and also in parameters of physical activity and endurance.

However if growth in functional activity of inhibiting systems and General Functional Condition of Central Nervous System, muscles relaxation characteristics, efficiency of CardioVascular System (CVS) activity and physical activity were not unexpected for us, as these effects were predicted at the working hypothesis formulation of research, the considerable growth in muscular retractive characteristics turned out a little bit unexpected. The matter is that, as it was already specified, the volunteers, who participated in experiments, were almost healthy (they were scientific employees with normal motor activity). That is why the following question arose: owing to which physiological mechanisms did the muscular retractive characteristics increase after rhythmic colour correction?

In order to answer this question it is necessary to remember that many movements, carried out with maximum speed, require making considerable efforts in a short time. Efficiency of such movements substantially depends on Retractive Rate (stress), force and speed of muscular relaxation. During the numerous researches of Individual Clonus (IC), executed on separate muscular fibres of birds, reptiles, mammal, etc. (Josephson, 1975; Smith et al., 1973; Ashler, Rigdway, 1968; Barany, 1967; Blinks Ct al., 1978; Eusebi Ct al., 1980; Guthe, 1982 etc.,) it is defined that Individual Clonus Rate, measured by the time passed from the electric stimulus till the moment of muscles half-relaxation, depends on plenty of factors: quantity of connected in series sarcometers, i.e. the length of muscular fibre, ATPhase actomyosin activity, ATPhase sarco-plasmic reticulum activity, and also the time, during which in sarcoplasma (in myofibril area) the supraliminal concentration of ions $Ca^{++}$ is supported, which, in turn, is defined by sarco-plasmic reticulum volume and by calcium pump capacity (Shigekawa Ct al., 1978; Dawson Ct al., 1980; Dynnik, 1985; Krolenko, 1985). And the speed of muscular fibre stress is not limited neither by diffusion of ions $Ca^{++}$, nor by the speed of emission $Ca^{++}$ from the end tanks, as the last process goes very quickly.

The main factor, limiting the rate of Individual retractive-relaxation cycle, is the calcium sequestration rate, affecting the Muscular Retractive Rate (MRR) and associated to the development rate of sarco-plasmic reticulum. Morphological research confirm the considerable differences in the structure of sarco-plasmic reticulum between fast and slow muscles. Thus, shortening the time of Individual Clonus, i.e. increasing the Stress and Relaxation Rate can be achieved by increase of volume, taken by sarco-plasmic reticulum due to the decrease of volume, taken by myofibril retractive organ. The consequence of quick-action increase can be the fall of muscular fibres specific force, which is defined by cross section of myofibril, composing these fibres (Gurfinkel, Levik, 1985). In some researches (Bruse Ct al., 1986) the positive correlation between isometric effort and the cross section area of muscles was found out.

If to follow this data, describing mainly the peripheral mechanisms, providing the increase of muscular retraction and relaxation rate, then the growth of retraction rate should be accompanied by the considerable morphological reconstructions, resulting in increase of sarco-plasmic reticulum capacity and, accordingly, to the reduction of muscles force. But muscles force in our experiments has increased.

Undoubtedly that in these processes not so much peripheral (because it is hardly possible to get the considerable morphological reconstructions in muscles structure during only 10 days of experiments), as the central mechanisms of voluntary movements regulation. It is known that at any voluntary muscles retraction and relaxation, besides the above listed factors, the rate of these processes and clonus force is defined by functional condition of the higher regulatory systems and the segmentary organ of nervous system, by supraspinal and esodic influences on alpha–motorneurons of spinal cord and, also, what is the most important, by the quantity and work synchronism of the moving organs, taking part in clonus process.

It is obvious that such considerable improvement of retractive (growth of Stress Rate for 33.7%, of maximum force - for 27.6%) and relaxation (growth for 30.4%) muscles characteristics is explained by considerable improvement of general functional Central Nervous System condition and, accordingly, its regulatory and control functions.

Testing task during check-ups, as it was specified above, required from examinees to fulfil testing movement with the maximum force and speed. In order to fulfil the task correctly the precise, well-organized and correct command from Central Nervous System to the executive organs (muscles) was necessary. In the beginning of experiment the control and regulatory Central Nervous System functions were not perfect at examinees, therefore not all of available moving organs could participate in the retractive action, or the inclusion sequence into the retractive action didn't provide the synchronism of their interaction. The consequence of it was the low parameters of Retractive Rate and maximum force of muscles.

At the end of the experiment the situation has changed. Due to the considerable improvement of regulatory and control Central Nervous System functions, the retractive action synchronously involved the maximum quantity of available in a muscle moving organs, what was the reason of high rate and the big force of muscular retractions.

**Starting from the above-stated, the high efficiency of "Virtual Scanner" system and its absolute availability for use not only in public health services (for treatment and prophylaxis of various pathological processes} is abundantly clear, but, also, for any kinds of sport and professional work, requiring normalisation of control functions of higher regulatory systems, improvement of inhibiting Central Nervous System control, increase of retractive and relaxation muscles characteristics, capacity of physiological protection mechanisms, efficiency of cardiovascular system activity, intellectual and physical activity, stress-resistance and survival rate in complex and extreme conditions of activity and of the environment.** Taking into account the minimal time expenses for complex diagnostics (not more than 10-15 minutes) and treatment or so-called informational correction (the session lasts 15-20 minutes), and also the main aim of informational correction - normalisation of control and regulatory brain functions, it is necessary to expect that system "Virtual Scanner" in the near future will find the adequate application in all areas of human activity, connected with big physical and psychoemotional load, the increased requirements to systems of movement regulation and coordination, stability to stress-generating and other negative factors (rescuers, firemen, choreography, ballet, sport, landing armies, riot squads, aircraft, astronautics etc.).

## FINDINGS

1. The special clinical research, which have been carried out on a large number of patients (370 people – diagnostics; 1672 people – treatment), have proven the high accuracy of diagnosis (on average 82.4% of concurrences to clinical diagnosis) and the high efficiency of treatment (on average 93.2% of recovery cases and considerable improvements) with the help of the "Virtual Scanner" system.

2. According to the data of electroencephalographical and polymyographical research it was established that "Virtual Scanner" system therapeutic sessions result in fast and considerable increase of adaptability (for 20.5% D < 0.001) and percentage of alpha rhythm (for 31.6% D < 0.001) in summary EEG, and also to the improvement of general functional Central Nervous System condition (for 7.2 % D < 0.001) due to increase of DRI (for 18.8% D < 0.001), functional Activity of Inhibiting Systems (AIS) (for 15.2% D < 0.01), considerable change in Balance of Nerve Processes (BNP) toward inhibiting processes (for 19.4% D < 0.001) and, thereafter, increasing inhibiting control from Central Nervous System side which is one of the major conditions for the control of the regulatory cerebral functions.

3. Efficiency increase of control and regulatory cerebrum activity under the influence of therapeutic sessions of "Virtual Scanner" system results in considerable increase of stress rate (for 33.7% D < 0.001), the maximum force (for 27.6% D < 0.001), relaxation rate (for 30.4% D < 0.001) and the general functional NeuroMuscular System condition (for 30% D < 0.001).

4. **The pronounced positive changes of Central Nervous System and NeuroMuscular System functional condition are accompanied by improved dynamics in physical activity and CVS functional condition.** After 20 "Virtual Scanner" system sessions, in comparison with the Initial Data, the Frequency of Cordial Clonus in quiescence (FCCq) and in period of rehabilitation (FCCr) authentically decreases for 8.9% (D < 0.001) and 5% (D < 0.01) accordingly. $N_p$ (work capacity) and speed endurance increased by 13.2% (D < 0.001) and 12.8% (D < C.01). Heart Activity Efficiency Factor (HAEF), Pulse Recovery Rate (PRR) and General Efficiency (GE) of organism systems raise for 15.6% (D < 0.001), 20% (D < 0.001) and 17.5% (D < 0.001) accordingly.

5. After 5, 10 and 20 "Virtual Scanner" sessions the substantial decrease of the characteristic, which shows the Possibility of Injury (IP) and Musculoskeletal system diseases, and also the heart overstress accordingly for 15% (D < 0.001), 16.8% (D < 0.001) and 18.1% (D < 0.001). **That allows concluding that "Virtual Scanner" system therapeutic sessions can become an effective overstress, injury and musculoskeletal system diseases preventive measure, and also for prevention of cordial overstress at hard physical and psycho-emotional load.**

6. Considerable improvement of retractive and relaxation muscle characteristics, increasing of physical activity, heart functioning efficiency, coordination in different organs and systems activity, which limit physical efficiency, and also reduction of injury possibility, musculoskeletal system diseases and cordial overstress is explained by improvement of overall functional Central Nervous System condition and, accordingly, of its control and regulator functions under the influence of "Virtual Scanner" system sessions.

7. "Virtual Scanner" is a high-performance system and absolutely suitable for wide application not only in public health service (for treatment and prophylaxis of different pathological processes), but **in any kinds of sport or professional human activity that requires effective correction of psychofunctional abnormalities, normalization of regulator systems control functions, improvement of inhibition Central Nervous System control, increasing of retractive and relaxation muscle characteristics, economy and effectivity of CardioVascular System activity, mental and physical activity, stress stability and human survival rate in complex and extreme conditions of activity or environment.**

8. Taking into account the minimum time spent for complex diagnostics (less than 10-15 minutes) and treatment (or so called informational correction) (session lasts 15-20 minutes), and also the main object of informational correction – normalisation of regulator and control of cerebrum functions, it is expected the "Virtual Scanner" system will be applicable in all areas of human activity concerned with hard physical and psycho-emotional load, increased requirements to regulating and movement coordination systems, physical activity, endurance,

stability to different stress-generative or confusing factors (sport, choreography, ballet, rescuers, firemen, landing troops, emergency platoons, aviation, cosmonautics and others).

**Yu.V.Vysochin**

# List of Abbreviations

| | |
|---|---|
| **AIS** | - Activity of Inhibiting Systems |
| **BNP** | - Balance of Nerve Processes |
| **BNP$_i$** | - Balance of Nerve Processes for inhibiting processes |
| **CIAT Type** | - Classification Index of strategy of long-term Adaptation strategy |
| **CNS** | - Central Nervous System |
| **CVS** | - CardioVascular System |
| **D** | - Distinctions consistency level |
| **DRE** | - Development Rate or force of Excitative process |
| **DRI** | - Development Rate and the force of Inhibiting processes |
| **EEG** | - ElectroEncephaloGraphy |
| **FCC$_q$** | - Frequency of Cordial Clonus in quiescence |
| **FCC$_r$** | - Frequency of Cordial Clonus in period of rehabilitation |
| **FCC$_m$** | - Frequency of Cordial Clonus maximum |
| **FS** | - Functional System |
| **GE** | - General Efficiency |
| **GFC$_{cns}$** | - General Functional Condition of CNS |
| **GFC$_m$** | - General Functional Condition of muscles |
| **GFC$_{cm}$** | - General Functional Condition of CNS and NMS |
| **HAEF** | - Heart Activity Efficiency Factor |
| **HSE** | - High-Speed Endurance |
| **IC** | - Individual Clonus |
| **IP** | - Injury Possibility |
| **IRFSP** | - General Inhibiting-Relaxation Functional System of urgent organism adaptation and Protection |
| **MRR** | - Muscular Retractive Rate |
| **MVF** | - Maximum Voluntary Force |
| **N$_p$** | - Work Capacity |
| **NMS** | - Nervous – Muscular System |
| **PhA** | - Physical Activity |
| **PMG** | - PolyMyoGraphy |
| **PRR** | - Pulse Recovery Rate |
| **RMRR** | - Rate of Motor Reaction Relaxation |
| **RMSR** | - Rate of Motor Stress Reaction |
| **RF** | - Russian Federation |
| **RR** | - Retractive Rate |
| **VSR** | - Voluntary Stress Rate |
| **VRR** | - Voluntary Relaxation Rate |

Quotes:

*"This is just phenomenal - working within the health service for so long as a square peg in a round hole has always been a difficulty but I have always thought that there was something out there that would revolutionise medical care".*

**"This is the future of medicine". – medical student**

**"The whole thing seems too advanced to be true and could be obtaining a Nobel Physics or Medical prize if it was true. The emotions related to hormones would have been discovered and that is the interaction of mind, heart and body. It will be too much to be true...."**

**"Thank you so much for your response and all the information. I have no doubt that your efforts will be rewarded. I think your explanation for how things are working is good. I may have an academic background but this does not mean that I am any better at explaining this remarkable phenomenon! I know that I would like to play with it much more".**

Diabetes GP, Diabetes Journal Club, Leicester General Hospital: *"I know about NeuroInformatics and what you are demonstrating has not yet been developed."*

Mother and Health Professional (Dentist): "I would not under normal circumstances comment upon the results of treatment after only 3 weeks but the improvement in my daughter's behaviour has been so clear and distinct that I feel obliged to say something."

**GP: 'I have practiced medicine in the UK since arriving in 1978. I have been waiting throughout my career for this technology'**

*'Since starting my therapy I can honestly say that I have not looked back. I have had an odd headache that's all. It's been a great relief. The aches and pains that I used to suffer due to spondylosis, rheumatism and arthritis are a lot better. I went to a hospital for a check-up on my arm just before Xmas 2004. The staff there were very pleased with the reduction in swelling and commented upon how well I looked. I told them that I could only put it down to the Virtual Scanning Therapy and explained what the treatment entailed. They were extremely interested in details because some of the staff and friends were also migraine sufferers.*

*Of course the people closest to me, my family, have seen the most dramatic change in my health. They have commented on the fact that I am far more relaxed and calmer. I am less likely to let situations upset me. I have become far more confident and have a more positive attitude to life in general. I must end this by also saying I am free of migraines after suffering from the age of 11 to 59 years. I just can't believe it".*

*'I have now finished the modules that I have on my computer. I have taken my time, partly because Christmas etc and a winter break intervened and partly because I still can get adverse effects from the modules, even after the module has finished. The worst one this time was the kidney one when I felt (and looked!) exhausted for more than a week.* **However the 'spiritual' one was a great success.** *I approached it with some trepidation, wondering how I would react to it.* **But I found it both soothing and invigorating and would happily do it again** *(incidentally two of the three colours were very similar to those in the duodenum module).*

I would like to continue with VS as I feel that I have definitely made progress and feel improved in myself generally and in specifics (eg my bladder irritability at night has diminished)'.

'.....if what you are claiming is accurate and true then the virtual scanner represents a revolution in diagnostic and therapeutic healthcare. I would therefore welcome the opportunity to possibly see and experience the scanner myself and be provided with the opportunity to ask questions about the technology and its applications......'

**'I have been amazed by the diagnosis which has proved absolutely accurate and has been pretty much confirmed by the medical tests which I have been having'.**

*'I went for the biopsy yesterday and it wasn't a traumatic experience. I expect to get an apppointment next week to see the surgeon for the results. I have noticed progress in myself in a number of things. I'm getting more things completed, rather than started and left which is a common pattern of mine. Nicely pointed out on the VS analysis. I haven't started the treatment for that yet so you may think it's unrelated. Also I have much more flexibility in both my left knee and ankle and the muscles seem to be working and supporting the joints more effectively. This is particularly noticeable on going up and down stairs. The skin on my left calf and ankle is now quiet and not irritated and healing well'.*

'A.............. had very poor reading and writing skills and found sequencing (i.e. the alphabet) very difficult. *He now has a reading and spelling age just above his chronological age. He now loves reading - getting him to stop is the hardest part!!* His fine motor skills (i.e. handwriting) are still poor but this has also improved. Perhaps the most exciting thing to me is that he can now say the alphabet all the way through with no problem what so ever. We are very pleased with his progress. Thanks'.

A parent, commenting upon his 21y.o. son

**'His short term memory has improved, he is more out-going in his personality, he no longer moves his lips when he reads, he is more communicative and initiates more conversations, he is more physically coordinated in his movements, his verbal responses are quicker and more confident. Apart from that there is nothing to report!'**

A 19y.o male university student:

*'My concentration has improved phenomenally. Whereas before I could concentrate for only 10-15 minutes, now I can easily concentrate for 2-3 hours at a time. Before you could follow me through the university by the pens which I left behind. Now I do not forget my pens'.*

Comments by book reviewers:

**'Its an absolute tour de force, brilliant' - Dr Keith Foster, CADUCEUS magazine**

"Virtual scanning is one of the most exciting, and innovative, diagnostic tools we have seen, and may herald the way forward in a healthcare culture without drugs."
— Bryan Hubbard, publisher, What Doctors Don't Tell You.

*Thank you for sending us the summary article about Virtual Scanning. We were wondering whether we are allowed to reprint this article in Virtual Medical Worlds Magazine? We think it would be of great interest to our readership. In case of your positive reaction, the article will appear in the July 2007 VMW issue.*
*- Virtual Medical Worlds Magazine*

I have read the draft and I agree with the other reviewers as you reported on the feedback you are receiving. It is a comprehensive volume in that it takes the reader from the first principles of human health - viewed holistically - and connects this to the virtual scanning principles, technology and research. It draws effectively on multidisciplinary perspectives to make a solid case. The technology is an exciting development and hopefully more research will be able to occur to add more statistical power to the argument for the efficacy of virtual scanning.

I look forward to the book being published and you are to be congratulated for your efforts and expertise.

Russell Renhard, Associate Professor, Quality Improvement Program
Centre for Quality Improvement Research and Practice
Australian Institute for Primary Care
LaTrobe Universit

This ground-breaking book illustrates that complementary health principles form the basis of Virtual Scanning technology which appears able to diagnose and treat the health of every system and organ in the body.

The book illustrates the origins of this world-leading technology, what it does and how it does it, and illustrates how cognition is directly related to health. It describes how mathematical modeling concepts are used to elucidate the relationships which exist between mind and body.

Virtual Scanning spans the theoretic divide between psychology and pathophysiology and defines how complementary health is associated with the processes which maintain our health whereas pathophysiology or biomedicine is focussed upon treating the symptoms of illness.

The book discusses how the physiological systems regulate the function of the organs and cells of the body and that the brain waves regulate their function. It illustrates how the the receipt of sensory data is responsible for the placebo effect and how the interaction of sensory data between people can be mathematically assessed.

The result is a fascinating book with conclusions which will advance our understanding of how the mind and body are related. It will revolutionise our attitude towards healthcare and will intrigue the lay person and medical practitioner.

ISBN: 978-0-9556213-0-7

Printed in the United Kingdom
by Lightning Source UK Ltd.
122211UK00001B/35-106/A

9 780955 621307